Math for Meds

Dosages & Solutions

Ninth Edition

Anna M. Curren, RN, MA

Former Associate Professor of Nursing
Long Beach City College
Long Beach, California

THOMSON

DELMAR LEARNING

Australia Canada Mexico Singapore Spain United Kingdom United States

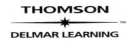

THOMSON

DELMAR LEARNING

Math for Meds: Dosages and Solutions, Ninth Edition
by Anna M. Curren, RN, MA

Vice President, Health Care Business Unit:
William Brottmiller

Editorial Director:
Cathy L. Esperti

Senior Acquisitions Editor:
Matthew Kane

Developmental Editor:
Maria D'Angelico

Editorial Assistant:
Erin Silk

Marketing Director:
Jennifer McAvey

Project Editor:
Daniel Branagh

Art & Design Specialist:
Robert Plante

Production Coordinator:
Bridget Lulay

Library of Congress Cataloging-in-Publication Data
Curren, Anna M.
   Math for meds : dosages & solutions / Anna M. Curren. — 9th ed.
      p. cm.
   Includes index.
   ISBN 1-4018-3122-2
   1. Pharmaceutical arithmetic — Programmed instruction. I. Title.
   RS57.C87 2004
   615'.14'01513--dc22

2004005982

NOTICE TO THE READER

Publisher does not warrant or guarantee any of the products described herein or perform any independent analysis in connection with any of the product information contained herein. Publisher does not assume, and expressly disclaims, any obligation to obtain and include information other than that provided to it by the manufacturer.

The reader is expressly warned to consider and adopt all safety precautions that might be indicated by the activities described herein and to avoid all potential hazards. By following the instructions contained herein, the reader willingly assumes all risks in connection with such instructions.

The publisher makes no representations or warranties of any kind, including but not limited to, the warranties of fitness for particular purpose or merchantability, nor are any such representations implied with respect to the material set forth herein, and the publisher takes no responsibility with respect to such material. The publisher shall not be liable for any special, consequential, or exemplary damages resulting, in whole or part, from the reader's use of, or reliance upon, this material.

Contents

SECTION 1 Refresher Math

SECTION 2 Introduction to Drug Measures

SECTION 3 Reading Medication Labels and Syringe Calibrations

SECTION **7** Pediatric Medication Calculations

Reviewers

Elizabeth Battalora, MSN, RN, CNOR
Assistant Professor of Nursing
Louisiana College
Pineville, LA

Suzanne Carpenter, MSN, RN
Associate Professor of Nursing
Our Lady of the Lake College
Baton Rouge, LA

Diane Creed-Kern, MSN, RN
Professor of Nursing
Moraine Valley Community College
Palos Hills, IL

Rebecca Gesler
Director of Nursing
St. Catherine College
Louisville, KY

Patricia A. Roper, MSN, RN
Professor of Nursing
Columbus State Community College
Columbus, OH

Susan T. Sanders, RN, MSN, CNAA
Director of Nursing Education
Motlow State Community College
Lynchburg, TN

Russell Shipley, MA, RN, MSN
Instructor
Department of Nursing
Laramie County Community College
Cheyenne, WY

Manufacturers

Abbott Laboratories, Abbott Park, IL
Aminophylline, Fentanyl, Sterile Water for Injection, Bacteriostatic Sodium, 0.9% Sodium Chloride, Various IV Solutions, Synthroid

Akorn, Inc., Buffalo Grove, IL
Inapsine

American Pharmaceutical Partners, Schaumberg, IL
Potassium Chloride, Sodium Bicarbonate, Heparin Sodium, Furosemide, Dexamethasone Sodium Phosphate, Calcium Gluconate Injection

Amgen Inc., Thousand Oaks, CA
Cyanocobalamin, Furosemide, Levothyroxine Sodium, Gentamicin Sulfate Injection

Apothecon, Princeton, NJ
Nafcillin

Astra Zeneca LP, Wilmington, DE
Nexium, Toprol XL

Aventis Pharmaceuticals, Bridgewater, NJ
Carafate, Diabeta, Lasix, Claforan, Trental

Baxter Healthcare Corporation, Round Lake, IL (Baxter and Continu-Flo are trademarks of Baxter International, Inc.)
5% Dextrose Injection, 0.45% Sodium Chloride Injection, Continu-Flo Solution Set, Duramorph, Morphine Sulfate Injection, Lidocaine HCl Injection, Methotrexate Injection, Meperidine HCl Injection, Naloxone, Robinul

Bayer Corporation, West Haven, CT
Cipro

Becton-Dickinson and Company, Franklin Lake, NJ
Insulin Syringes, Tuberculin Syringe, Intravenous Syringes, Needleless Syringe System

Eisai, Inc., Teaneck, NJ
Aricept

Eli Lilly and Company, Indianapolis, IN
Humulin R, Humulin L, Humulin 50/50, Humulin 70/30, Humulin N, Humulin U, Humalog, Keflex, Tazidime, Oncovin, V-Cillin K, Nebcin, Vancocin, Kefzol, Ceclor, Regular Iletin, NPH Iletin

Endo Pharmaceutical, Chadds Ford, PA
Percocet, Narcan, Nubain

ESI Lederle, Division of Wyeth, Philadelphia, PA (Labels courtesy of ESI Lederle, a Business Unit of Wyeth Pharmaceuticals)
Robinul, Reglan, Hep-Lock, Heparin

GlaxoSmithKline, Research Triangle Park, NC (Labels reproduced with permission of GlaxoSmithKline)
Dyazide, Thorazine, Augmentin, Eskalith, Amoxil, Stelazine, Tazicef, Ticar, Ancef, Lanoxin, Zantac, Fortaz, Zofran

ICN Pharmaceuticals, Inc. (The following drugs are distributed by ICN Pharmaceuticals, Inc.)
Librium, Special Muscular Diluent

King Pharmaceuticals, Inc.
Bicillin C-R

Knoll Pharmaceuticals, Mt. Olive, NJ
Synthroid

Luitpold Pharmaceuticals, Shirley, NJ
Epinephrine Injection, Furosemide Injection

McNeil Consumer Health, Raritan, NJ (Courtesy of McNeil Consumer and Specialty Pharmaceuticals)
Haldol, Tylenol

Merck & Co. Inc., North Wales, PA (Labels used with permission of Merck & Co., Inc.)
Prinivil, Vasotec, Aldomet, Blocadren

Monarch Pharmaceuticals, Bristol, TN
Procanbid

Novartis Pharmaceuticals Corporation, Summit, NJ
Lopressor, Brethine

Novo Nordisk Pharmaceuticals, Inc., Princeton, NJ
Novolin 70/30, Novolin R, Novolin L, Novolin, N NPH

Ortho-McNeil Pharmaceuticals, Raritan, NJ
Haldol

Pfizer, Inc., New York, NY (Labels reproduced with permission of Pfizer, Inc.)
Antivert, Vistaril, Pfizerpen, Zithromax, Unasyn, Lopid, Nitrostat, Terramycin, Dilantin, Procardia, Glucotrol, Feldene, Minipress

Pharmaceutical Associates, Inc., Tampa, FL
Potassium Chloride Solution

Pharmacia Corporation, Peapack, NJ, and Kalamazoo, MI
Solu-Medrol, Micronase, Calan, Xanax, Halcion, Cleocin Phosphate, Lomotil, Theo-24, Flagyl, Aldactone, Heparin Sodium, Depo-Provera, Vantin, Bacitracin for Injection, Amphocin, Azulphidine

Roche
    Librium

Roxane Laboratories, Inc., Columbus, OH (Labels used with permission of Roxane Laboratories, Inc.)
    Furosemide Oral Solution, Dexamethasone

Schering Laboratories, Kenilworth, NJ
    Proventil, Claritin D

Schwarz Pharma, Inc., Milwaukee, WI
    Dilatrate SR, Verelan

G.D. Searle & Co., Chicago, IL
    Aldactone, Calan SR, Flagyl, Lomotil, Lactulose

UCB Pharma, Inc., Smyrna, GA
    Lortab

Wyeth-Ayerst Laboratories, St. Davids, PA (Courtesy of Wyeth Pharmaceuticals)
    Robitussin, Robinul, Inderal, Phenergan

Zeneca Pharmaceuticals, Wilmington, DE
    Nolvadex, Oral Sorbitrate

Preface

This ninth edition of *Math for Meds* comes to press celebrating its thirty-first year as North America's leading dosage and solutions text. It continues to fill the instructional needs not only of the full range of nursing programs, but also of allied health programs as diverse as veterinarian, paramedical, and radiologic technology. In the past thirty-one years *Math for Meds* has participated in the education of close to a million learners, and the total of number of learners using the text has continued to rise yearly.

APPROACH

This edition represents an important milestone in dosage and solutions instruction. Because the Board of Nurse Examiners has changed its policy to approve use of calculators, safety in calculator use specific to dosage calculations has been included. The addition of calculators as a tool does not, however, eliminate the need for basic math competency in common and decimal fraction calculations. Dosage calculations, contrary to the innate fear still extant in many learners, are not difficult and can very often be done more quickly and safely manually. *Math for Meds* continues to address this need.

ORGANIZATION AND UNIQUE FEATURES

Math for Meds allows for self-paced study, progressing from basic to more complex information. Examples and review tests are used throughout to aid comprehension, and running answers allow the learner to receive immediate feedback on deficits and strengths. A key icon is used throughout the chapters to allow learners to easily identify important information. The most up-to date equipment and safety devices are depicted in color, and, finally, real, full-color drug labels are included with the problem sets.

CHANGES TO THE NINTH EDITION

An amazing number of changes are necessary in each text revision. New and changed equipment and drugs are but a few of the factors that mandate updating. Educators generously continue to gift their time and expertise, as do hundreds of experts in the private sector. All suggestions and innovations are thoroughly evaluated and, where pertinent, appropriately incorporated. A new CD-ROM accompanies this edition of *Math for Meds*, bringing an important additional tool to calculation instruction. "Directions to the Learner" is retained as an integral component of instruction, as is the Refresher Math PreTest.

Suggestions from educators continue to be my most important revision tool. I encourage comments from both educators and learners, which can be sent care of Thomson Delmar Learning.

Anna M. Curren
San Diego, CA

How to Use This Book

This text accommodates the needs of diverse learners through its step-by-step building block approach. It begins with a basic math pretest and progresses through elementary mathematical concepts such as working with fractions and decimals. It then begins familiarizing the user with drug labels and common drug measures and moves on to dosage calculations starting with the easiest and progressing to more complex problems. Each concept is explained and illustrated with examples. The user then has an opportunity to practice problems and is provided with answers that immediately follow the problem sets. This approach has been a successful tool for 31 years. Through dedicated study of this text, the user will build confidence and skill in performing dosage calculations.

PROBLEM SETS

Each chapter includes problem sets that allow the user to practice each concept with answers that directly follow for immediate feedback.

KEY POINTS

 When two insulins are combined in the same syringe, the regular (shortest acting) insulin is drawn up first.

A key icon designates important hints and reminders to help the user with calculations and to highlight important safety considerations.

EXAMPLES

EXAMPLE 2 The dosage strength available is **25 mg in 1.5 mL**. A dosage of **20 mg** has been ordered.

$$25 \text{ mg} : 1.5 \text{ mL} = 20 \text{ mg} : X \text{ mL}$$ make sure the units are written in the same sequence: mg : mL = mg : mL

$$25 : 1.5 = 20 : X$$ drop the measurement units

$$25X = 1.5 \times 20$$ multiply the extremes; then the means; keep X on the left

$$= \frac{30}{25}$$ divide by the number in front of X

$$= \frac{30}{25} = 1.2$$ reduce the common denominator by 5, then divide the final fraction, 6 by 5

$$X = \textbf{1.2 mL}$$

The dosage ordered, 20 mg, is a smaller amount of drug than the strength available, 25 mg (in 1.5 mL). So the answer should be smaller than 1.5 mL, and it is, 1.2 mL. This answer is logical.

Each concept is explicated using step-by-step examples of calculations with a mathematical illustration and a step-by-step narrative explanation.

SUMMARY SELF-TESTS

A comprehensive test is included at the end of each chapter to review all of the concepts presented in the chapter

COMBINED SYRINGE AND LABEL QUESTIONS

Problems require the user to perform dosage calculations and then indicate correct dosages on real-life syringes. Combined questions ensure that knowledge is integrated and applied.

LABELS

Actual, full-color labels are used to support the problems. The problems challenge the user to read and interpret information on the labels.

SYRINGE PHOTOS

Photos of real syringes are depicted in actual size to allow the user to practice reading intricate calibrations.

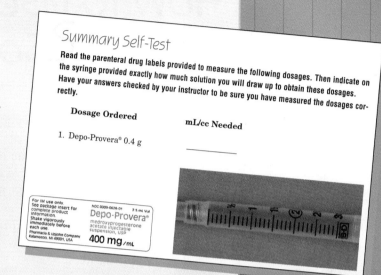

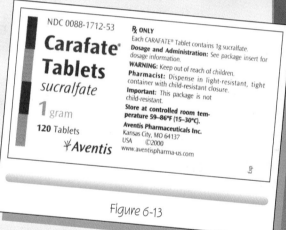

Figure 6-13

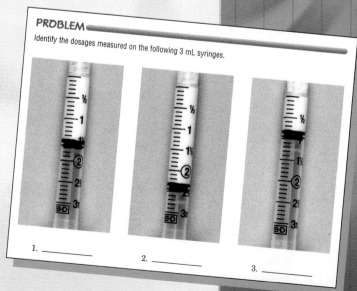

How to Use the Practice Software

We hope you enjoy the interactive CD that accompanies this book. Every attempt has been made to make it a fun, attractive, and effective learning environment for the user. Careful attention was paid to providing step-by-step solutions in a consistent format. Through the use of this software, the user will continuously expand skills and confidence in performing dosage calculations.

ORGANIZATION AND FEATURES

Main Menu

The main menu is organized by units and chapters that correspond to the units and chapters in the core book. The user can simultaneously view the names of each Unit, Chapter, Problem Set, and Summary Self-Test to select a topic to practice.

Practice Problems

Each chapter includes practice problems that incorporate labels and syringes for the most realistic and challenging practice experience. Practice problems allow the user two tries to obtain the correct answer. If the correct answer is not obtained on the second try, the answer and solution will appear on the screen.

Scoring

Most of the problems are scored so the user can assess strengths and weaknesses and determine which topics need further study.

Labels and Syringes

Real, full-color labels are provided to aid recognition and readability of information needed to perform a calculation. Photos of real syringes are also provided.

Interactive Syringes

Some questions include the use of interactive syringes. Users can actually use their mouse to click and drag the syringe plunger to the correct syringe measurement. All syringes are duplicated in actual size.

Summary Self-Tests

Comprehensive tests follow each chapter. The user has one opportunity to answer correctly to simulate a true testing environment. Answers and solutions are provided.

Directions to the Learner

Welcome to what we anticipate will be one of the most enjoyable texts you have ever used. *Math for Meds* is about to reassure you that math is nothing to be afraid of; that even the most difficult clinical calculations you encounter will present no problem for you; and that, on completion of your instruction, you will have the calculation skills you need to practice safely in your profession. You don't have to be a math expert to use this text. All that is required is average ability and a desire to learn. If you have not used your math skills for a number of years, you will still have no difficulty because the refresher math section will quickly bring you up to date. *Math for Meds* lets you move at your own pace through the content, which ranges from easy to thought provoking. Hundreds of examples and problems will keep your learning on track and you will enjoy learning from *Math for Meds*. Here are the tips you need to get started.

1. Gather a calculator, pencil or pen, and plenty of scratch paper.

2. Record the answers to calculations in your text as well as on the scratch paper. It makes checking your answers against those we provide much easier.

3. As you work your way through the chapters do exactly as you are instructed to do, and no more. Programmed learning proceeds in small steps, and jumping ahead may cause confusion. All chapters are designed to let you move at your own speed and if you already know some of the basics, you will move through them more quickly than you can imagine.

4. Start by completing the math pretest. This will alert you to those areas in the refresher math section that you will need to pay particular attention to. Some of the items in the pretest and refresher math section were designed to be completed without using a calculator, but the choice is entirely yours; when you need one, use one. You must remember, however, that calculator settings may vary. All answers in this text were checked with a calculator set to hundredths. If you use one with a different setting, you may experience differences in your answers in the number representing the hundredths or tenths.

5. Once you have completed your instruction, keep *Math for Meds* in your personal library. As you move to different clinical areas during your career, you will encounter different types of calculations. A quick refresher with *Math for Meds* will be invaluable when that occurs.

REFRESHER MATH PRETEST

If you can complete the following pretest with 100% accuracy, you may wish to bypass the Refresher Math section of this text, because all the pertinent math concepts are covered in the test items included. You should be aware, however, that this section offers many memory cues and shortcuts for solving clinical calculations without a calculator that will be used throughout the text.

Identify the decimal fraction with the highest value in each of the following.

1. a) 4.4   b) 2.85   c) 5.3   _____
2. a) 6.3   b) 5.73   c) 4.4   _____
3. a) 0.18   b) 0.62   c) 0.35   _____
4. a) 0.2   b) 0.125   c) 0.3   _____
5. a) 0.15   b) 0.11   c) 0.14   _____
6. a) 4.27   b) 4.31   c) 4.09   _____

Add the following decimals.

7. $0.2 + 2.23$ = _____
8. $1.5 + 0.07$ = _____
9. $6.45 + 12.1 + 9.54$ = _____
10. $0.35 + 8.37 + 5.15$ = _____

Subtract the following decimals.

11. $3.1 - 0.67$ = _____
12. $12.41 - 2.11$ = _____
13. $2.235 - 0.094$ = _____
14. $4.65 - 0.7$ = _____

15. If tablets with a strength of 0.2 mg are available and 0.6 mg is ordered, how many tablets must you give? _____

16. If tablets are labeled 0.8 mg and 0.4 mg is ordered, how many tablets must you give? _____

17. If the available tablets have a strength of 1.25 mg and 2.5 mg is ordered, how many tablets must you give? _____

18. If 0.125 mg is ordered and the tablets available are labeled 0.25 mg, how many tablets must you give? _____

Express the following numbers to the nearest tenth.

19. 2.17 = _____
20. 0.15 = _____
21. 3.77 = _____
22. 4.62 = _____
23. 11.74 = _____
24. 5.26 = _____

Express the following to the nearest hundredth.

25. 1.357 = _____
26. 7.413 = _____
27. 10.105 = _____
28. 3.775 = _____
29. 0.176 = _____
30. Define "product."

_____
_____

Multiply the following decimals. Express your answers to the nearest tenth.

31. 0.7×1.2 = _____
32. 1.8×2.6 = _____
33. $5.1 \times 0.25 \times 1.1$ = _____
34. 3.3×3.75 = _____

Divide the following fractions. Express your answers to the nearest hundredth.

35. $16.3 \div 3.2$ = _____
36. $15.1 \div 1.1$ = _____
37. $2 \div 0.75$ = _____
38. $4.17 \div 2.7$ = _____
39. Define "numerator."

_____
_____

40. Define "denominator."

_____
_____

41. Define "highest common denominator."

_____
_____

Solve the following equations. Express your answers to the nearest tenth.

42. $\dfrac{1}{4} \times \dfrac{2}{3}$ = _____

43. $\dfrac{240}{170} \times \dfrac{135}{300}$ = _____

44. $\dfrac{0.2}{1.75} \times \dfrac{1.5}{0.2}$ = _____

45. $\dfrac{2.1}{3.6} \times \dfrac{1.7}{1.3}$ = _____

46. $\dfrac{0.26}{0.2} \times \dfrac{3.3}{1.2}$ = _____

47. $\dfrac{750}{1} \times \dfrac{300}{50} \times \dfrac{7}{2}$ = _____

48. $\dfrac{50}{1} \times \dfrac{60}{240} \times \dfrac{1}{900} \times \dfrac{400}{1}$ = _____

49. $\dfrac{35,000}{750} \times \dfrac{35}{1}$ = _____

50. $\dfrac{50}{2} \times \dfrac{450}{40} \times \dfrac{1}{900} \times \dfrac{114}{1}$ = _____

Answers
1. c
2. a
3. b
4. c
5. a
6. b
7. 2.43
8. 1.57
9. 28.09
10. 13.87
11. 2.43
12. 10.3
13. 2.141
14. 3.95
15. 3 tab
16. ½ tab
17. 2 tab
18. ½ tab
19. 2.2
20. 0.2
21. 3.8
22. 4.6
23. 11.7
24. 5.3
25. 1.36
26. 7.41
27. 10.11
28. 3.78
29. 0.18
30. The answer obtained from the multiplication of two or more numbers
31. 0.8
32. 4.7
33. 1.4
34. 12.4
35. 5.09
36. 13.73
37. 2.67
38. 1.54
39. The top number in a common fraction
40. The bottom number in a common fraction
41. The highest number that can be divided into two numbers to reduce them to their lowest terms (values)
42. 0.2
43. 0.6
44. 0.9
45. 0.8
46. 3.6
47. 15,750
48. 5.6
49. 1633.3
50. 35.6

SECTION 1

Refresher Math

Relative Value, Addition and Subtraction of Decimals

In the course of administering medications, you will be dealing with decimal fraction dosages on a daily basis. The first two chapters of this text provide a complete and easy refresher of everything you need to know about decimals, including safety measures when you do calculations both manually and with a calculator. We'll start with a review of the range of decimal values you will see in dosages. This will enable you to immediately recognize which of two or more numbers has the highest (and lowest) value—a skill you will use constantly in your professional career.

RELATIVE VALUE OF DECIMALS

The most helpful fact to remember about decimals is that **our monetary system of dollars and cents is a decimal system**. The whole numbers in dosages have the same relative value as dollars, and decimal fractions have the same value as cents: **the higher the number, the higher the value**. If you keep this constantly in mind, you will already have learned the most important safety measure of dealing with decimals.

The range of drug dosages, which includes decimal fractions, stretches from millions on the whole number side to thousandths on the decimal side. Refer to the decimal scale in Figure 1-1, and locate the decimal point, which is slightly to the right on this scale. Notice first the whole numbers on the left of the scale, which rise increasingly in value from ones (units) to millions, which is the largest whole number drug dosage in use.

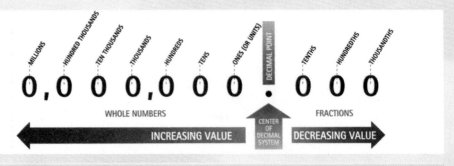

Figure 1-1

The first key point in determining relative value of decimals is the presence of whole numbers. The higher the whole number, the higher the value.

EXAMPLE 1 | 10.1 is higher than 9.15

EXAMPLE 2 | 3.2 is higher than 2.99

EXAMPLE 3 | 7.01 is higher than 6.99

PROBLEM

Identify the number with the highest value in each of the following.

1. a) 3.5   b) 2.7   c) 4.2   _____

2. a) 6.15   b) 5.95   c) 4.54   _____

3. a) 12.02   b) 10.19   c) 11.04   _____

4. a) 2.5   b) 1.75   c) 0.75   _____

5. a) 4.3   b) 2.75   c) 5.1   _____

6. a) 6.15   b) 7.4   c) 5.95   _____

Answers **1.** c **2.** a **3.** a **4.** a **5.** c **6.** b

If, however, the whole numbers are the same, for example, **10**.2 and **10**.7, or there are no whole numbers, for example, **0**.25 and **0**.35, **then the fraction will determine the relative value**. Let's take a closer look at the fractional side of the scale (refer to Figure 1-2).

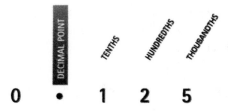

Figure 1-2

It is necessary to consider only three figures after the decimal point on the fractional side because drug dosages measured as decimal fractions do not contain more than three digits, for example, 0.125 mg. First notice that a **zero is used to replace the whole number** in this decimal fraction and in all other dosages that do not contain a whole number.

 If a decimal fraction is not preceded by a whole number, a zero is used in front of the decimal point to emphasize that the number is a fraction.

EXAMPLE | **0.125   0.1   0.45**

Look once again at Figure 1-2. The numbers on the right of the decimal point represent **tenths**, **hundredths**, and **thousandths** in that order. When you see a decimal fraction in which the **whole numbers are the same**, or there are **no whole numbers**, stop and look first at the number representing **tenths**.

 The fraction with the highest number representing tenths has the higher value.

| EXAMPLE 1 | 0.3 is higher than 0.27 |

| EXAMPLE 2 | 0.4 is higher than 0.29 |

| EXAMPLE 3 | 1.2 is higher than 1.19 |

PROBLEM

Which of the following decimals has the highest value?

1. a) 0.4   b) 0.2   c) 0.5   _____

2. a) 2.73   b) 2.61   c) 2.87   _____

3. a) 0.19   b) 0.61   c) 0.34   _____

4. a) 3.5   b) 3.75   c) 3.25   _____

5. a) 0.3   b) 0.25   c) 0.4   _____

6. a) 1.35   b) 1.29   c) 1.4   _____

Answers **1.** c. **2.** c **3.** b **4.** b **5.** c **6.** c

If in decimal fractions the numbers representing **the tenths are identical**, for example, 0.25 and 0.27, then **the number representing the hundredths will determine the relative value**.

 The decimal fraction with the higher number representing hundredths will have the higher value when the tenths are identical.

| EXAMPLE 1 | 0.27 is higher than 0.25 |

| EXAMPLE 2 | 0.15 is higher than 0.1 (0.1 is the same as 0.10) |

 Extra zeros on the end of decimal fractions are omitted in drug dosages because they can easily be misread.

| EXAMPLE 3 | 2.25 is higher than 2.2 (same as 2.20) |

| EXAMPLE 4 | 9.77 is higher than 9.7 (same as 9.70) |

PROBLEM

Which of the following decimals has the highest value?

1. a) 0.12	b) 0.15	c) 0.17	_____
2. a) 1.21	b) 1.24	c) 1.23	_____
3. a) 0.37	b) 0.32	c) 0.36	_____
4. a) 3.27	b) 3.25	c) 3.21	_____
5. a) 0.16	b) 0.11	c) 0.19	_____
6. a) 4.23	b) 4.2	c) 4.09	_____

Answers **1.** c **2.** b **3.** a **4.** a **5.** c **6.** a

 The number of figures on the right of the decimal point is not an indication of relative value. Always look at the figure representing the tenths first, and if these are identical, the hundredths, to determine which has the higher value.

PROBLEM

Which of the following fractions has the higher value?

a) 0.125   b) 0.25

Answer The correct answer is b) 0.25. The decimal fraction that has the higher number representing the **tenths** has the higher value. **2** is higher than **1**; therefore 0.**25** has a higher value than 0.**125**. Medication errors have been made in this **identical** decimal fraction; so remember it well.

This completes your introduction to the relative value of decimals. The key points just reviewed will cover all situations in dosage calculations where you will have to recognize high and low values. Therefore, you are now ready to test yourself more extensively on this information.

PROBLEM

Identify the decimal with the highest value in each of the following.

1. a) 0.24	b) 0.5	c) 0.125	_____
2. a) 0.4	b) 0.45	c) 0.5	_____
3. a) 7.5	b) 6.25	c) 4.75	_____
4. a) 0.3	b) 0.25	c) 0.35	_____
5. a) 1.125	b) 1.75	c) 1.5	_____
6. a) 4.5	b) 4.75	c) 4.25	_____
7. a) 0.1	b) 0.01	c) 0.04	_____
8. a) 5.75	b) 6.25	c) 6.5	_____
9. a) 0.6	b) 0.16	c) 0.06	_____
10. a) 3.55	b) 2.95	c) 3.7	_____

Answers **1.** b **2.** c **3.** a **4.** c **5.** b **6.** b **7.** a **8.** c **9.** a **10.** c

ADDITION AND SUBTRACTION OF DECIMALS

Complicated addition and subtraction of decimals should be done with a calculator, but, on occasion, time can be saved by doing simple dosage calculations without one. Let's start by looking at a few key points that will make manual solution safer.

 When you write the numbers down, line up the decimal points.

EXAMPLE | To add 0.25 and 0.27

$$
\begin{array}{l}
0.25 \\
+0.27 \text{ is safe}
\end{array}
\qquad
\begin{array}{l}
0.25 \\
0.27 \text{ may be unsafe; it could lead to errors.}
\end{array}
$$

 Always add or subtract from right to left.

If you decide to write the numbers down, **don't confuse yourself by trying to "eyeball" the answer**. Also write any numbers carried, or rewrite those reduced by borrowing if you find this helpful.

EXAMPLE 1 | When adding 0.25 and 0.27

$$
\begin{array}{r}
1 \\
0.25 \\
+0.27 \\
\hline
0.52
\end{array}
$$
add the 5 and 7 first, then the 2, 2, and the 1 you carried. Work from right to left.

EXAMPLE 2 | When subtracting 0.63 from 0.71

$$
\begin{array}{r}
6\,1 \\
0.7\!\!\!\diagup1 \\
-0.63 \\
\hline
0.08
\end{array}
$$
borrow 1 from 7 and rewrite as 6, write the borrowed 1. Subtract 3 from 11. Subtract 6 from 6. Work from right to left.

 Add zeros as necessary to make the fractions of equal length.

This does not alter the value of the fractions and it helps prevent confusion and mistakes.

EXAMPLE | When subtracting 0.125 from 0.25

$$
\begin{array}{l}
0.25 \\
0.125
\end{array}
\quad \text{becomes} \quad
\begin{array}{l}
0.250 \\
0.125
\end{array}
\qquad \text{Answer} = \mathbf{0.125}
$$

If you follow these simple rules and make them a habit, you will automatically reduce calculation errors. The problems on the following page will give you an excellent opportunity to practice them.

PROBLEM

Add the following decimals.

1. 0.25 + 0.55 = _____

2. 0.1 + 2.25 = _____

3. 1.74 + 0.76 = _____

4. 1.4 + 0.02 = _____

5. 2.3 + 1.45 = _____

6. 3.75 + 1.05 = _____

7. 6.35 + 2.05 = _____

8. 5.57 + 4.03 = _____

9. 0.33 + 2.42 = _____

10. 1.44 + 3.06 = _____

Subtract the following decimals.

11. 1.25 − 1.125 = _____

12. 3.25 − 0.65 = _____

13. 2.3 − 1.45 = _____

14. 0.02 − 0.01 = _____

15. 5.5 − 2.5 = _____

16. 7.33 − 4.03 = _____

17. 4.25 − 1.75 = _____

18. 0.07 − 0.035 = _____

19. 0.235 − 0.12 = _____

20. 5.75 − 0.95 = _____

Answers **1.** 0.8 **2.** 2.35 **3.** 2.5 **4.** 1.42 **5.** 3.75 **6.** 4.8 **7.** 8.4 **8.** 9.6 **9.** 2.75 **10.** 4.5 **11.** 0.125 **12.** 2.6 **13.** 0.85 **14.** 0.01 **15.** 3 **16.** 3.3 **17.** 2.5 **18.** 0.035 **19.** 0.115 **20.** 4.8 **Note:** If you did not add a zero before the decimal point in answers that do not contain a whole number, or failed to eliminate unnecessary zeros from the end of decimal fractions, your answers are incorrect.

USING A CALCULATOR FOR ADDITION AND SUBTRACTION

Calculators vary in how plus or minus signs must be entered and in the number of fractions they display after the decimal point, so the first precaution in calculator use is to be sure you know how to use the one available to you. If you find yourself in a situation where you must do frequent calculations, it would be wise to buy and use your own. The next precaution, and this is critical, is to enter the decimal numbers correctly, which includes **entering the decimal points**. This is not as simple as it sounds, and it is here that most dosage errors occur. Be aware that **calculator entry errors may be repetitive, so visually check each entry before entering the next**.

If you enter the numbers correctly, a calculator will normally **add a zero when a whole number is not present** in the answer and **eliminate excess zeros at the end of the answer**.

Summary

This concludes the refresher on relative value, addition and subtraction of simple decimals. The important points to remember from this chapter are:

- If the decimal fraction contains a whole number, the value of the whole number is the first determiner of relative value.

- If the fraction does not include a whole number, a zero is placed in front of the decimal point to emphasize it.

- If there is no whole number, or if the whole numbers are the same, the number representing the tenths in the decimal fraction will be the next determiner of relative value.

- If the tenths in decimal fractions are identical, the number representing hundredths will determine relative value.

- When adding or subtracting decimal fractions, first line up the decimal points, then add or subtract from right to left.

- Extra zeros on the end of decimal fractions can be a source of error and are routinely eliminated.

Summary Self-Test

Choose the decimal with the highest value from each of the following.

1. a) 2.45   b) 2.57   c) 2.19   _____

2. a) 3.07   b) 3.17   c) 3.71   _____

3. a) 0.12   b) 0.02   c) 0.01   _____

4. a) 5.31   b) 5.35   c) 6.01   _____

5. a) 4.5   b) 4.51   c) 4.15   _____

6. a) 0.015   b) 0.15   c) 0.1   _____

7. a) 1.3   b) 1.25   c) 1.35   _____

8. a) 0.1   b) 0.2   c) 0.25   _____

9. a) 0.125   b) 0.1   c) 0.05   _____

10. a) 13.7   b) 13.5   c) 13.25   _____

11. If you have medication tablets whose strength is 0.1 mg and you must give 0.3 mg, you will need

    a) 1 tablet   b) less than 1 tablet   c) more than 1 tablet   _____

12. If you have tablets with a strength of 0.25 mg and you must give 0.125 mg, you will need

    a) 1 tablet   b) less than 1 tablet   c) more than 1 tablet   _____

13. If you have an order to give a dosage of 7.5 mg and the tablets have a strength of 3.75 mg, you will need

    a) 1 tablet   b) less than 1 tablet   c) more than 1 tablet   _____

14. If the order is to give 0.5 mg and the tablet strength is 0.5 mg, you will give

    a) 1 tablet   b) less than 1 tablet   c) more than 1 tablet   _____

15. The order is to give 0.5 mg and the tablets have a strength of 0.25 mg. You must give

    a) 1 tablet   b) less than 1 tablet   c) more than 1 tablet   _____

Add the following decimals using a calculator.

16. $1.31 + 0.4 =$ _____   18. $2.5 + 0.75 =$ _____

17. $0.15 + 0.25 =$ _____   19. $3.2 + 2.17 =$ _____

20. 1.3 + 1.04 = _____   22. 0.5 + 0.5 = _____

21. 4.7 + 3.03 = _____   23. 5.4 + 2.6 = _____

24. You have just given two tablets with a dosage strength of 3.5 mg each. What was the total dosage administered? _____

25. You are to give your patient one tablet labeled 0.5 mg and one labeled 0.25 mg. What is the total dosage of these two tablets? _____

26. If you give two tablets labeled 0.02 mg, what total dosage will you administer? _____

27. You are to give one tablet labeled 0.8 mg and two tablets labeled 0.4 mg. What is the total dosage? _____

28. You have two tablets: one is labeled 0.15 mg and the other 0.3 mg. What is the total dosage of these two tablets? _____

Subtract the following decimals using a calculator.

29. 4.32 − 3.1 = _____   33. 1.3 − 0.02 = _____

30. 2.1 − 1.91 = _____   34. 0.2 − 0.07 = _____

31. 3.73 − 1.93 = _____   35. 3.95 − 0.35 = _____

32. 5.75 − 4.05 = _____   36. 1.9 − 0.08 = _____

37. Your patient is to receive a dosage of 7.5 mg and you have only one tablet labeled 3.75 mg. How many more milligrams must you give? _____

38. You have a tablet labeled 0.02 mg and your patient is to receive 0.06 mg. How many more milligrams must you give? _____

39. The tablet available is labeled 0.5 mg but you must give a dosage of 1.5 mg. How many more milligrams will you need to obtain the correct dosage? _____

40. Your patient is to receive a dosage of 1.2 mg and you have one tablet labeled 0.6 mg. What additional dosage in milligrams will you need? _____

41. You must give your patient a dosage of 2.2 mg but you have only two tablets labeled 0.55 mg. What additional dosage in milligrams will you need? _____

Determine how many tablets will be needed to give the following dosages.

42. Tablets are labeled 0.01 mg. You must give 0.02 mg. _____

43. Tablets are labeled 2.5 mg. You must give 5 mg. _____

44. Tablets are labeled 0.25 mg. Give 0.125 mg. _____

45. Tablets are 0.5 mg. Give 1.5 mg. _____

46. A dosage of 1.8 mg is ordered. Tablets are 0.6 mg. _____

47. Tablets available are 0.04 mg. You are to give 0.02 mg. _____

48. The dosage ordered is 3.5 mg. The tablets available are 1.75 mg. _____

49. Prepare a dosage of 3.2 mg using tablets with a strength of 1.6 mg. _____

50. You have tablets labeled 0.25 mg, and a dosage of 0.375 mg is ordered. _____

Answers	11. c	22. 1	33. 1.28	44. ½ tab
1. b	12. b	23. 8	34. 0.13	45. 3 tab
2. c	13. c	24. 7 mg	35. 3.6	46. 3 tab
3. a	14. a	25. 0.75 mg	36. 1.82	47. ½ tab
4. c	15. c	26. 0.04 mg	37. 3.75 mg	48. 2 tab
5. b	16. 1.71	27. 1.6 mg	38. 0.04 mg	49. 2 tab
6. b	17. 0.4	28. 0.45 mg	39. 1 mg	50. 1½ tab
7. c	18. 3.25	29. 1.22	40. 0.6 mg	
8. c	19. 5.37	30. 0.19	41. 1.1 mg	
9. a	20. 2.34	31. 1.8	42. 2 tab	
10. a	21. 7.73	32. 1.7	43. 2 tab	

Note: If you did not add a zero before the decimal point in answers that did not contain a whole number, or failed to eliminate unnecessary zeros from the end of decimal fractions, your answers are incorrect.

Multiplication and Division of Decimals

Multiplication and division of dosages containing decimals may be routinely done using a calculator. For the purpose of review, however, this chapter starts with a refresher on the terminology of both multiplication and division that will be used in later chapters, as well as a refresher on simple multiplications that may be done manually without a calculator.

MULTIPLICATION OF DECIMALS WITHOUT USING A CALCULATOR

The main precaution in non-calculator multiplication of decimals is the **placement of the decimal point in the answer,** which is called the **product**.

 The decimal point in the product of decimal fractions is placed the same number of places to the left in the product as the total of numbers after the decimal points in the fractions multiplied.

> EXAMPLE 1 | Multiply 0.35 by 0.5.

Begin by lining up the numbers to be multiplied on the right side, because this is safer. Then disregard the decimals during the multiplication.

$$\begin{array}{r} 0.35 \\ \times\ \underline{0.5} \\ 175 \end{array}$$

0.35 has two numbers after the decimal and 0.5 has one. Place the decimal point three places to the left in the product to make it .175, then add a zero (0) in front of the fraction to emphasize it.

Answer = **0.175**

Objectives

The learner will:

1. define product, numerator, and denominator

2. multiply decimal fractions

3. reduce fractions using common denominators

4. divide fractions and express answers to the nearest tenth and hundredth using a calculator

Prerequisite

Chapter 1

EXAMPLE 2 | Multiply 1.61 by 0.2.

$$
\begin{array}{r}
1.61 \\
\times \quad 0.2 \\
\hline
322
\end{array}
$$

1.61 has two numbers after the decimal point and 0.2 has one. Place the decimal point three places to the left in the product, so that 322 becomes .322, then add a zero in front of the fraction to emphasize it.

Answer = **0.322**

 If the product contains insufficient numbers for correct placement of the decimal point, add as many zeros as necessary to the left of the product to correct this.

EXAMPLE 3 | Multiply 1.5 by 0.06.

$$
\begin{array}{r}
1.5 \\
\times \quad 0.06 \\
\hline
90
\end{array}
$$

1.5 has one number after the decimal point and 0.06 has two. To place the decimal three places to the left in the product, a zero must be added, making it 0.090. The excess zero is then eliminated from the end of the fraction; thus 0.090 becomes 0.09.

Answer = **0.09**

EXAMPLE 4 | Multiply 0.21 by 0.32.

$$
\begin{array}{r}
0.21 \\
\times \quad 0.32 \\
\hline
42 \\
\times \quad 63 \\
\hline
672
\end{array}
$$

In this example 0.21 has two numbers after the decimal point and 0.32 also has two. Add a zero in front of the product to allow correct placement of the decimal point, making it .0672, then add a zero in front of the fraction to emphasize it.

Answer = **0.0672**

EXAMPLE 5 | Multiply 0.12 by 0.2.

$$
\begin{array}{r}
0.12 \\
\times \quad 0.2 \\
\hline
24
\end{array}
$$

In this example there are a total of three numbers after the decimal points in 0.12 and 0.2. Add a zero in front of the product for correct decimal placement in the answer, making it .024, then add a zero in front of .024 to emphasize the fraction.

Answer = **0.024**

PROBLEM

Multiply the following decimal fractions without using a calculator.

1. 0.45×0.2 = _____   4. 0.7×0.04 = _____

2. 0.35×0.12 = _____   5. 0.4×0.17 = _____

3. 1.3×0.05 = _____   6. 2.14×0.03 = _____

Answers **1.** 0.09 **2.** 0.042 **3.** 0.065 **4.** 0.028 **5.** 0.068 **6.** 0.0642

DIVISION OF DECIMALS

A calculator should be used for all complicated divisions involving dosages. However, let's start by reviewing the terminology of common fraction division and **three important precalculator** steps that may make final division easier: **elimination of decimal points, reduction of fractions**, and **reduction of numbers ending in zero**. The following is a sample of a common fraction division seen in dosages:

EXAMPLE 1 $\quad \dfrac{0.25}{0.125} = \dfrac{\text{numerator}}{\text{denominator}}$

You'll recall that the **top number** in a common fraction is called the **numerator**, whereas the **bottom number** is called the **denominator**. If you have trouble remembering which is which, think of **D**, for **down**, for **denominator**. The denominator is on the bottom. With this basic terminology reviewed, we are now ready to look at the preliminary math steps that are used to simplify a fraction before calculator division.

ELIMINATION OF DECIMAL POINTS

Decimal points can be eliminated from the numbers in a decimal fraction without changing its value.

 To eliminate the decimal points from decimal fractions, move them the same number of places to the right in a numerator and a denominator until they are eliminated from both. Zeros may have to be added to accomplish this.

EXAMPLE 1 $\quad \dfrac{0.25}{0.125}$ becomes $\dfrac{250}{125}$

The decimal point must be moved three places to the right in the denominator 0.125 to make it 125. Therefore, it must be moved three places to the right in the numerator 0.25, which requires the addition of one zero to make it 250.

EXAMPLE 2 $\quad \dfrac{0.3}{0.15}$ becomes $\dfrac{30}{15}$

The decimal point must be moved two places in 0.15 to make it 15 so it must be moved two places in 0.3, which requires the addition of one zero to become 30.

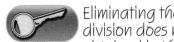 EXAMPLE 3 | $\dfrac{1.5}{2}$ becomes $\dfrac{15}{20}$

Move the decimal point one place in 1.5 to make it 15; add one zero to 2 to make it 20.

EXAMPLE 4 | $\dfrac{4.5}{0.95}$ becomes $\dfrac{450}{95}$

Eliminating the decimal points from a decimal fraction before final division does not alter the value of the fraction or the answer obtained in the final division.

PROBLEM

Eliminate the decimal points from the following decimal fractions.

1. $\dfrac{17.5}{2}$ = _____

2. $\dfrac{0.5}{25}$ = _____

3. $\dfrac{6.3}{0.6}$ = _____

4. $\dfrac{3.76}{0.4}$ = _____

5. $\dfrac{8.4}{0.7}$ = _____

6. $\dfrac{0.1}{0.05}$ = _____

7. $\dfrac{0.9}{0.03}$ = _____

8. $\dfrac{10.75}{2.5}$ = _____

9. $\dfrac{0.4}{0.04}$ = _____

10. $\dfrac{1.2}{0.4}$ = _____

Answers 1. $\dfrac{175}{20}$ 2. $\dfrac{5}{250}$ 3. $\dfrac{63}{6}$ 4. $\dfrac{376}{40}$ 5. $\dfrac{84}{7}$ 6. $\dfrac{10}{5}$ 7. $\dfrac{90}{3}$ 8. $\dfrac{1075}{250}$ 9. $\dfrac{40}{4}$ 10. $\dfrac{12}{4}$

REDUCTION OF FRACTIONS

Once the decimal points are eliminated, a second simplification step is to reduce the numbers as far as possible using common denominators.

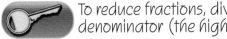 To reduce fractions, divide both numbers by their highest common denominator (the highest number that will divide into both).

The **highest common denominator** is usually **2, 3, 4, 5, or multiples of these numbers**, such as 6, 8, 25, and so on.

EXAMPLE 1 | $\dfrac{175}{20}$ The highest common denominator is 5

$$\dfrac{\cancel{175}}{\cancel{20}} = \dfrac{35}{4}$$

EXAMPLE 2 | $\dfrac{63}{6}$ The highest common denominator is 3

$$\dfrac{\cancel{63}}{\cancel{6}} = \dfrac{21}{2}$$

EXAMPLE 3 | $\dfrac{1075}{250}$ The highest common denominator is 25

$$\dfrac{\cancel{1075}}{\cancel{250}} = \dfrac{43}{10}$$

There is a second way you could have reduced the fraction in example 3, and it is equally as correct. Divide by 5, then 5 again.

$$\dfrac{\cancel{1075}}{\cancel{250}} = \dfrac{\cancel{215}}{\cancel{50}} = \dfrac{43}{10}$$

 If the highest common denominator is difficult to determine, reduce several times by using smaller common denominators.

EXAMPLE 4 | $\dfrac{376}{40} = \dfrac{47}{5}$ Reduce by 8

or divide by 4, then 2 $\dfrac{\cancel{376}}{\cancel{40}} = \dfrac{\cancel{94}}{\cancel{10}} = \dfrac{47}{5}$

or divide by 2, 2, then 2 $\dfrac{\cancel{376}}{\cancel{40}} = \dfrac{\cancel{188}}{\cancel{20}} = \dfrac{\cancel{94}}{\cancel{10}} = \dfrac{47}{5}$

Remember that **simple numbers are easiest to work with**, and the time spent in extra reductions may be well worth the payoff in safety.

PROBLEM

Reduce the following fractions as much as possible in preparation for final division.

1. $\dfrac{84}{8}$ = _____   6. $\dfrac{40}{14}$ = _____

2. $\dfrac{20}{16}$ = _____   7. $\dfrac{82}{28}$ = _____

3. $\dfrac{250}{325}$ = _____   8. $\dfrac{100}{75}$ = _____

4. $\dfrac{96}{34}$ = _____   9. $\dfrac{50}{75}$ = _____

5. $\dfrac{175}{20}$ = _____   10. $\dfrac{60}{88}$ = _____

Answers **1.** $\dfrac{21}{2}$ **2.** $\dfrac{5}{4}$ **3.** $\dfrac{10}{13}$ **4.** $\dfrac{48}{17}$ **5.** $\dfrac{35}{4}$ **6.** $\dfrac{20}{7}$ **7.** $\dfrac{41}{14}$ **8.** $\dfrac{4}{3}$ **9.** $\dfrac{2}{3}$ **10.** $\dfrac{15}{22}$

REDUCTION OF NUMBERS ENDING IN ZERO

The third type of simplification is not solely related to decimal fractions but is best covered at this time. This concerns reductions when both numbers in the fraction end with zeros.

EXAMPLE $\dfrac{800}{250}$

 Fractions that end in a zero or zeros may initially be reduced by crossing off the same number of zeros in both a numerator and a denominator.

EXAMPLE 1 $\dfrac{800}{250}$

In this fraction the numerator, 800, has two zeros and the denominator, 250, has one zero. The number of zeros crossed off must be the same in both numerator and denominator, so only one zero can be eliminated from each.

$$\frac{80\cancel{0}}{25\cancel{0}} = \frac{80}{25} \quad \text{Reduce by 5} = \frac{16}{5}$$

EXAMPLE 2 $\dfrac{24\cancel{00}}{20\cancel{00}} = \dfrac{24}{20}$ Reduce by 4 $= \dfrac{6}{5}$

Two zeros can be eliminated from the denominator and the numerator in this fraction.

EXAMPLE 3 $\dfrac{15\cancel{000}}{30\cancel{000}} = \dfrac{15}{30}$ Reduce by 5 $= \dfrac{3}{6}$

In this fraction three zeros can be eliminated.

PROBLEM

Reduce the following fractions to their lowest terms in preparation for final division.

1. $\dfrac{50}{250}$ = _____   6. $\dfrac{110}{100}$ = _____

2. $\dfrac{120}{50}$ = _____   7. $\dfrac{200{,}000}{150{,}000}$ = _____

3. $\dfrac{2500}{1500}$ = _____   8. $\dfrac{1000}{800}$ = _____

4. $\dfrac{1{,}000{,}000}{750{,}000}$ = _____   9. $\dfrac{60}{40}$ = _____

5. $\dfrac{800}{150}$ = _____   10. $\dfrac{150}{200}$ = _____

Answers **1.** $\frac{1}{5}$ **2.** $\frac{12}{5}$ **3.** $\frac{5}{3}$ **4.** $\frac{4}{3}$ **5.** $\frac{16}{3}$ **6.** $\frac{11}{10}$ **7.** $\frac{4}{3}$ **8.** $\frac{5}{4}$ **9.** $\frac{3}{2}$ **10.** $\frac{3}{4}$

EXPRESSING TO THE NEAREST TENTH

When a fraction is reduced as much as possible, it is ready for final division. This is done by **dividing the numerator by the denominator**. Answers are most often rounded off and expressed as decimal numbers to the nearest tenth. If the division is simple it can be done manually, or you may use a calculator.

 To express an answer to the nearest tenth, the division is carried to hundredths (two places after the decimal). When the number representing hundredths is 5 or larger, the number representing tenths is increased by one.

EXAMPLE 1 $\dfrac{0.35}{0.4}$ = 0.35 ÷ 0.4 = 0.87

Answer = **0.9**

The number representing hundredths is 7, so the number representing tenths is increased by one: 0.87 becomes 0.9.

EXAMPLE 2 $\dfrac{0.5}{0.3}$ = 0.5 ÷ 0.3 = 1.66 = **1.7**

The number representing hundredths, 6, is larger than 5, so 1.66 becomes 1.7

EXAMPLE 3 $\dfrac{0.16}{0.3}$ = 0.53 = **0.5**

The number representing hundredths, 3, is less than 5, so the number representing tenths, 5, remains unchanged.

EXAMPLE 4 $\dfrac{0.2}{0.3}$ = 0.66 = **0.7**

EXAMPLE 5 An answer of 1.42 remains **1.4**

EXAMPLE 6 An answer of 1.86 becomes **1.9**

PROBLEM

Use a calculator to divide the following decimal numbers. Express your answers to the nearest tenth.

1. $\dfrac{5.1}{2.3}$ = _____

2. $\dfrac{0.9}{0.7}$ = _____

3. $\dfrac{3.7}{2}$ = _____

4. $\dfrac{6}{1.3}$ = _____

5. $\dfrac{1.5}{2.1}$ = _____

6. $\dfrac{2.7}{1.1}$ = _____

7. $\dfrac{4.2}{5}$ = _____

8. $\dfrac{0.5}{2.5}$ = _____

9. $\dfrac{5.2}{0.91}$ = _____

10. $\dfrac{2.4}{2.7}$ = _____

Answers **1.** 2.2 **2.** 1.3 **3.** 1.9 **4.** 4.6 **5.** 0.7 **6.** 2.5 **7.** 0.8 **8.** 0.2 **9.** 5.7 **10.** 0.9

EXPRESSING TO THE NEAREST HUNDREDTH

Some drugs are administered in dosages carried to the nearest hundredth. This is common in pediatric dosages and in drugs that alter the body's vital function, for example, heart rate.

 To express an answer to the nearest hundredth, the division is carried to thousandths (three places after the decimal point). When the number representing thousandths is 5 or larger, the number representing hundredths is increased by one.

EXAMPLE 1 | 0.736 becomes **0.74**

The number representing thousandths, 6, is larger than 5, so the number representing hundredths, 3, is increased by one to become 4.

EXAMPLE 2 | 0.777 becomes **0.78**

EXAMPLE 3 | 0.373 remains **0.37**

The number representing thousandths, 3, is less than 5, so the number representing hundredths, 7, remains unchanged.

EXAMPLE 4 | 0.934 remains **0.93**

PROBLEM

Express the following numbers to the nearest hundredth.

1. 0.175 = _____
2. 0.344 = _____
3. 1.853 = _____
4. 0.306 = _____
5. 3.015 = _____
6. 2.154 = _____

7. 1.081 = _____
8. 1.327 = _____
9. 0.739 = _____
10. 0.733 = _____
11. 2.072 = _____
12. 0.089 = _____

Answers **1.** 0.18 **2.** 0.34 **3.** 1.85 **4.** 0.31 **5.** 3.02 **6.** 2.15 **7.** 1.08 **8.** 1.33 **9.** 0.74 **10.** 0.73 **11.** 2.07 **12.** 0.09

Summary

This concludes the chapter on multiplication and division of decimals. The important points to remember from this chapter are:

- When decimal fractions are multiplied, the decimal point is placed the same number of places to the left in the product as the total of numbers after the decimal points in the fractions multiplied.

- Zeros must be placed in front of a product if it contains insufficient numbers for correct placement of the decimal point.

- To simplify decimal fractions before calculator division, the preliminary steps of eliminating the decimal points and reducing the numbers by common denominators can be used.

- A calculator may be used for division of fractions.

- To express to tenths, increase the answer by one if the number representing the hundredths is 5 or larger.

- To express to hundredths, increase the answer by one if the number representing the thousandths is 5 or larger.

- When a calculator is used, it will automatically add a zero in front of a decimal fraction and eliminate unnecessary zeros from the end of a fraction.

Summary Self-Test

Multiply the following decimals. A calculator may be used.

1. $1.49 \times 0.05 =$ _____

2. $0.15 \times 3.04 =$ _____

3. $0.025 \times 3.5 =$ _____

4. $0.55 \times 2.5 =$ _____

5. $1.31 \times 2.07 =$ _____

6. $5.3 \times 1.02 =$ _____

7. $0.35 \times 1.25 =$ _____

8. $4.32 \times 0.05 =$ _____

9. $0.2 \times 0.02 =$ _____

10. $0.4 \times 1.75 =$ _____

11. You are to administer four tablets with a dosage strength of 0.04 mg each. What total dosage are you giving? _____

12. You have given 2½ (2.5) tablets with a strength of 1.25 mg per tablet. What total dosage is this? _____

13. The tablets your patient is to receive are labeled 0.1 mg and you are to give 3½ (3.5) tablets. What total dosage is this? _____

14. You gave your patient 3 tablets labeled 0.75 mg each, and he was to receive a total of 2.25 mg. Did he receive the correct dosage? _____

15. The tablets available for your patient are labeled 12.5 mg, and you are to give 4½ (4.5) tablets. What total dosage will this be? _____

16. Your patient is to receive a dosage of 4.5 mg. The tablets available are labeled 3.5 mg, and there are 2½ tablets in his medication drawer. Is this a correct dosage? _____

Use a calculator to divide the following fractions. Express your answers to the nearest tenth.

17. $\dfrac{1.3}{0.7}$ = _____

18. $\dfrac{1.9}{3.2}$ = _____

19. $\dfrac{32.5}{9}$ = _____

20. $\dfrac{0.04}{0.1}$ = _____

21. $\dfrac{1.45}{1.2}$ = _____

22. $\dfrac{250}{1000}$ = _____

23. $\dfrac{0.8}{0.09}$ = _____

24. $\dfrac{2,000,000}{1,500,000}$ = _____

25. $\dfrac{4.1}{2.05}$ = _____

26. $\dfrac{7.3}{12}$ = _____

27. $\dfrac{150,000}{120,000}$ = _____

28. $\dfrac{0.15}{0.08}$ = _____

29. $\dfrac{2700}{900}$ = _____

30. $\dfrac{0.25}{0.15}$ = _____

Use a calculator to divide the following fractions. Express your answers to the nearest hundredth.

31. $\dfrac{900}{1700}$ = _____

32. $\dfrac{0.125}{0.3}$ = _____

33. $\dfrac{1450}{1500}$ = _____

34. $\dfrac{65}{175}$ = _____

35. $\dfrac{0.6}{1.35}$ = _____

36. $\dfrac{0.04}{0.12}$ = _____

37. $\dfrac{750}{10,000}$ = _____

38. $\dfrac{0.65}{0.8}$ = _____

39. $\dfrac{3.01}{4.2}$ = _____

40. $\dfrac{4.5}{6.1}$ = _____

41. $\dfrac{0.13}{0.25}$ = _____

42. $\dfrac{0.25}{0.7}$ = _____

43. $\dfrac{3.3}{5.1}$ = _____

44. $\dfrac{0.19}{0.7}$ = _____

45. $\dfrac{1.1}{1.3}$ = _____

46. $\dfrac{3}{4.1}$ = _____

47. $\dfrac{62}{240}$ = _____

48. $\dfrac{280,000}{300,000}$ = _____

49. $\dfrac{115}{255}$ = _____

50. $\dfrac{10}{14.3}$ = _____

Answers

1. 0.0745	**11.** 0.16 mg	**22.** 0.3	**33.** 0.97	**44.** 0.27
2. 0.456	**12.** 3.125 mg	**23.** 8.9	**34.** 0.37	**45.** 0.85
3. 0.0875	**13.** 0.35 mg	**24.** 1.3	**35.** 0.44	**46.** 0.73
4. 1.375	**14.** Yes	**25.** 2	**36.** 0.33	**47.** 0.26
5. 2.7117	**15.** 56.25 mg	**26.** 0.6	**37.** 0.08	**48.** 0.93
6. 5.406	**16.** No	**27.** 1.3	**38.** 0.81	**49.** 0.45
7. 0.4375	**17.** 1.9	**28.** 1.9	**39.** 0.72	**50.** 0.7
8. 0.216	**18.** 0.6	**29.** 3	**40.** 0.74	
9. 0.004	**19.** 3.6	**30.** 1.7	**41.** 0.52	
10. 0.7	**20.** 0.4	**31.** 0.53	**42.** 0.36	
	21. 1.2	**32.** 0.42	**43.** 0.65	

3

Solving Common Fraction Equations

The majority of clinical drug dosage calculations involve solving an equation containing one to five common fractions. Two examples are:

$$\frac{2}{5} \times \frac{3}{4} \quad \text{and} \quad \frac{20}{1} \times \frac{1000}{60,000} \times \frac{1200}{1} \times \frac{1}{60}$$

In this chapter you will practice solving equations that contain whole and decimal number common fractions. The examples that follow include simplifying the fractions before calculator use as you learned to do in Chapter 2. Answers are most often expressed to the nearest tenth, but practice is also provided in expressing to the nearest hundredth and, in some calculations, whole numbers.

 Common fraction equations are solved by dividing the numerators by the denominators.

It is very important that you **do the math** of the following examples yourself and **compare it** with the math provided. Simply reading the examples will not help you understand why initial reduction of the fractions can often be helpful, nor will it help you develop an appreciation of why large number and decimal calculator entries require particular care. So take the time to do each example very carefully.

WHOLE NUMBER EQUATIONS

Two options are available to solve any equation: calculator use throughout, or initial reduction of the fractions before final calculator division. Experiment with both options, then choose the one you feel most comfortable with.

 Calculator solution of equations is most safely done by concentrating only on the entries to be made, not the totals that register and change throughout the calculation.

Note: Answers in all of the examples are expressed to the nearest tenth and hundredth.

EXAMPLE 1 | **Option 1: Calculator Use Throughout**

$$\frac{2}{5} \times \frac{3}{4}$$

$2 \times 3 \div 5 \div 4$ multiply the numerators, 2 and 3, divide by the
denominators, 5 then 4, in continuous entries

$= 0.3$

Answer $=$ **0.3 (tenth)** or **0.3 (hundredth)**

Option 2: Initial Reduction of Fractions

$$\frac{2}{5} \times \frac{3}{4}$$

$$\frac{{}^{1}\cancel{2}}{5} \times \frac{3}{\cancel{4}_{2}}$$ divide the numerator, 2, and the denominator, 4, by 2 (to
become 1 and 2)

$3 \div 5 \div 2$ use the calculator to divide the remaining numerator, 3, by
the remaining denominators, 5 and 2

$= 0.3$

Answer $=$ **0.3 (tenth)** or **0.3 (hundredth)**

 Initial reduction of fractions in an equation can simplify final
calculator entries, especially if the numbers are large, contain
decimal fractions, or zeros.

EXAMPLE 2 | **Option 1: Calculator Use Throughout**

$$\frac{250}{175} \times \frac{150}{325}$$

$250 \times 150 \div 175 \div 325$ multiply the numerators, 250 and 150, then
divide by the denominators, 175 and 325

$= 0.659$

Answer $=$ **0.7 (tenth)** or **0.66 (hundredth)**

Option 2: Initial Reduction of Fractions

$$\frac{250}{175} \times \frac{150}{325}$$

$$\frac{\overset{10}{\cancel{250}}}{\underset{7}{\cancel{175}}} \times \frac{\overset{6}{\cancel{150}}}{\underset{13}{\cancel{325}}}$$ divide the numerator, 250, and the denominator,
175, by 25 (to become 10 and 7); divide the
numerator, 150, and denominator, 325, by 25 (to
become 6 and 13)

$10 \times 6 \div 7 \div 13$ use the calculator to multiply the numerators, 10 and
6, then divide by the denominators, 7 and 13

$= 0.659$

Answer $=$ **0.7 (tenth)** or **0.66 (hundredth)**

EXAMPLE 3 | **Option 1: Calculator Use Throughout**

$$\frac{7}{50} \times \frac{25}{3} \times \frac{120}{32}$$

$7 \times 25 \times 120 \div 50 \div 3 \div 32$ multiply the numerators, 7, 25, and 120, then divide by the denominators, 50, 3, and 32

$= 4.375$

Answer = **4.4 (tenth)** or **4.38 (hundredth)**

Option 2: Initial Reduction of Fractions

$$\frac{7}{50} \times \frac{25}{3} \times \frac{120}{32}$$

$$\frac{7}{\underset{2}{\cancel{50}}} \times \frac{\overset{1}{\cancel{25}}}{3} \times \frac{\overset{15}{\cancel{120}}}{\underset{4}{\cancel{32}}}$$ divide 25 and 50 by 25; divide 120 and 32 by 8

$7 \times 15 \div 2 \div 3 \div 4$

$= 4.375$

Answer = **4.4 (tenth)** or **4.38 (hundredth)**

EXAMPLE 4 | **Option 1: Calculator Use Throughout**

$$\frac{20}{1} \times \frac{1000}{60,000} \times \frac{1200}{1} \times \frac{1}{60}$$

$20 \times 1000 \times 1200 \div 60,000 \div 60$

$= 6.666$

Answer = **6.7 (tenth)** or **6.67 (hundredth)**

Option 2: Initial Reduction of Fractions

$$\frac{20}{1} \times \frac{1000}{60,000} \times \frac{1200}{1} \times \frac{1}{60}$$

$$\frac{\overset{1}{\cancel{20}}}{1} \times \frac{1000}{\underset{3}{\cancel{60,000}}} \times \frac{\overset{20}{\cancel{1200}}}{1} \times \frac{1}{\underset{1}{\cancel{60}}}$$ reduce 1000 and 60,000 by eliminating three zeros from each; divide 20 and 60 by 20; divide 1200 and 60 by 60

$20 \div 3$ divide the remaining numerator, 20, by the remaining denominator, 3

$= 6.666$

Answer = **6.7 (tenth)** or **6.67 (hundredth)**

EXAMPLE 5 | **Option 1: Calculator Use Throughout**

$$\frac{2000}{1500} \times \frac{2500}{3000}$$

$$2000 \times 2500 \div 1500 \div 3000$$

$$= 1.111$$

Answer = **1.1 (tenth)** or **1.11 (hundredth)**

Option 2: Initial Reduction of Fractions

$$\frac{2000}{1500} \times \frac{2500}{3000}$$

$$\frac{\cancel{2000}}{\underset{3}{\cancel{1500}}} \times \frac{\overset{5}{\cancel{2500}}}{\cancel{3000}}$$ eliminate three zeros in 2000 and 3000; eliminate two zeros in 2500, 1500, 3000, and 1500; divide 25 and 15 by 5

$$2 \times 5 \div 3 \div 3$$

$$= 1.111$$

Answer = **1.1 (tenth)** or **1.11 (hundredth)**

PROBLEM

Solve the following equations. Express your answers to the nearest tenth and hundredth. A calculator may be used.

1. $\dfrac{3}{8} \times \dfrac{6}{3}$　　　　　　　= _____

2. $\dfrac{3}{4} \times \dfrac{10}{2}$　　　　　　　= _____

3. $\dfrac{3}{5} \times \dfrac{1050}{40}$　　　　　　　= _____

4. $\dfrac{10}{1} \times \dfrac{750}{40,000} \times \dfrac{1000}{1} \times \dfrac{1}{60}$　= _____

5. $\dfrac{12}{1} \times \dfrac{500}{2700} \times \dfrac{2000}{1} \times \dfrac{1}{60}$　= _____

6. $\dfrac{1500}{750} \times \dfrac{350}{600}$　　　　　　= _____

7. $\dfrac{1000}{2700} \times \dfrac{1300}{500} \times \dfrac{70}{50}$　　= _____

8. $\dfrac{15}{1} \times \dfrac{2500}{20,000} \times \dfrac{1000}{1} \times \dfrac{1}{60}$　= _____

Answers **1.** 0.8; 0.75 **2.** 3.8; 3.75 **3.** 15.8; 15.75 **4.** 3.1; 3.13 **5.** 74.1; 74.07 **6.** 1.2; 1.17 **7.** 1.3; 1.35 **8.** 31.3; 31.25

DECIMAL FRACTION EQUATIONS

Decimal fraction equations raise an instant warning flag in calculations, because it is here that most dosage errors occur. As with whole number equations, simplifying the numbers, first by eliminating decimal points then reducing the numbers, is an option. However, if you elect to do the entire calculation with a calculator, be sure to take your time to enter the decimal points very carefully. Double-check all calculator entries and answers.

 Extreme care must be taken with calculator entry of decimal numbers to include the decimal point, and answers must be routinely double-checked.

EXAMPLE 1 | **Option 1: Calculator Use Throughout**

$$\frac{0.3}{1.65} \times \frac{2.5}{1}$$

$0.3 \times 2.5 \div 165$ multiply 0.3 by 2.5, then divide by 1.65

$= 0.454$

Answer $=$ **0.5 (tenth)** or **0.45 (hundredth)**

Option 2: Initial Elimination of Decimal Points and Reduction of Fractions

$$\frac{0.3}{1.65} \times \frac{2.5}{1}$$

$$\frac{30}{165} \times \frac{25}{10}$$ move the decimal point two places in 0.3 and 1.65 (to become 30 and 165), and one place in 2.5 and 1 (to become 25 and 10)

$$\frac{\overset{3}{\cancel{30}}}{\underset{33}{\cancel{165}}} \times \frac{\overset{5}{\cancel{25}}}{\underset{1}{\cancel{10}}}$$ divide 30 and 10 by 10; divide 25 and 165 by 5

$$\frac{\overset{1}{\cancel{3}}}{\underset{11}{\cancel{35}}} \times \frac{5}{1}$$ divide 3 and 33 by 3

$5 \div 11$ divide the remaining numerator, 5, by the denominator, 11

$= 0.454$

Answer $=$ **0.5 (tenth)** or **0.45 (hundredth)**

EXAMPLE 2 | **Option 1: Calculator Use Throughout**

$$\frac{0.3}{1.2} \times \frac{2.1}{0.15}$$

$0.3 \times 2.1 \div 1.2 \div 0.15$ multiply 0.3 by 2.1, then divide by 1.2 and 0.15

= 3.5

Answer = **3.5 (tenth)** or **3.5 (hundredth)**

**Option 2: Initial Elimination of Decimal Points and
Reduction of Fractions**

$$\frac{0.3}{1.2} \times \frac{2.1}{0.15}$$

$$\frac{3}{12} \times \frac{210}{15}$$ eliminate the decimal points by moving them one place in 0.3 and 1.2 (to become 3 and 12), and two places in 2.1 and 0.15 (to become 210 and 15)

$$\frac{\overset{1}{\cancel{3}}}{\underset{4}{\cancel{12}}} \times \frac{\overset{42}{\cancel{210}}}{\underset{3}{\cancel{15}}}$$ divide 3 and 12 by 3; divide 210 and 15 by 5

$$\frac{1}{\underset{2}{\cancel{4}}} \times \frac{\overset{21}{\cancel{42}}}{3}$$ divide 42 and 4 by 2

$$21 \div 2 \div 3$$ use a calculator to divide the numerator, 21, by 2 then by 3

= 3.5

Answer = **3.5 (tenth)** or **3.5 (hundredth)**

EXAMPLE 3   **Option 1: Calculator Use Throughout**

$$\frac{0.15}{0.17} \times \frac{3.1}{2}$$

$$0.15 \times 3.1 \div 0.17 \div 2$$ multiply 0.15 by 3.1, divide by 0.17 then by 2

= 1.367

Answer = **1.4 (tenth)** or **1.37 (hundredth)**

**Option 2: Initial Elimination of Decimal Points and
Reduction of Fractions**

$$\frac{0.15}{0.17} \times \frac{3.1}{2}$$

$$\frac{15}{17} \times \frac{31}{20}$$ move the decimal point two places in 0.15 and 0.17; move it one place in 3.1 and 2 (requires adding a zero to 2)

$$\frac{\overset{3}{\cancel{15}}}{17} \times \frac{31}{\underset{4}{\cancel{20}}}$$ divide 15 and 20 by 5

$$3 \times 31 \div 17 \div 4$$ complete with a calculator: 3 × 31 ÷ 17 ÷ 4

= 1.367

Answer = **1.4 (tenth)** or **1.37 (hundredth)**

EXAMPLE 4 | **Option 1: Calculator Use Throughout**

$$\frac{2.5}{1.5} \times \frac{1.2}{1.1}$$

$2.5 \times 1.2 \div 1.5 \div 1.1$ multiply 2.5 by 1.2, divide by 1.5 then by 1.1

$= 1.818$

Answer $= $ **1.8 (tenth)** or **1.82 (hundredth)**

Option 2: Initial Elimination of Decimal Points and Reduction of Fractions

$$\frac{2.5}{1.5} \times \frac{1.2}{1.1}$$

$$\frac{25}{15} \times \frac{12}{11}$$ move the decimal point one place in 2.5 and 1.5; move it one place in 1.2 and 1.1

$$\frac{\overset{5}{\cancel{25}}}{\underset{3}{\cancel{15}}} \times \frac{12}{11}$$ divide 25 and 15 by 5

$$\frac{5}{\underset{1}{\cancel{3}}} \times \frac{\overset{4}{\cancel{12}}}{11}$$ divide 12 and 3 by 3

$5 \times 4 \div 11$ complete with a calculator: $5 \times 4 \div 11$

$= 1.818$

Answer $= $ **1.8 (tenth)** or **1.82 (hundredth)**

PROBLEM

Solve the following equations. Express your answers to the nearest tenth and hundredth. A calculator may be used.

1. $\dfrac{2.1}{1.15} \times \dfrac{0.9}{1.2} = $ _____

2. $\dfrac{3.1}{2.7} \times \dfrac{2.2}{1.4} = $ _____

3. $\dfrac{0.3}{1.2} \times \dfrac{3}{2.1} = $ _____

4. $\dfrac{0.17}{0.3} \times \dfrac{2.5}{1.5} = $ _____

5. $\dfrac{1.75}{0.95} \times \dfrac{1.5}{2} = $ _____

6. $\dfrac{0.75}{1.15} \times \dfrac{3}{1.25} = $ _____

7. $\dfrac{10.2}{1.5} \times \dfrac{2}{5.1} = $ _____

8. $\dfrac{0.125}{0.25} \times \dfrac{2.5}{1.5} = $ _____

9. $\dfrac{0.9}{0.3} \times \dfrac{1.2}{1.4} = $ _____

10. $\dfrac{0.35}{1.7} \times \dfrac{2.5}{0.7} = $ _____

Answers **1.** 1.4; 1.37 **2.** 1.8; 1.8 **3.** 0.4; 0.36 **4.** 0.9; 0.94 **5.** 1.4; 1.38 **6.** 1.6; 1.57 **7.** 2.7; 2.67 **8.** 0.8; 0.83 **9.** 2.6; 2.57 **10.** 0.7; 0.74

MULTIPLE NUMBER EQUATIONS

The calculation steps already practiced are also used for multiple number equations. Reduction of numbers may be of particular benefit here, because calculations of this type sometimes have large numbers that either cancel or reduce dramatically.

Note: Answers are expressed to the nearest whole number in the examples and problems that follow to replicate actual clinical calculations.

EXAMPLE 1 | **Option 1: Calculator Use Throughout**

$$\frac{60}{1} \times \frac{1000}{4} \times \frac{1}{1000} \times \frac{6}{1}$$

$60 \times 1000 \times 6 \div 4 \div 1000$ multiply 60 by 1000, then by 6; divide by 4 and 1000

$= 90$

Answer = **90**

Option 2: Initial Reduction of Fractions

$$\frac{60}{1} \times \frac{1000}{4} \times \frac{1}{1000} \times \frac{6}{1}$$

$$\frac{60}{1} \times \frac{\overset{1}{\cancel{1000}}}{\underset{2}{\cancel{4}}} \times \frac{1}{\underset{1}{\cancel{1000}}} \times \frac{\overset{3}{\cancel{6}}}{1}$$ eliminate 1000 from a numerator and denominator; divide 6 and 4 by 2

$60 \times 3 \div 2$ multiply 60 by 3; divide by 2

$= 90$

Answer = **90**

EXAMPLE 2 | **Option 1: Calculator Use Throughout**

$$\frac{1}{60} \times \frac{1}{12} \times \frac{10}{1} \times \frac{750}{1}$$

$10 \times 750 \div 60 \div 12$ multiply 10 by 750; divide by 60, then by 12

$= 9.86$ round to whole number

Answer = **10**

Option 2: Initial Reduction of Fractions

$$\frac{1}{60} \times \frac{1}{12} \times \frac{10}{1} \times \frac{750}{1}$$

$$\frac{1}{\underset{6}{\cancel{60}}} \times \frac{1}{\underset{6}{\cancel{12}}} \times \frac{\overset{1}{\cancel{10}}}{1} \times \frac{\overset{375}{\cancel{750}}}{1}$$ divide 10 and 60 by 10; divide 750 and 12 by 2

$375 \div 6 \div 6$ use a calculator to divide 375 by 6, then again by 6

$= 9.86$ round to whole number

Answer = **10**

EXAMPLE 3 | **Option 1: Calculator Use Throughout**

$$\frac{20}{1} \times \frac{75}{1} \times \frac{1}{60}$$

$20 \times 75 \div 60$ multiply 20 by 75; divide by 60

$= 25$

Answer $= $ **25**

Option 2: Initial Reduction of Fractions

$$\frac{20}{1} \times \frac{75}{1} \times \frac{1}{60}$$

$$\overset{1}{\cancel{20}} \times \overset{25}{\cancel{75}} \times \frac{1}{\underset{\underset{1}{\cancel{3}}}{\cancel{60}}}$$ divide 20 and 60 by 20 to become 1 and 3; divide 75 and 3 by 3 to become 25 and 1

$= 25$

Answer $= $ **25**

EXAMPLE 4 | **Option 1: Calculator Use Throughout**

$$\frac{2}{0.5} \times \frac{1}{100} \times \frac{275}{1}$$

$2 \times 275 \div 0.5 \div 100$ multiply 2 by 275; divide by 0.5 and 100

$= 11$

Answer $= $ **11**

Option 2: Initial Reduction of Fractions

$$\frac{2}{0.5} \times \frac{1}{100} \times \frac{275}{1}$$

$$\frac{20}{5} \times \frac{1}{100} \times \frac{275}{1}$$ eliminate the decimal point by moving it one place in 0.5, and one place in 2, which requires adding a zero to 2 (to become 5 and 20)

$$\frac{\overset{1}{\cancel{20}}}{\underset{1}{\cancel{5}}} \times \frac{1}{\underset{5}{\cancel{100}}} \times \frac{\overset{55}{\cancel{275}}}{1}$$ divide 20 and 100 by 20; divide 275 and 5 by 5

$$\frac{1}{\underset{1}{\cancel{5}}} \times \frac{\overset{11}{\cancel{55}}}{1}$$ divide 5 and 55 by 5

$= 11$

Answer $= $ **11**

PROBLEM

Solve the following equations. Express answers to the nearest whole number.

1. $\dfrac{15}{1} \times \dfrac{350}{5} \times \dfrac{1}{60}$ = _____

2. $\dfrac{1}{32} \times \dfrac{60}{1} \times \dfrac{7.5}{3.1}$ = _____

3. $\dfrac{10}{1} \times \dfrac{2500}{24} \times \dfrac{1}{60}$ = _____

4. $\dfrac{1.7}{2.3} \times \dfrac{15.3}{12.1} \times \dfrac{6.2}{0.3}$ = _____

5. $\dfrac{20}{1} \times \dfrac{1200}{16} \times \dfrac{1}{60}$ = _____

Answers **1.** 18 **2.** 5 **3.** 17 **4.** 19 **5.** 25

Summary

This concludes the chapter on solving common fraction equations. The important points to remember from this chapter are:

- Most dosage calculations consist of an equation containing one to five common fractions.
- In common fraction math, the numerators must be multiplied then divided by the denominators.
- Numbers in an equation may initially be reduced to simplify final multiplication and division.
- If an equation contains decimal fractions, the decimal points may be eliminated from numerators and denominators without altering the value.
- Zeros may be eliminated from the same number of numerators and denominators without altering the value.
- A calculator may be used to multiply and divide in an equation.
- Answers may be expressed as whole numbers or to the nearest tenth or hundredth depending on the calculation being done.

Summary Self-Test

Solve the following equations. Express your answers to the nearest tenth and hundredth. A calculator may be used.

1. $\dfrac{0.8}{0.65} \times \dfrac{1.2}{1}$ = _____

2. $\dfrac{350}{1000} \times \dfrac{4.4}{1}$ = _____

3. $\dfrac{0.35}{1.3} \times \dfrac{4.5}{1}$ = _____

4. $\dfrac{0.4}{1.5} \times \dfrac{2.3}{1}$ = _____

5. $\dfrac{1}{75} \times \dfrac{500}{1}$ = _____

6. $\dfrac{0.15}{0.12} \times \dfrac{1.45}{1}$ = _____

7. $\dfrac{100,000}{80,000} \times \dfrac{1.7}{1}$ = _____

8. $\dfrac{1.45}{2.1} \times \dfrac{1.5}{1}$ = _____

9. $\dfrac{1550}{500} \times \dfrac{0.5}{1}$ = _____

10. $\dfrac{4}{0.375} \times \dfrac{0.25}{1}$ = _____

11. $\dfrac{0.08}{0.1} \times \dfrac{2.1}{1}$ = _____

12. $\dfrac{1.5}{1.25} \times \dfrac{1.45}{1}$ = _____

13. $\dfrac{0.5}{0.15} \times \dfrac{0.35}{1}$ = _____

14. $\dfrac{300,000}{200,000} \times \dfrac{1.7}{1}$ = _____

15. $\dfrac{13.5}{10} \times \dfrac{1.8}{1}$ = _____

16. $\dfrac{1,000,000}{800,000} \times \dfrac{1.4}{1}$ = _____

17. $\dfrac{1.3}{0.2} \times \dfrac{0.25}{1}$ = _____

18. $\dfrac{1.5}{0.1} \times \dfrac{0.25}{1}$ = _____

19. $\dfrac{1.9}{3.5} \times \dfrac{3.2}{1.4}$ = _____

20. $\dfrac{15,000}{7500} \times \dfrac{3.5}{1.2}$ = _____

21. $\dfrac{4.7}{1.3} \times \dfrac{50}{20} \times \dfrac{4}{25} \times \dfrac{8.2}{2.1}$ = _____

22. $\dfrac{40}{24} \times \dfrac{250}{5} \times \dfrac{0.375}{7.5}$ = _____

23. $\dfrac{6.9}{21.6} \times \dfrac{250}{5} \times \dfrac{0.75}{2.1}$ = _____

24. $\dfrac{1}{60} \times \dfrac{1}{25} \times \dfrac{10}{1} \times \dfrac{1000}{1}$ = _____

25. $\dfrac{50.5}{22.75} \times \dfrac{4.7}{6.3} \times \dfrac{31.7}{10.2}$ = _____

Solve the following equations. Express your answers to the nearest whole number. A calculator may be used.

26. $\dfrac{104}{95} \times \dfrac{20}{15} \times \dfrac{63}{1.6}$ = _____

27. $\dfrac{40,000}{10,000} \times \dfrac{30}{1} \times \dfrac{3.7}{12.5}$ = _____

28. $\dfrac{60}{1} \times \dfrac{500}{50} \times \dfrac{1}{1000} \times \dfrac{116}{1}$ = _____

29. $\dfrac{1.5}{0.6} \times \dfrac{10}{14} \times \dfrac{3.2}{5.3} \times \dfrac{100}{2}$ = _____

30. $\dfrac{60}{1} \times \dfrac{50}{250} \times \dfrac{1}{100} \times \dfrac{455}{1}$ = _____

31. $\dfrac{33.7}{15.9} \times \dfrac{19.2}{2.6} \times \dfrac{2.9}{3.85}$ = _____

32. $\dfrac{20}{4} \times \dfrac{100}{88} \times \dfrac{1200}{250} \times \dfrac{10}{30}$ = _____

33. $\dfrac{14}{7.9} \times \dfrac{88}{8}$ = _____

34. $\dfrac{10}{1} \times \dfrac{325}{1.5} \times \dfrac{1}{60}$ = _____

35. $\dfrac{60}{1} \times \dfrac{300}{400} \times \dfrac{1}{800} \times \dfrac{400}{1}$ = _____

36. $\dfrac{3.7}{1.3} \times \dfrac{12}{8} \times \dfrac{3.1}{7.4} \times \dfrac{5}{1}$ = _____

37. $\dfrac{20}{2} \times \dfrac{125}{25} \times \dfrac{2}{750} \times \dfrac{216}{1}$ = _____

38. $\dfrac{4}{3} \times \dfrac{45}{1} \times \dfrac{22.5}{37.8}$ = _____

39. $\dfrac{7.5}{12.3} \times \dfrac{55}{5} \times \dfrac{23.2}{1.2}$ = _____

40. $\dfrac{1000}{1} \times \dfrac{50}{250} \times \dfrac{20}{1} \times \dfrac{1}{60}$ = _____

41. $\dfrac{15}{1} \times \dfrac{1000}{4000} \times \dfrac{800}{1} \times \dfrac{1}{60}$ = _____

42. $\dfrac{15}{1} \times \dfrac{500}{3} \times \dfrac{1}{60}$ = _____

43. $\dfrac{25}{3} \times \dfrac{750}{8} \times \dfrac{0.1}{1}$ = _____

44. $\dfrac{40}{2} \times \dfrac{250}{50} \times \dfrac{1}{800} \times \dfrac{154}{1}$ = _____

45. $\dfrac{33}{4} \times \dfrac{75}{40} \times \dfrac{2}{150} \times \dfrac{432}{1}$ = _____

46. $\dfrac{22.5}{7} \times \dfrac{100}{5} \times \dfrac{1}{700} \times \dfrac{3}{80} \times \dfrac{3150}{1}$ = _____

47. $\dfrac{100}{250} \times \dfrac{50}{1} \times \dfrac{27.5}{1.375}$ = _____

48. $\dfrac{2.2}{0.25} \times \dfrac{3.6}{1} \times \dfrac{3.7}{7.1}$ = _____

49. $\dfrac{1.3}{0.21} \times \dfrac{0.3}{2} \times \dfrac{10.1}{0.75}$ = _____

50. $\dfrac{27.5}{10} \times \dfrac{40}{7} \times \dfrac{8.5}{1.9}$ = _____

Answers

1. 1.5; 1.48	**11.** 1.7; 1.68	**22.** 4.2; 4.17	**33.** 19	**44.** 19
2. 1.5; 1.54	**12.** 1.7; 1.74	**23.** 5.7; 5.7	**34.** 36	**45.** 89
3. 1.2; 1.21	**13.** 1.2; 1.17	**24.** 6.7; 6.67	**35.** 23	**46.** 11
4. 0.6; 0.61	**14.** 2.6; 2.55	**25.** 5.1; 5.15	**36.** 9	**47.** 400
5. 6.7; 6.67	**15.** 2.4; 2.43	**26.** 57	**37.** 29	**48.** 17
6. 1.8; 1.81	**16.** 1.8; 1.75	**27.** 36	**38.** 36	**49.** 13
7. 2.1; 2.13	**17.** 1.6; 1.63	**28.** 70	**39.** 130	**50.** 70
8. 1; 1.04	**18.** 1.9; 1.88	**29.** 54	**40.** 67	
9. 1.6; 1.55	**19.** 1.2; 1.24	**30.** 55	**41.** 50	
10. 2.7; 2.67	**20.** 5.8; 5.83	**31.** 12	**42.** 42	
	21. 5.6; 5.65	**32.** 9	**43.** 78	

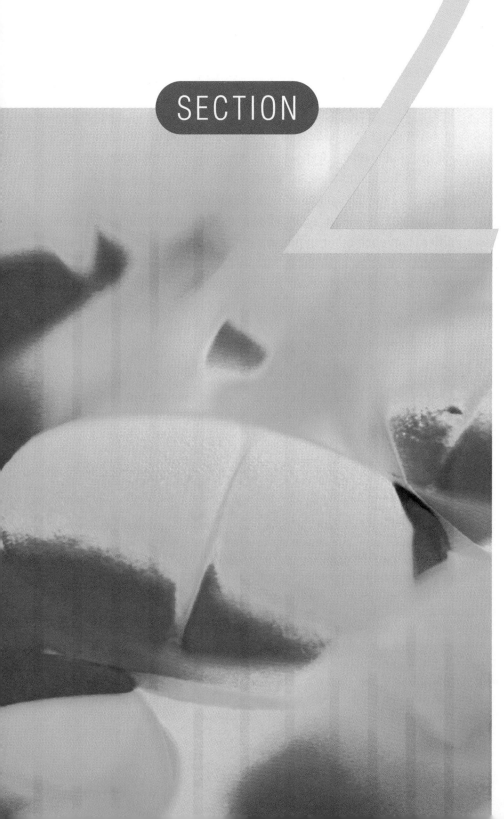

Introduction to Drug Measures

4 Metric, International (SI) System

Objectives

The learner will:

1. list the commonly used units of measure in the metric system

2. distinguish between the official abbreviations and variations in common use

3. express metric weights and volumes using correct notation rules

4. convert metric weights and volumes within the system

The major system of weights and measures used in medicine is the metric/international/SI (from the French Système International). The metric system was invented in France in 1875, and takes its name from the meter, a length roughly equivalent to a yard, from which all other units of measure in the system are derived. The strength of the metric system lies in its simplicity, because **all units of measure differ from each other in powers of ten (10). Conversions between units in the system are accomplished by simply moving a decimal point.**

Although it is not necessary for you to know the entire metric system to administer medications safely, you must understand its basic structure and become familiar with the units of measure you will be using.

BASIC UNITS OF THE METRIC/SI SYSTEM

Three types of metric measures are in common use: those for **length**, **volume** (or capacity), and **weight**. The basic units or beginning points of these three measures are:

> **length — meter**
> **volume — liter**
> **weight — gram**

You must memorize these basic units: do so now if you do not already know them. In addition to these basic units, there are both larger and smaller units of measure for length, volume, and weight. Let's compare this concept with something familiar. The pound is a unit of weight that we use every day. A smaller unit of measure is the ounce, a larger, the ton. **However, all are units measuring weight**.

In the same way, there are smaller and larger units than the basic meter, liter, and gram. In the metric system, however, there is one very important advantage: **all other units, whether larger or smaller than the basic units, have the name of the basic unit incorporated in them**. So when you see a unit of metric measure there is no doubt what it is measuring: **meter–length**, **liter–volume**, **gram–weight**.

PROBLEM

Identify the following metric measures with their appropriate category of weight, length, or volume.

1. milligram   _____

2. centimeter   _____

3. milliliter   _____

4. millimeter   _____

5. kilogram   _____

6. microgram   _____

Answers **1.** weight **2.** length **3.** volume **4.** length **5.** weight **6.** weight

METRIC/SI PREFIXES

Prefixes are used in combination with the names of the basic units to identify larger and smaller units of measure. The same prefixes are used with all three measures. Therefore, there is a kilo**meter**, kilo**gram**, and a kilo**liter**. Prefixes also change the value of each of the basic units by the same amount. For example, the prefix "kilo" identifies a unit of measure that is larger than (or multiplies) the basic unit by 1000. Therefore,

1 kilometer	=	1000 meters
1 kilogram	=	1000 grams
1 kiloliter	=	1000 liters

Kilo is the only prefix you will be using that identifies a measure **larger** than the basic unit. Kilograms are frequently used as a measure for body weight, especially for infants and children.

You will see only three measures **smaller** than the basic unit in common use. The prefixes for these are:

centi—as in centimeter
milli—as in milligram
micro—as in microgram

Therefore, you will actually be working with only four prefixes: **kilo**, which identifies a larger unit of measure than the basics; and **centi**, **milli**, and **micro**, which identify smaller units than the basics.

METRIC/SI ABBREVIATIONS

In actual use the units of measure are abbreviated.

 The basic units are abbreviated to their first initial and printed in small letters, with the exception of liter, which is capitalized.

gram is abbreviated **g**
liter is abbreviated **L**
meter is abbreviated **m**

The abbreviations for the prefixes used in combination with the basic units are all printed using small letters.

> kilo is **k** (as in kilogram—kg)
> centi is **c** (as in centimeter—cm)
> milli is **m** (as in milligram—mg)
> micro is **mc** (as in microgram—mcg)

Micro has an additional abbreviation, the symbol µ, which is used in combination with the basic unit, as in microgram, **µg**.

Although you will occasionally see the **symbol µg** on drug labels for microgram you should be aware that it has an **inherent safety risk**. When handprinted it is very easy for microgram (*ug*) to be mistaken for milligram (*mg*). These units differ from each other in value by 1000 (1 mg = 1000 mcg), and misreading these dosages could be critical.

 To ensure safety when transcribing orders by hand, always use the abbreviation mc to designate micro rather than its symbol.

In combination, liter remains capitalized. Therefore, milliliter is **mL**, and kiloliter **kL**.

PROBLEM

Print the abbreviations for the following metric units.

1. microgram   _____
2. liter   _____
3. kilogram   _____
4. milliliter   _____
5. centimeter   _____
6. milligram   _____
7. meter   _____
8. kiloliter   _____
9. millimeter   _____
10. gram   _____

Answers **1.** mcg **2.** L **3.** kg **4.** mL **5.** cm **6.** mg **7.** m **8.** kL **9.** mm **10.** g

VARIATIONS OF METRIC/SI ABBREVIATIONS

Although the metric system was invented in 1875, it was not until 1960, nearly 100 years later, that a standard system of abbreviations, the **International System of Units**, was adopted. Therefore, a variety of unofficial abbreviations are still occasionally used. Most of the variations were designed to prevent confusion with the much older apothecaries' system, which was in common use at that time in drug dosages. The major difference is that gram was abbreviated **Gm**, in an effort to differentiate it from the apothecaries' grain, **gr**. This, of course, led to milligram and microgram being abbreviated **mgm**, and **mcgm**. Liter was routinely abbreviated small **l**, and milliliter, **ml**. You may still see these abbreviations used, particularly ml, even on drug labels, but do not fall into the habit of using them yourself. **They are officially obsolete**.

 The abbreviations Gm, mgm, mcgm, and ml are officially obsolete and should not be used.

METRIC/SI NOTATION RULES

The easiest way to remember the rules of metric **notations**, in which **a unit of measure is expressed with a quantity**, is to memorize some prototypes (examples) that incorporate all the rules. Then if you get confused, you can stop and think and remember the correct way to write them. For the metric system the notations for one-half, one, and one and one-half milliliters will incorporate all the rules you must know.

Prototype Notations: **0.5 mL   1 mL   1.5 mL**

RULE 1 | **The quantity is written in Arabic numerals, 1, 2, 3, 4, etc.**

example: 0.5   1   1.5

RULE 2 | **The numerals representing the quantity are placed in front of the abbreviations.**

example: 0.5 mL   1 mL   1.5 mL   (not mL 0.5, etc.)

RULE 3 | **A full space is used between the numeral and the abbreviation.**

example: 0.5 mL   1 mL   1.5 mL   (not 0.5mL, etc.)

RULE 4 | **Fractional parts of a unit are expressed as decimal fractions.**

example: 0.5 mL   1 mL   (not ½ mL, 1½ mL, etc.)

RULE 5 | **A zero is placed in front of the decimal when it is not preceded by a whole number to emphasize the decimal point.**

example: 0.5 mL   1 mL   1.5 mL   (not 0.50 mL, 1.0 mL, 1.50 mL)

So once again, as examples of the rules of metric notations, memorize the prototypes 0.5 mL—1 mL—1.5 mL. Just refer back to these in your memory if you get confused, and you will be able to write the notations correctly.

PROBLEM

Write the following metric measures using official abbreviations and notation rules.

1. two grams   _____

2. five hundred milliliters   _____

3. five-tenths of a liter   _____

4. two-tenths of a milligram   _____

5. five-hundredths of a gram   _____

6. two and five-tenths kilograms   _____

7. one hundred micrograms   _____

8. two and three-tenths milliliters   _____

9. seven-tenths of a milliliter   _____

10. three-tenths of a milligram   _____

11. two and four-tenths liters   _____

12. seventeen and five-tenths kilograms   _____

13. nine hundredths of a milligram   _____

14. ten and two-tenths micrograms   _____

15. four-hundredths of a gram   _____

Answers **1.** 2 g **2.** 500 mL **3.** 0.5 L **4.** 0.2 mg **5.** 0.05 g **6.** 2.5 kg **7.** 100 mcg **8.** 2.3 mL **9.** 0.7 mL **10.** 0.3 mg
11. 2.4 L **12.** 17.5 kg **13.** 0.09 mg **14.** 10.2 mcg **15.** 0.04 g

CONVERSION BETWEEN METRIC/SI UNITS

When you administer medications, you will routinely be **converting units of measure within the metric system**, for example, g to mg, and mg to mcg. Learning the relative value of the units you will be working with is the first prerequisite to accurate conversions. There are only four metric **weights** commonly used in medicine. From **highest** to **lowest** value these are:

kg	=	kilogram
g	=	gram
mg	=	milligram
mcg	=	microgram

Only two units of **volume** are frequently used. From **highest** to **lowest** value these are:

L	=	liter
mL	=	milliliter

 Each of the metric measures used in medication dosages differs from the next by 1000.

1 kg	=	1000 g
1 g	=	1000 mg
1 mg	=	1000 mcg
1 L	=	1000 mL (1000 cc)

 The abbreviations for milliliter (mL) and cubic centimeter (cc) are used interchangeably. A cc is actually the amount of physical space that a 1 mL volume occupies, but the two measures are considered identical.

Once again, from highest to lowest value the units are, for weight: kg—g—mg—mcg; for volume: L—mL (cc). Each unit differs in value from the next by 1000, and **all conversions will be between touching units of measure**, for example, g to mg, mg to mcg, L to mL.

PROBLEM

Indicate if the following statements are true or false.

1. T F	1000 cc	=	1000 L	6. T F	1 kg	= 1000 g
2. T F	1000 mg	=	1 g	7. T F	1 mg	= 1000 g
3. T F	1000 mL	=	1000 cc	8. T F	1000 mcg	= 1 mg
4. T F	1000 mg	=	1 mcg	9. T F	1000 mL	= 1 L
5. T F	1000 mcg	=	1 g	10. T F	3 cc	= 3 mL

Answers **1.** F **2.** T **3.** T **4.** F **5.** F **6.** T **7.** F **8.** T **9.** T **10.** T

Because the metric system is a decimal system, **conversions between the units are accomplished by moving the decimal point**. Also, because each unit of measure in common use differs from the next by 1000, if you know one conversion, you know them all.

How far do you move the decimal point? Here is an unforgettable memory cue that can be used with **all** metric conversions. There are **three zeros in 1000**. The decimal point moves **three places**, the **same number of places as the zeros** in the conversion.

 In metric conversions between touching units of measure differing by 1000 the decimal point is moved three places, the same as the number of zeros in 1000.

This rule holds true for **all** decimal conversions in the metric system. If the difference in value is **10**, which has **one zero**, it will move **one place**. If the difference is **100**, which has **two zeros**, it will move **two places**. When the difference is **1000**, as it is in dosage conversions, which has **three zeros**, the decimal point moves **three places**.

Which way do you move the decimal point? If you are converting **down** the scale to a **smaller** unit of measure, for example, g to mg or L to mL, the **quantity must get larger**. So the decimal point must move three places to the **right**.

EXAMPLE 1 | 0.5 g = _____ mg

You are converting **down** the scale from **g to mg** so the quantity must be **larger**. Move the decimal point **three places to the right**. To do this, you must **add two zeros** to the end of the quantity and **eliminate the zero in front** of it. The larger 500 mg quantity indicates that you have moved the decimal point in the correct direction.

Answer   **0.5 g = 500 mg**

EXAMPLE 2 | 2.5 L = _____ mL

You are converting **down** the scale from **L to mL** so the quantity must be **larger**. Move the decimal point **three places to the right**. To do this, you must **add two zeros**. The larger 2500 mL quantity indicates that you have moved the decimal point in the correct direction.

Answer   **2.5 L = 2500 mL**

PROBLEM

Convert the following metric measures.

1. 7 mg   = _____ mcg   6. 1.5 mg   = _____ mcg

2. 1.7 L   = _____ mL   7. 0.7 g   = _____ mg

3. 3.2 g   = _____ mg   8. 0.3 L   = _____ mL

4. 0.03 kg   = _____ g   9. 7 kg   = _____ g

5. 0.4 mg   = _____ mcg   10. 0.01 mg   = _____ mcg

Answers **1.** 7000 mcg **2.** 1700 mL **3.** 3200 mg **4.** 30 g **5.** 400 mcg **6.** 1500 mcg **7.** 700 mg **8.** 300 mL **9.** 7000 g **10.** 10 mcg

In metric conversions **up the scale**, from **smaller to larger units** of measurement, such as mL to L, the quantity will be **smaller**. The decimal point is moved **three places to the left**.

EXAMPLE 1 | 200 mL = _____ L

You are converting **up** the scale from **mL to L** so the quantity will be **smaller**. Move the decimal point **three places left. Eliminate two zeros at the end** of the 200 mL quantity and **add a zero in front of** the decimal point to make it 0.2 L.

Answer   **200 mL = 0.2 L**

EXAMPLE 2 | 500 mcg = _____ mg

You are converting **up** the scale from **mcg to mg** so the quantity will be **smaller**. Move the decimal point **three places to the left. Eliminate two zeros at the end** of 500 and **add a zero in front of** the decimal point.

Answer   **500 mcg = 0.5 mg**

PROBLEM

Convert the following metric measures.

1. 3500 mL   = _____ L   6. 250 mcg   = _____ mg

2. 520 mg   = _____ g   7. 1200 mg   = _____ g

3. 1800 mcg   = _____ mg   8. 600 mL   = _____ L

4. 750 cc   = _____ L   9. 100 mg   = _____ g

5. 150 mg   = _____ g   10. 950 mcg   = _____ mg

Answers **1.** 3.5 L **2.** 0.52 g **3.** 1.8 mg **4.** 0.75 L **5.** 0.15 g **6.** 0.25 mg **7.** 1.2 g **8.** 0.6 L **9.** 0.1 g **10.** 0.95 mg

COMMON ERRORS IN METRIC/SI DOSAGES

Most errors in metric dosages occur when a dosage or calculation contains a decimal. So let's take a close look at some basic safety rules that can reduce the possibility of error.

The first way to prevent errors is to make sure orders are interpreted and transcribed correctly. Doctors do not always write orders in the safest manner, and you must learn to question everything that looks suspicious. A common error is **failure to write a zero in front of the decimal point** in decimal fractions, for example, .2 mg instead of 0.2 mg. This makes the decimal easy to miss. This error can be eliminated by strict adherence to the rule of placing a zero in front of decimal fractions. Regardless of the presence of a zero in a written order, make sure one is added when it is transferred to a medication administration record or patient chart.

 Fractional dosages in the metric system must be transcribed with a zero in front of the decimal point to draw attention to it.

The next most common error is **to include zeros where they should not be**, for example, .20 mg. An order written like this can easily be misread as 20 mg. Or, consider a dosage written 2.0 mg. The same potential for error exists. There is an unnecessary zero included in the order.

 Unnecessary zeros must be eliminated when metric dosages are transcribed.

The third error to watch for is in **calculations where decimal fractions are involved**. The presence of a decimal point in a calculation should raise a warning flag to slow down and double-check all math. Use your reasoning powers. If you misplace a decimal point, you are going to get an answer a minimum of ten times too much, or too little. **Learn to question quantities than seem unreasonable**. A 1 mL dosage makes sense if you are calculating an IM injection. A 0.1 mL or 10 mL (or a 10 tab) dosage does not, and this is the type of error you might see. Be alert when assessing answers, and determine if they seem reasonable.

 Question answers to calculations that seem unreasonably large or small.

The final error to be aware of is in **conversions within the metric system**. Errors in conversions can be eliminated by thinking **three**. All conversions between the g, mg, and mcg measures used in dosages are accomplished by moving the decimal point **three** places. Always, and forever. There are not many things you can use the words "always" and "forever" for, but converting between these units of measure in the metric system is one of those rare instances.

 Conversions between g, mg, and mcg units of measure in metric dosages require moving the decimal point three places.

If you are constantly mindful of these problem areas, you can be an outstandingly safe clinical practitioner.

Summary

This concludes the refresher on the metric system. The important points to remember from this chapter are:

- The meter, liter, and gram are the basic units of metric measure.
- Larger and smaller units than the basics are identified by the use of prefixes.
- The larger unit you will be seeing is the kilo, whose prefix is k.
- The smaller units you will be seeing are milli–m, micro–mc, and centi–c.
- Each prefix changes the value of the basic unit by the same amount.
- Converting from one unit to another within the system is accomplished by moving the decimal point.
- When you convert down the scale to smaller units of measurement, the quantity will get larger.
- To convert down the scale from larger to smaller units, the decimal point is moved to the right.
- When you convert up the scale to larger units of measurement, the quantity will get smaller.
- To convert up the scale from smaller to larger units, the decimal point is moved to the left.
- Conversions between g, mg, and mcg, and mL, L all require moving the decimal point three places.
- Fractional dosages are transcribed with a zero in front of the decimal point.
- Unnecessary zeros are eliminated from dosages.

Summary Self-Test

List the basic units of measure of the metric system and indicate what type of measure they are used for.

1. _____   _____

   _____   _____

   _____   _____

Which of the following are official metric/SI abbreviations?

2. a) L   e) mg

   b) g   f) kg

   c) kL   g) ml

   d) mgm   h) G

   _____

Express the following measures using official metric abbreviations and notation rules.

3. six-hundredths of a milligram _____

4. three hundred and ten milliliters _____

5. three-tenths of a kilogram _____

6. four-tenths of a cubic centimeter _____

7. one and five-tenths grams _____

8. one-hundredths of a gram _____

9. four thousand milliliters _____

10. one and two-tenths milligrams _____

List the four commonly used units of weight and the two of volume, from highest to lowest value.

11. _____ _____ _____

_____ _____ _____

Convert the following metric measures.

12. 160 mg = _.16_ g

13. 10 kg = _10,000._ g

14. 1500 µg = _____ mg

15. 750 mg = _.75_ g

16. 200 mL = _____ L

17. 0.3 g = _300_ mg

18. 0.05 g = _____ mg

19. 0.15 g = _____ mg

20. 1.2 L = _____ mL

21. 15 mL = _____ cc

22. 2 mg = _____ mcg

23. 900 mcg = _____ mg

24. 2.1 L = _____ mL

25. 475 mL = _____ L

26. 0.9 cc = _____ mL

27. 300 mg = _____ g

28. 2.5 mg = _____ mcg

29. 1 kL = _____ L

30. 3 L = _____ cc

31. 10 cc = _____ mL

32. 0.7 mg = _____ mcg

33. 4 g = _____ mg

34. 1000 mL = _____ L

35. 2.5 mL = _____ cc

36. 1000 mg = _____ g

37. 0.2 mg = _____ mcg

38. 2000 g = _____ kg

39. 1.4 g = _____ mg

40. 2.5 L = _____ cc

Answers
1. gram-weight; liter-volume; meter-length
2. a, b, c, e, f
3. 0.06 mg
4. 310 mL
5. 0.3 kg
6. 0.4 cc
7. 1.5 g
8. 0.01 g
9. 4000 mL
10. 1.2 mg
11. kg, g, mg, mcg, L, mL
12. 0.16 g
13. 10,000 g
14. 1.5 mg
15. 0.75 g
16. 0.2 L
17. 300 mg
18. 50 mg
19. 150 mg
20. 1200 mL
21. 15 cc
22. 2000 mcg
23. 0.9 mg
24. 2100 mL
25. 0.475 L
26. 0.9 mL
27. 0.3 g
28. 2500 mcg
29. 1000 L
30. 3000 cc
31. 10 mL
32. 700 mcg
33. 4000 mg
34. 1 L
35. 2.5 cc
36. 1 g
37. 200 mcg
38. 2 kg
39. 1400 mg
40. 2500 cc

5

Additional Drug Measures: Unit, Percentage, Milliequivalent, Ratio, Apothecary, Household

Objectives

The learner will recognize dosages:

1. measured in units
2. measured as percentages
3. using ratio strengths
4. in milliequivalents
5. in apothecary measures
6. in household measures

Although metric measures predominate in medications, there are several other measures frequently used, particularly in parenteral solutions, that are important for you to know. In addition you must be able to recognize several measures in the apothecaries' and household systems, because you may occasionally see these.

INTERNATIONAL UNITS (U)

A number of drugs are measured in International Units. Insulin, penicillin, and heparin are commonly seen examples. A unit **measures a drug in terms of its action**, not its physical weight. Units are **abbreviated U**, and are written using **Arabic numerals in front of the symbol**, with a space between, for example, 2000 U, or 1,000,000 U. **Commas are not used in a quantity unless it has at least five numbers**, for example, 45,000 U. Some facilities require that the "U" abbreviation not be used. If this is the policy, the word "units" is written instead.

PROBLEM

Express the following unit dosages using their official abbreviation.

1. two hundred and fifty thousand units   _____
2. ten units   _____
3. five thousand units   _____
4. forty-four units   _____
5. forty thousand units   _____
6. one million units   _____
7. one thousand units   _____
8. twenty-five hundred units   _____
9. thirty-four units   _____
10. one hundred units   _____

Answers   **1.** 250,000 U   **2.** 10 U   **3.** 5000 U   **4.** 44 U   **5.** 40,000 U   **6.** 1,000,000 U   **7.** 1000 U   **8.** 2500 U   **9.** 34 U
10. 100 U

PERCENTAGE (%) MEASURES

Percentage strengths are used extensively in intravenous solutions and somewhat less commonly for a variety of other medications, including eye and topical (for external use) ointments. **Percentage (%) means parts per hundred. The higher the percentage strength, the stronger the solution or ointment**.

 In solutions, percent represents the number of grams of drug per 100 mL (cc) of solution.

EXAMPLE 1	100 mL of a 1% solution will contain 1 g of drug
EXAMPLE 2	100 mL of a 2% solution will contain 2 g of drug
EXAMPLE 3	50 mL of a 1% solution will contain 0.5 g of drug
EXAMPLE 4	200 mL of a 2% solution will contain 4 g of drug

 This is not a calculation you will have to do. The examples are included only to point out that percentage solutions contain a significant amount of drug or other solute, and reading percentage labels requires the same care as other drug dosages.

MILLIEQUIVALENT (mEq) MEASURES

Milliequivalents (**mEq**) is **an expression of the number of grams of a drug contained in 1 mL of a normal solution**. This is a definition that may be quite understandable to a pharmacist or chemist, but you need not memorize it. Milliequivalent dosages are written using **Arabic numbers**, with the **abbreviation following**, for example, 30 mEq. You will see milliequivalents used in a variety of oral and parenteral solutions, potassium chloride being a common example.

PROBLEM

Express the following milliequivalent dosages using correct abbreviations.

1. sixty milliequivalents   _____

2. fifteen milliequivalents   _____

3. forty milliequivalents   _____

4. one milliequivalents   _____

5. fifty milliequivalents   _____

6. eighty milliequivalents   _____

7. fifty-five milliequivalents   _____

8. seventy milliequivalents   _____

9. thirty milliequivalents   _____

10. twenty milliequivalents   _____

Answers **1.** 60 mEq **2.** 15 mEq **3.** 40 mEq **4.** 1 mEq **5.** 50 mEq **6.** 80 mEq **7.** 55 mEq **8.** 70 mEq **9.** 30 mEq **10.** 20 mEq

RATIO MEASURES

Ratio strengths are used primarily in solutions. They represent **parts of drug per parts of solution**, for example, 1 : 1000 (one part drug to 1000 parts solution).

EXAMPLE 1	A 1 : 100 strength solution has 1 part drug in 100 parts solution
EXAMPLE 2	A 1 : 5 solution contains 1 part drug in 5 parts solution
EXAMPLE 3	A solution that is 1 part drug in 2 parts solution would be written 1 : 2

The **less solution** a drug is dissolved in, the **stronger the solution**. For example, a ratio strength of 1 : 10 (1 part drug to 10 parts solution) is much stronger than a 1 : 100 (1 part drug in 100 parts solution).

Ratio strengths are always expressed in their **simplest terms**. For example, 2 : 10 would be incorrect, because it can be reduced to 1 : 5. Dosages expressed using ratio strengths are not common, but you do need to know what they represent.

PROBLEM

Express the following solution strengths as ratios.

1. 1 part drug to 200 parts solution _____

2. 1 part drug to 4 parts solution _____

3. 1 part drug to 7 parts solution _____

Identify the strongest solution in each of the following.

4. a) 1 : 20   b) 1 : 200   c) 1 : 2   _____

5. a) 1 : 50   b) 1 : 20   c) 1 : 100   _____

6. a) 1 : 1000   b) 1 : 5000   c) 1 : 2000   _____

Answers **1.** 1 : 200 **2.** 1 : 4 **3.** 1 : 7 **4.** c **5.** b **6.** a

APOTHECARY AND HOUSEHOLD MEASURES

Apothecary and household measures are the oldest of the drug measurements. Apothecary measures are seldom used today, but you must be aware of their existence, just in case one is. Apothecary dosages are also rarely seen on medication labels, other than for older drugs such as phenobarbital and aspirin. Even if a drug label contains an apothecary dosage, it will always be in conjunction with the metric dosage equivalent.

There is only one apothecary measure for weight, the grain, and three for volume (liquids), the minim, dram, and ounce. Their abbreviations/symbols are:

WEIGHT	VOLUME		
grain gr	minim m min		
	dram ℥ dr fluid dram		
	ounce ℥ oz fluid ounce		

You may have difficulty remembering the difference between the symbols for dram and ounce, so let's take a minute to clarify these. **An ounce equals 30 mL**, or a full medication cup in case it's easier for you to relate to that. It is the larger of the two measures and the symbol is likewise larger, having an extra loop on top. In fact, it almost looks like oz written carelessly ℥. **A dram equals 4 mL**. It just covers the bottom of a medication cup and is therefore very small compared with an ounce. Its symbol is also smaller, ʒ. It is important not to confuse these symbols because the large difference in measures, 30 mL for ounce as opposed to 4 mL for dram, could make errors very serious.

$$\text{Once again:} \quad \text{ounce} = ℥ = 30 \text{ mL}$$

$$\text{dram} = ʒ = 4 \text{ mL}$$

A **minim** is approximately equal to a **drop**, so it is a very small measure.

 Minim dosages are rarely seen, except as calibrations on some syringes and medication cups. They are gradually being removed from all medicinal supplies to eliminate this confusing dosage and its abbreviation.

1 minum = m or min = 1 drop

Three **household** measures are still occasionally used.

tablespoon—T or tbs   teaspoon—t or tsp   drop—gtt

Memorize these if you are not already familiar with them. Be careful not to confuse the single letter abbreviations for table and teaspoon. A tablespoon is larger (15 mL) and is printed with a capital T; the teaspoon, which is smaller (5 mL), is printed with a small t.

$$\text{Once again:} \quad \text{tablespoon} = \text{T or tbs} = 15 \text{ mL}$$

$$\text{teaspoon} = \text{t or tsp} = 5 \text{ mL}$$

PROBLEM

Write the symbols and/or abbreviations for the following measures.

1. minim   _____   _____

2. teaspoon   _____   _____

3. ounce   _____   _____

4. grain   _____   _____

5. dram   _____   _____

6. drop   _____   _____

7. tablespoon   _____   _____

Answers **1.** min, m **2.** t, tsp **3.** ℥, oz **4.** gr **5.** ʒ, dr **6.** gtt **7.** T, tbs

Do not continue with the remaining apothecary system instruction until you have checked with your instructor, who will advise you if any of the clinical facilities you will be utilizing require your learning this material. If you are to omit this section, turn now to page 52 for the chapter Summary.

APOTHECARY/HOUSEHOLD NOTATIONS

The best overall description of apothecary notations is that they are the exact opposite of metric notations. The symbol/abbreviation is placed in front of the quantity, which may be expressed in Arabic numbers, for example, gr 2, or Roman numerals, for example, gr II. Do you need a refresher in Roman numerals? One to ten are: I, II, III, IV, V, VI, VII, VIII, IX, X. In both systems fractional dosages may be expressed as common fractions, for example, gr ½, except that **the symbol s̄s̄ may also be used for one half**, gr s̄s̄. All or none of these rules may be followed, so if you do see an apothecary notation don't expect consistency.

APOTHECARY/HOUSEHOLD TO METRIC/SI EQUIVALENTS TABLE

When an order is written in apothecary or household measures, it will have to be converted to metric because very few drug labels contain apothecary or household dosages. There are two recommended ways to do this. The first is to use an **equivalents table**. Most medication rooms/carts should have one. So let's begin by looking at the equivalents table in Figure 5-1. Notice that **liquid** equivalents are on the **left**, and **weights** are on the **right**.

APOTHECARY / HOUSEHOLD / METRIC EQUIVALENTS							
Liquid				Weight			
oz	mL	min	mL	gr	mg	gr	mg
1 = 30		45 = 3		15 = 1000		1/4 = 15	
½ = 15		30 = 2		10 = 600		1/6 = 10	
		15 = 1		7½ = 500		1/8 = 7.5	
dr	mL	12 = 0.75		5 = 300		1/10 = 6	
2½ = 10		10 = 0.6		4 = 250		1/15 = 4	
2 = 8		8 = 0.5		3 = 200		1/20 = 3	
1¼ = 5		5 = 0.3		2½ = 150		1/30 = 2	
1 = 4		4 = 0.25		2 = 120		1/40 = 1.5	
		3 = 0.2		1½ = 100		1/60 = 1	
1 min = 1 gtt		1½ = 0.1		1 = 60		1/100 = 0.6	
1T = 15 mL		1 = 0.06		3/4 = 45		1/120 = 0.5	
1t = 5 mL		¾ = 0.05		1/2 = 30		1/150 = 0.4	
		½ = 0.03		1/3 = 20		1/200 = 0.3	
						1/250 = 0.25	

Figure 5-1

The numbers on this equivalents table, as on most equivalents tables, are **small and close together**. This contributes to the **most common error** in the use of equivalents tables, which is to **misread from one column to another**. For example, if you are converting gr ⅛ to mg, it is not impossible to incorrectly read one line above the correct equivalent, 10 mg, or one line below, 6 mg. To eliminate this possibility

always use a guide to read from one column to the other. Use any straight-edge available and you will see immediately that gr ⅛ is equivalent to 7.5 mg. Very simple, very safe.

PROBLEM

Use the equivalents table in Figure 5-1 to determine the following equivalent measures.

1. gr ¼   = _____ mg

2. 30 mL   = oz _____

3. 100 mg = gr _____

4. gr ⅙   = _____ mg

5. 60 mg = gr _____

6. 4 mL   = dr _____

7. gr 7½ = _____ mg

8. oz ½   = _____ mL

9. 300 mg = gr _____

10. 15 mg   = gr _____

11. gr 1/100 = _____ mg

12. 0.4 mg = gr _____

13. 2 min   = _____ gtt

14. 30 mg   = gr _____

15. 10 mL   = _____ t

16. 2 T   = _____ mL

Answers **1.** 15 mg **2.** oz 1 **3.** gr 1½ **4.** 10 mg **5.** gr 1 **6.** dr 1 **7.** 500 mg **8.** 15 mL **9.** gr 5 **10.** gr ¼ **11.** 0.6 mg **12.** gr 1/150 **13.** 2 gtt **14.** gr ½ **15.** 2 t **16.** 30 mL

THE APOTHECARY/METRIC CONVERSION CLOCK

The second way to remember conversions is to visualize an "apothecary/metric clock." Because 60 mg equals gr 1, and there are 60 minutes in one hour, mg can be used to represent minutes, and fractions of the hour to represent gr. Refer to Figure 5-2 to see how this works for conversions.

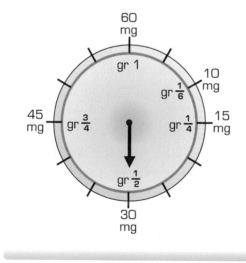

Figure 5-2

As you can see on this "clock," 60 mg (representing 60 minutes) equals gr 1 (1 hour). It then follows that 30 mg equals gr ½, 10 mg equals gr ⅙ and so on. Two hours (gr 2) = 120 mg, and gr 5 = 300 mg. One additional equivalent to remember that does not correspond exactly to the clock is gr 15, which equals 1000 mg (1 gram).

A few moments ago you also learned that 1 oz = 30 mL, 1 dr = 4 mL, 1 T = 15 mL, 1 tsp = 5 mL. Use these equivalents now in the following problems.

PROBLEM

Convert the following to equivalent measures.

1. gr ¾   = _____ mg   6. 300 mg   = gr _____

2. gr ¼   = _____ mg   7. gr ⅙   = _____ mg

3. ½ oz   = _____ mL   8. 10 mL   = _____ t

4. gr 15   = _____ mg   9. dr 1   = _____ mL

5. 8 mL   = dr _____   10. 2 T   = _____ mL

Answers **1.** 45 mg   **2.** 15 mg   **3.** 15 mL   **4.** 1000 mg   **5.** dr 2   **6.** gr 5   **7.** 10 mg   **8.** 2 t   **9.** 4 mL   **10.** 30 mL

Summary

This concludes your introduction to the additional measures you will see used in dosages and in solutions. The important points to remember from this chapter are:

- International units, abbreviated U, measure a drug by its action rather than its weight.

- Percentage (%) strengths are frequently used in solutions and ointments.

- Percent represents grams of drug per 100 mL of solution.

- The higher the percentage strength, the stronger the solution.

- Milliequivalent is abbreviated mEq and is a frequently used measure in solutions.

- Ratio strengths represent parts of drug per parts of solution.

- Apothecary measures are so infrequently used that they should be immediately converted to metric measures to prevent medication errors.

- The larger ℥ symbol represents ounce, the smaller ℨ, dram.

- T or tbs is the abbreviation for tablespoon (15 mL); t or tsp for teaspoon (5 mL).

- Do not confuse the apothecary minim, which is abbreviated m, with metric measures.

Summary Self-Test

Express the following dosages using official symbols/abbreviations.

1. three hundred thousand units   _____

2. forty-five units   _____

3. ten percent   _____

4. two and a half percent   _____

5. forty milliequivalents   _____

6. a one in two thousand ratio   _____

7. two ounces   _____

8. three drams   _____

9. one tablespoon   _____

10. two thousand units   _____

11. five teaspoons   _____

12. nine-tenths percent   _____

13. ten units   _____

14. a one in two ratio   _____

15. five percent   _____

16. twenty milliequivalents   _____

17. fourteen units   _____

18. twenty percent   _____

19. two million units   _____

20. one hundred thousand units   _____

Answers

1. 300,000 U
2. 45 U
3. 10%
4. 2.5%
5. 40 mEq

6. 1 : 2000
7. 2 oz, ℥ II
   (varies)
8. ℥ III, 3 dr
   (varies)

9. 1 T, 1 tbs
   (varies)
10. 2000 U
11. 5 tsp, 5 t
   (varies)
12. 0.9%

13. 10 U
14. 1 : 2
15. 5%
16. 20 mEq
17. 14 U
18. 20%

19. 2,000,000 U
20. 100,000 U

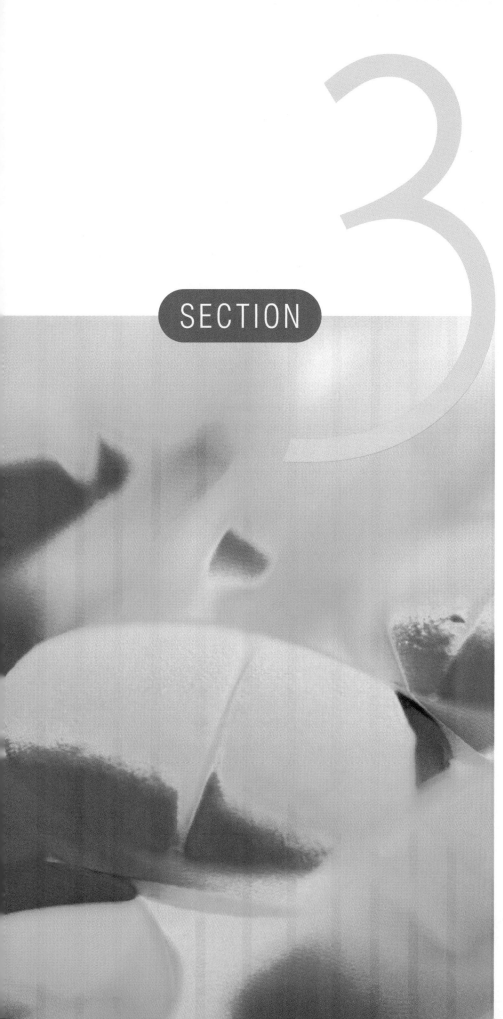

6

Reading Oral Medication Labels

Medication labels contain a variety of information that ranges from simple to complex. In this chapter, you will be introduced to labels of oral medications, which are generally the least complicated. With this instruction, you will be able to locate drugs and calculate simple dosages without confusion, as well as understand the more complicated labels presented in later chapters.

We will begin with labels for solid drug preparations. These include tablets; scored tablets (which contain an indented marking to make breakage for partial dosages possible); enteric coated tablets (which delay absorption until the drug reaches the small intestine); capsules (powdered or oily drugs in a gelatin cover); and sustained or controlled release capsules (action spread over a prolonged period of time, for example, 12 hours). See illustrations in Figure 6-1.

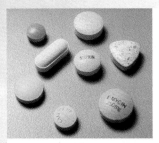
Tablets

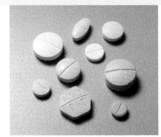
Scored Tablets

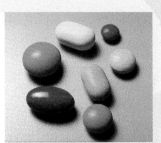
Enteric Coated Tablets

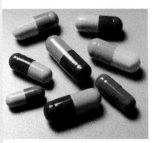
Capsules

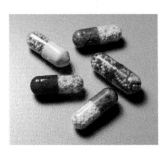
Controlled Release Capsules

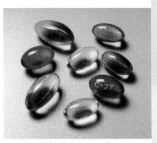
Gelatin Capsules

Figure 6-1

TABLET AND CAPSULE LABELS

The most common type of label you will see in the hospital setting is the **unit dosage label**, in which each tablet or capsule is packaged separately. However, the dosage on both unit and multiple dose labels is identical.

EXAMPLE 1

Look at the Lanoxin® label in Figure 6-2. The first thing to notice is that this drug has two names. The first, Lanoxin, is its **trade name**, which is identified by the ® registration symbol. Trade names are usually capitalized and printed first on the label. The name in smaller print, digoxin, is the **generic** or **official name** of the drug. Each drug has only one official name but may have several trade names, each for the exclusive use of the company that manufactures it. It is important to remember, however, that most labels do contain **both** names, because drugs may be ordered by either name depending on hospital policy or physician preference. You will frequently need to cross-check trade and generic names for accurate drug identification.

Next on the label is the **dosage strength**, 250 mcg or 0.25 mg. The dosage is often representative of the **average dosage strength, the dosage given to the average patient at one time**. This label also identifies the manufacturer of this drug, GlaxoSmithKline.

Notice that "1000 Tablets" is printed at the top left of this label. This is the total number of tablets in the bottle. Be careful not to confuse the quantity of tablets or capsules in a container with the dosage strength. **The dosage strength always has a unit of measure associated with it**, in this case mcg and mg. Because label designs vary widely, this is an important point to remember.

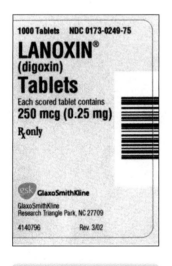

Figure 6-2

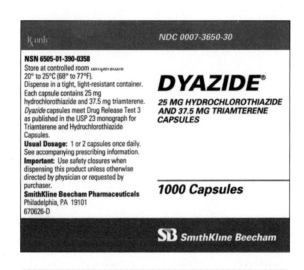

Figure 6-3

EXAMPLE 2

The Dyazide® label in Figure 6-3 is for a medication that contains two different drugs, hydrochlorothiazide 25 mg and triamterene 37.5 mg, both of which are generic drug names. Medications that contain more than one drug would be ordered by trade name, in this case Dyazide, and number of capsules or tablets to be given, rather than by dosage. The total of Dyazide capsules in this package, 1000, is listed near the bottom of the label, as is the drug manufacturer, SmithKline Beecham. On the left is information about storage and dosage, which, as a rule in routine medication administration, would not be necessary to read.

 Tablets and capsules that contain more than one drug are ordered by trade name and number of tablets or capsules to be given, rather than by dosage.

EXAMPLE 3

The small unit dosage (single dose) label in Figure 6-4 bears only one name, pheno-barbital, which is actually the generic name of the drug. This labeling is common with drugs that have been in use for many years. The official (generic) name was so well established that drug manufacturers did not try to promote their own trade names. Also notice that immediately after the drug name are the initials **U.S.P.** This is the abbreviation for **U**nited **S**tates **P**harmacopeia, one of the two official national listings of drugs. The other is the **N**ational **F**ormulary, **N.F.** You will see U.S.P. and N.F. on drug labels and must not confuse them with other initials that identify additional drugs or specific action of drugs in a preparation.

Next, notice that this label gives the dosage strength of phenobarbital in both metric and apothecaries' units of measure, 15 mg and gr 1/4. Finally, on the right of the label, printed sideways, are the letters "Exp." This represents "expiration," the last date when the drug should be used. **Make a habit of checking the expiration dates on labels.**

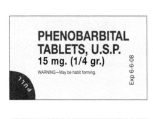

Figure 6-4

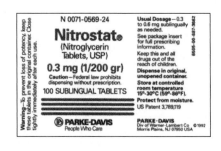

Figure 6-5

PROBLEM

Refer to the label in Figure 6-5 and answer the following questions about this drug.

1. What is the generic name? _____

2. What is the trade name? _____

3. What is the dosage strength in metric units? _____

4. What is the dosage strength in apothecary measures? _____

Answers **1.** nitroglycerin **2.** Nitrostat® **3.** 0.3 mg **4.** 1/200 gr

PROBLEM

Refer to the label in Figure 6-6 and answer the following questions about this drug.

1. What is the generic name? _____

2. What is the trade name? _____

3. What is the dosage strength? _____

4. What company manufactured this drug? _____

5. How many tablets are in this container? _____

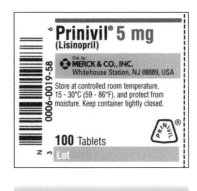

Figure 6-6

Answers   **1.** lisinopril   **2.** Prinivil®   **3.** 5 mg   **4.** Merck & Co., Inc.   **5.** 100 tablets

Refer to the Sinemet® label in Figure 6-7. Sinemet is another example of a combined drug tablet. The generic names of the drugs it contains are carbidopa and levodopa. These are listed on the label in several places: directly under the trade name, then with the **amount** of each drug in the fine print near the bottom of the label. Also notice the box to the right of the trade name, which contains the numbers 25–100. This again is the amount of carbidopa—25 mg, and levodopa—100 mg. Contrast this with the Sinemet labels in Figures 6-8 and 6-9.

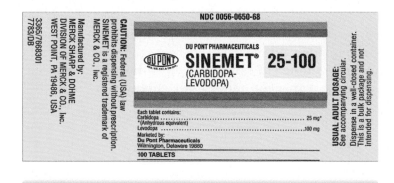

Figure 6-7

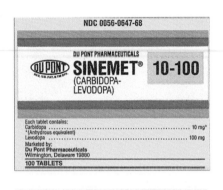

Figure 6-8

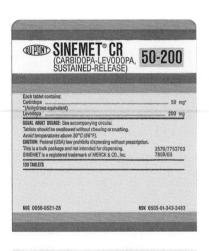

Figure 6-9

In Figure 6-8 the dosage strengths are different. A box to the right of the trade name identifies the strengths of carbidopa and levodopa as 10 mg and 100 mg, respectively, actually a lower dosage. And finally, Figure 6-9 is a label for Sinemet **CR**, a **c**ontrolled **r**elease or sustained release tablet, with yet another dosage strength of 50–200, carbidopa 50 mg, levodopa 200 mg. Unlike the previous combined drug tablet discussed, an order for Sinemet **must** include the dosage because it is available in several strengths.

 Extra numbers after a drug name may be used to identify the dosage strengths of more than one drug in a preparation, and extra initials may be used to identify a special drug action.

TABLET/CAPSULE DOSAGE CALCULATION

When the time comes for you to administer medications, you will have to read a medication record or Kardex to prepare the dosage. This will tell you the name and amount of drug to be given, but **it will not tell you how many tablets or capsules contain this dosage**. This you must calculate yourself. However, this is not difficult. Most tablets/capsules are prepared in average dosage strengths, and most orders will involve giving one half to three tablets (or one to three capsules, since capsules cannot be broken in half). **Learn to question orders for more than three tablets or capsules**. Although some drugs require multiple tablets, most do not, and **an unusual number of tablets or capsules could be a warning of an error in prescribing, transcribing, or your calculations**.

 Regardless of the source of an error, if you give a wrong drug or dosage you are legally responsible for it.

Let's look at some sample orders and do some actual dosage calculations. **Assume that both tablets in our problems are scored and can be broken in half.**

PROBLEM

Refer to the Thorazine® label in Figure 6-10 and answer the following questions.

1. What is the dosage strength? _____

2. If you have an order for 100 mg give _____

3. If you have an order for 150 mg give _____

4. If 300 mg are ordered give _____

5. What is the generic name of this drug? _____

6. What is the total number of tablets in this package? _____

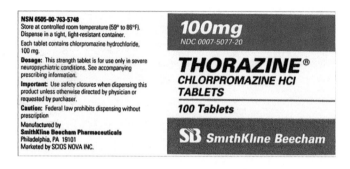

Figure 6-10

Answers **1.** 100 mg **2.** 1 tab **3.** 1½ tab **4.** 3 tab **5.** chlorpromazine HCl **6.** 100 tablets

PROBLEM

Refer to the Aricept® label in Figure 6-11 and answer the following questions.

1. What is the dosage strength? _____

2. If 10 mg is ordered give _____

3. If 2.5 mg is ordered give _____

4. If 5 mg is ordered give _____

5. What is the generic name of this drug? _____

6. What is the total number of tablets in this package? _____

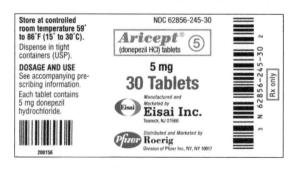

Figure 6-11

Answers **1.** 5 mg **2.** 2 tab **3.** ½ tab **4.** 1 tab **5.** donepezil HCl **6.** 30 tablets

It is not uncommon to have a drug **ordered** in one unit of metric measure, for example, mg, and discover that it is **labeled** in another measure, for example, g. It will then be necessary to **convert the units to calculate the dosage**. This is not difficult because conversions will always be between touching units of measure: g and mg, or mg and mcg. Converting is a matter of moving the decimal point three places.

EXAMPLE 1

Refer to the Halcion® label in Figure 6-12. A dosage of 250 mcg has been ordered. The label reads 0.25 mg. Convert the mg to mcg and you can mentally verify that these dosages are identical. Give 1 tablet.

EXAMPLE 2

Refer to the Carafate® label in Figure 6-13. Carafate 2000 mg is ordered. The label reads 1 gram, so you must give 2 tablets (1 tab = 1000 mg, so 2000 mg requires 2 tab).

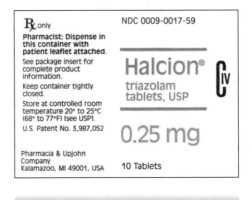

Figure 6-12

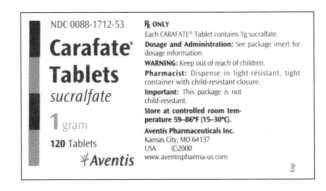

Figure 6-13

PROBLEM

Locate the appropriate labels for the following dosages, and indicate how many tablets or capsules are needed to give them. Assume all tablets are scored.

1. verapamil HCl 0.12 g   _____ cap

2. Micronase® 2500 mcg   _____ tab

3. Dilatrate®-SR 0.04 g   _____ cap

4. terbutaline sulfate 5000 mcg   _____ tab

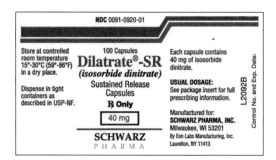

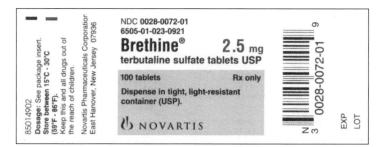

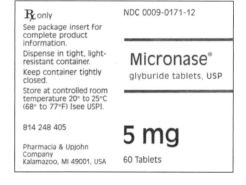

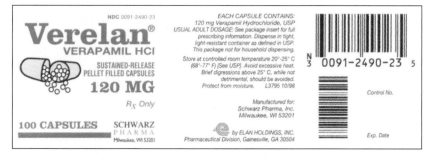

PROBLEM

Locate the appropriate labels for the following drug orders and indicate the number of tablets/capsules that will be required to administer the dosages ordered. Assume that all tablets are scored. Notice that both generic and trade names are used for the orders, and a label may be used in more than one problem.

1. isosorbide dinitrate 80 mg _____ cap

2. sulfasalazine 0.5 g _____ tab

3. sulfasalazine 1 g _____ tab

4. hydrochlorothiazide 25 mg _____ tab

5. chlordiazepoxide HCl 50 mg _____ cap

6. Stelazine® 7.5 mg _____ tab

7. Minipress® 2 mg _____ cap

8. methyldopa 500 mg _____ tab

9. levothyroxine Na 0.2 mg _____ tab

10. DiaBeta® 3.75 mg _____ tab

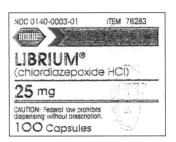

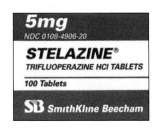

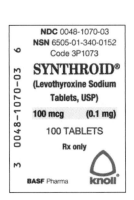

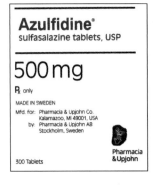

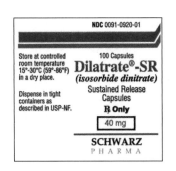

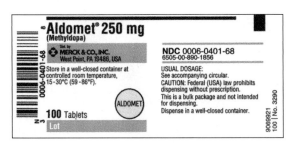

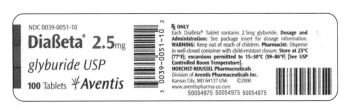

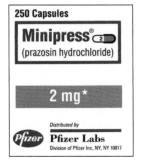

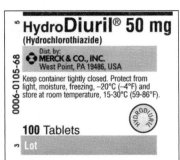

ORAL SOLUTION LABELS

In liquid drug preparations the weight of the drug is contained in a certain **volume of solution**, most frequently, mL or cc's. Let's review dosages in some solid and liquid drug preparations to illustrate the difference.

EXAMPLE 1 | **Solid:** 250 mg in **1 tablet**   **Liquid:** 250 mg in **5 mL**

EXAMPLE 2 | **Solid:** 100 mg in **1 capsule**   **Liquid:** 100 mg in **10 mL**

Solution strength can also be expressed in ounces, drams, teaspoons, or tablespoons, but these measures are less common. Look at the following solution labels so that you can become familiar with them.

EXAMPLE 3

Refer to the Lomotil® label in Figure 6-14. The information it contains will be familiar. Lomotil is the trade name, diphenoxylate is the generic or official name. The dosage strength is **2.5 mg per 5 mL**. As with solid drugs, the medication record will tell you the **dosage of the drug** to be administered, but rarely will it specify **the volume that contains this dosage**.

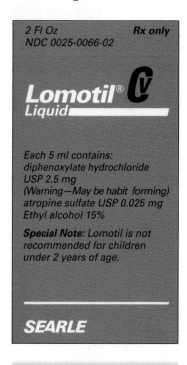

2 Fl Oz
NDC 0025-0066-02   **Rx only**

Lomotil® Cᵥ
Liquid

Each 5 ml contains:
diphenoxylate hydrochloride
USP 2.5 mg
(Warning—May be habit forming)
atropine sulfate USP 0.025 mg
Ethyl alcohol 15%

Special Note: Lomotil is not
recommended for children
under 2 years of age.

SEARLE

Figure 6-14

PROBLEM

Refer to the Lomotil label in Figure 6-14 again, and calculate the following dosages.

1. The order is for diphenoxylate 2.5 mg. Give _____

2. The order is for Lomotil 5 mg. Give   _____

Answers **1.** 5 mL **2.** 10 mL   If you did not express your answers as mL, they are incorrect. **Numbers have no meaning unless they are expressed with a unit of measure**, in this case, mL.

PROBLEM

Refer to the Amoxil® label in Figure 6-15, and calculate the following dosages.

1. The order is for amoxicillin susp. 250 mg.   _____

2. Amoxil 125 mg has been ordered.   _____

3. amoxicillin 375 mg has been ordered.   _____

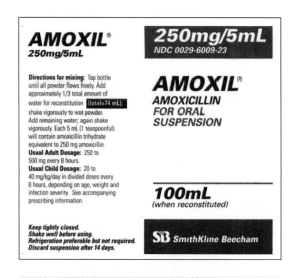

Figure 6-15

PROBLEM

Refer to the solution labels in Figures 6-16 and 6-17 and calculate the following dosages.

1. Prozac® soln. 10 mg   _____

2. cefaclor susp. 187 mg   _____

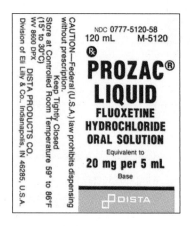

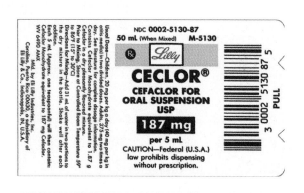

Figure 6-16   Figure 6-17

3. Ceclor® susp. 374 mg _____

4. fluoxetine HCl soln. 30 mg _____

5. Prozac® soln. 40 mg _____

6. fluoxetine HCl soln. 20 mg _____

Answers **1.** 2.5 mL **2.** 5 mL **3.** 10 mL **4.** 7.5 mL **5.** 10 mL **6.** 5 mL

MEASUREMENT OF ORAL SOLUTIONS

Oral solutions can be measured using a **calibrated medicine cup** such as the one shown in Figure 6-18, which contains calibrations in mL (cc), tbs, tsp, dr, and oz. To pour accurately hold the cup at eye level, then line up the measure you need and pour until the medication is level with the desired dosage.

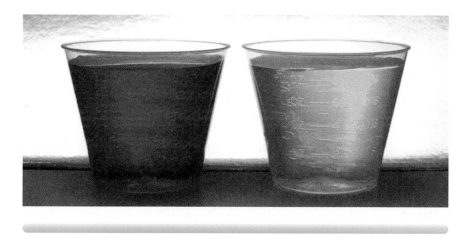

Figure 6-18

Solutions can also be measured using specially calibrated **oral syringes** such as those illustrated in Figures 6-19 and 6-20. Oral syringes have safety features built into their design to prevent their being mistaken for hypodermic syringes. One of these features is **color**, as illustrated in Figure 6-19 (hypodermic syringes are not colored, although their packaging and needle covers may be to aid in identification). A second feature is the syringe tip, which is a **different size** and **shape**, and is often **off center** (termed **eccentric**). Figure 6-20 illustrates an eccentric oral syringe tip.

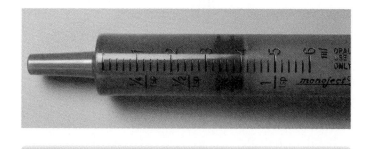

Figure 6-19

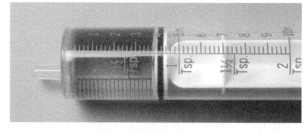

Figure 6-20

Hypodermic syringes (without a needle) can also be used to measure and administer oral dosages. The main concern with correct syringe identification is that oral syringes, which are **not sterile**, not be confused and used for hypodermic medications, which **are sterile**. This mistake has been made, in spite of the fact that hypodermic needles do not fit correctly on oral syringes. The precaution, therefore, does need to be stressed.

Oral solutions may also be ordered as drops (gtt), and when this is the case the dropper is usually attached to the bottle stopper. It is also common for medicine droppers to be calibrated, for example in mL, or by actual dosage, 125 mg, etc. (see Figure 20-2 on page 289).

Summary

This concludes the chapter on reading oral medication labels. The important points to remember from this chapter are:

- Most labels contain both generic and trade names.

- Dosages are clearly printed on the label, except for preparations containing multiple drugs, which will list the name and dosage of each drug.

- Multiple dosage medications will be ordered by trade name and number of tablets/capsules to be given.

- The letters U.S.P. (United States Pharmacopeia) and N.F. (National Formulary) on drug labels identify their official generic listings.

- Additional letters that follow a drug name are used to identify additional drugs in the preparation or a special action of the drug.

- Most dosages of oral medications will involve giving one half to three tablets (1–3 capsules, which cannot be broken in half).

- Check drug expiration dates before use.

- Oral solution dosages may be measured in cc, mL, oz, tsp, tbs, dr, or gtt.

- For accurate measurement, oral solutions are poured and measured at eye level when a medicine cup is used.

- Liquid oral medications may be measured and administered using an oral medication syringe or hypodermic syringe (without the needle).

- Care must be taken not to use oral syringes for hypodermic medication preparation because these are not sterile.

Summary Self-Test

Locate the appropriate label for each of the following drug orders, and indicate the number of tablets/capsules or mL/cc that will be required to administer them. Assume that all tablets are scored and can be broken in half.

PART I

1. Glucotrol® 15 mg   _____

2. dexamethasone 4 mg   _____

3. Sorbitrate® 60 mg   _____

4. Trental® 0.2 g   _____

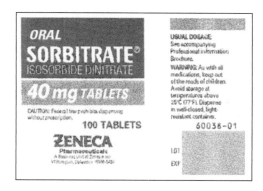

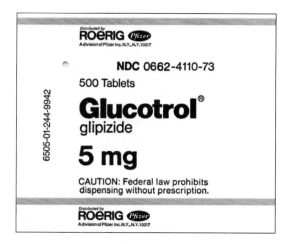

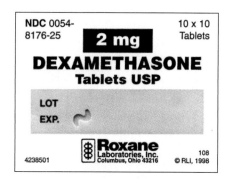

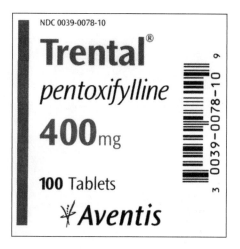

PART II

5. piroxicam 20 mg   _____

6. amoxicillin susp. 250 mg   _____

7. Lortab® 5/500 2 tab   _____

8. Calan® SR 240 mg   _____

9. alprazolam 750 mcg   _____

10. gabapentin 0.2 g   _____

11. Procanbid® 1 g   _____

12. lithium 0.3 g   _____

13. timolol maleate 30 mg   _____

14. triazolam 500 mcg   _____

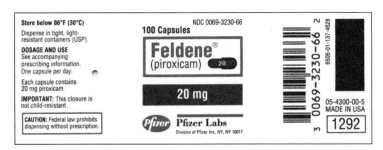

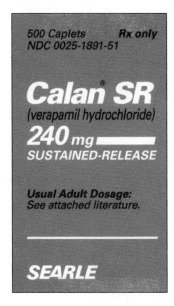

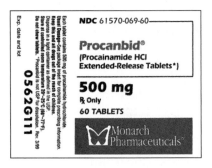

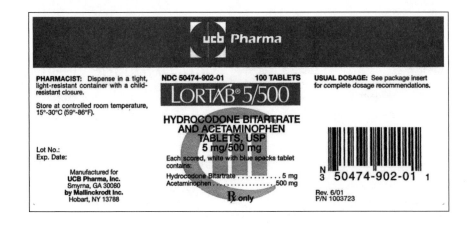

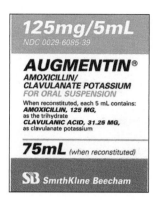

125mg/5mL
NDC 0029-6085-39

AUGMENTIN®
AMOXICILLIN/
CLAVULANATE POTASSIUM
FOR ORAL SUSPENSION

When reconstituted, each 5 mL contains:
AMOXICILLIN, 125 MG,
as the trihydrate
CLAVULANIC ACID, 31.25 MG,
as clavulanate potassium

75mL *(when reconstituted)*

SB *SmithKline Beecham*

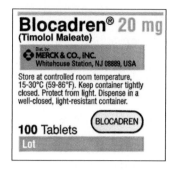

Blocadren® 20 mg
(Timolol Maleate)

Dist. by:
MERCK & CO., INC.
Whitehouse Station, NJ 08889, USA

Store at controlled room temperature,
15-30°C (59-86°F). Keep container tightly
closed. Protect from light. Dispense in a
well-closed, light-resistant container.

100 Tablets   (BLOCADREN)

Lot

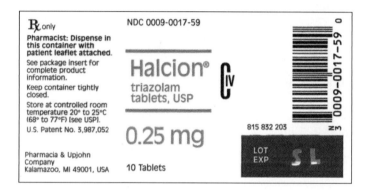

℞ only
**Pharmacist: Dispense in
this container with
patient leaflet attached.**
See package insert for
complete product
information.
Keep container tightly
closed.
Store at controlled room
temperature 20° to 25°C
(68° to 77°F) [see USP].
U.S. Patent No. 3,987,052

Pharmacia & Upjohn
Company
Kalamazoo, MI 49001, USA

NDC 0009-0017-59

Halcion® **C**IV
triazolam
tablets, USP

0.25 mg

10 Tablets

815 832 203

0009-0017-59 0

LOT
EXP

N 0071-0803-24

Neurontin®
(gabapentin)
capsules
100 mg
℞ only
100 CAPSULES

Store at controlled room temperature 15–30°C
(59–86°F).

Ⓟ **PARKE-DAVIS**

NSN 6505-00-482-8058
Store between 15° and 30°C (59° and 86°F).
Dispense in a tight container. Each capsule
contains lithium carbonate, 300 mg.
Usual Dosage: 1 or 2 capsules t.i.d.
See accompanying prescribing information.
Important: Use safety closures when
dispensing this product unless otherwise
directed by physician or requested by
purchaser.
Manufactured by
International Processing Corporation,
Winchester, KY 40391 for
SmithKline Beecham Pharmaceuticals,
Philadelphia, PA 19101
Marketed by Scios Inc.   ℞ only

300mg
NDC 0007-4007-20

ESKALITH®
**LITHIUM CARBONATE
CAPSULES**

100 Capsules

SB *SmithKline Beecham*

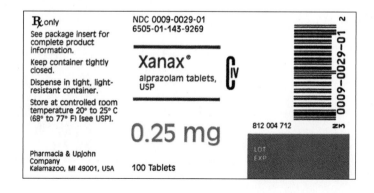

℞ only
See package insert for
complete product
information.
Keep container tightly
closed.
Dispense in tight, light-
resistant container.
Store at controlled room
temperature 20° to 25° C
(68° to 77° F) [see USP].

Pharmacia & Upjohn
Company
Kalamazoo, MI 49001, USA

NDC 0009-0029-01
6505-01-143-9269

Xanax® **C**IV
alprazolam tablets,
USP

0.25 mg

100 Tablets

812 004 712

0009-0029-01 2

LOT
EXP

PART III

15. acetaminophen 650 mg   _____

16. Aldactone® 75 mg   _____

17. meclizine HCl 50 mg   _____

18. cefaclor 0.5 g   _____

19. ciprofloxacin HCl 0.375 g   _____

20. metoprolol tartrate 0.15 g   _____

21. nifedipine 10 mg   _____

22. furosemide 10 mg   _____

23. Lasix® 30 mg   _____

24. dexamethasone 3 mg   _____

25. Librium® 75 mg   _____

26. terbutaline sulfate 5 mg   _____

27. Toprol-XL 0.1 g   _____

28. Synthroid® 225 mcg   _____

29. DiaBeta® 5000 mcg   _____

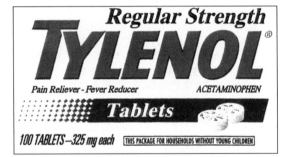

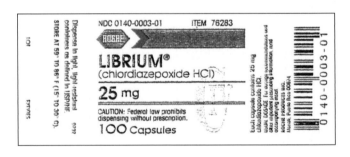

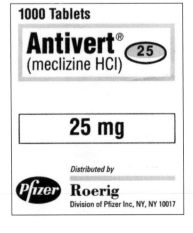

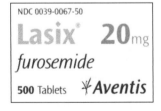

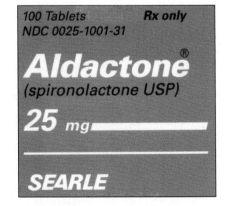

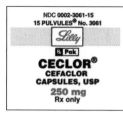

NDC 0002-3061-15
15 PULVULES® No. 3061
Lilly
℞ Pak
CECLOR®
CEFACLOR
CAPSULES, USP
250 mg
Rx only

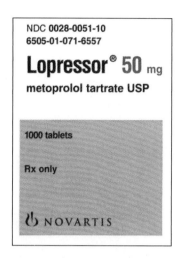

NDC 0028-0051-10
6505-01-071-6557

Lopressor® 50 mg

metoprolol tartrate USP

1000 tablets

Rx only

ひ NOVARTIS

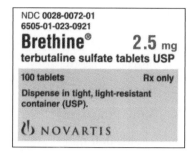

NDC 0028-0072-01
6505-01-023-0921

Brethine® 2.5 mg

terbutaline sulfate tablets USP

100 tablets   Rx only

Dispense in tight, light-resistant
container (USP).

ひ NOVARTIS

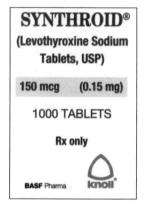

SYNTHROID®

(Levothyroxine Sodium
Tablets, USP)

150 mcg   (0.15 mg)

1000 TABLETS

Rx only

BASF Pharma   knoll®

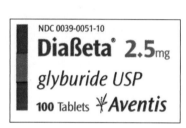

NDC 0039-0051-10

Diaßeta® 2.5mg

glyburide USP

100 Tablets ⚕*Aventis*

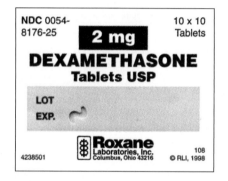

NDC 0054-
8176-25   **2 mg**   10 x 10
Tablets

DEXAMETHASONE
Tablets USP

LOT

EXP.

⊛ **Roxane**
Laboratories, Inc.
Columbus, Ohio 43216

4238501   108
© RLI, 1998

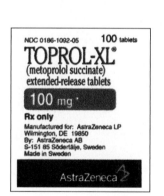

NDC 0186-1092-05   **100** tablets

TOPROL-XL®
(metoprolol succinate)
extended-release tablets

100 mg ·

Rx only

Manufactured for: AstraZeneca LP
Wilmington, DE 19850
By: AstraZeneca AB
S-151 85 Södertälje, Sweden
Made in Sweden

AstraZeneca

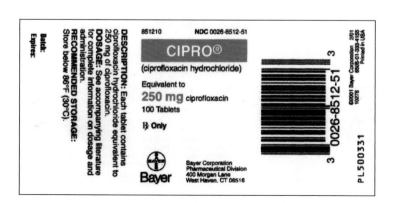

Batch:
Expires:

Store below 86°F (30°C).
RECOMMENDED STORAGE:
administration.
for complete information on dosage and
DOSAGE: See accompanying literature
250 mg of ciprofloxacin.
ciprofloxacin hydrochloride equivalent to
DESCRIPTION: Each tablet contains

851210   NDC 0026-8512-51

CIPRO®

(ciprofloxacin hydrochloride)

Equivalent to
250 mg ciprofloxacin
100 Tablets

℞ Only

Bayer Corporation
Pharmaceutical Division
400 Morgan Lane
West Haven, CT 06516

Bayer

©2001 Bayer Corporation 2/01
6505-01-530-4155
10278   Printed in USA

3 0026-8512-51 3

PL500331

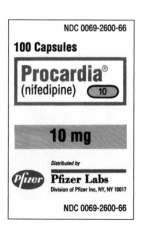

NDC 0069-2600-66

100 Capsules

Procardia®
(nifedipine)   10

10 mg

Distributed by

Pfizer **Pfizer Labs**
Division of Pfizer Inc, NY, NY 10017

NDC 0069-2600-66

PART IV

30. amoxicillin susp. 0.25 g   _____

31. Percocet® 2 tab   _____

32. metronidazole 0.75 g   _____

33. piroxicam 40 mg   _____

34. Lopid® 300 mg   _____

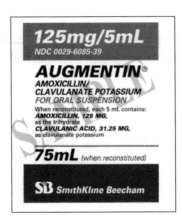

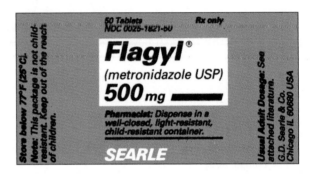

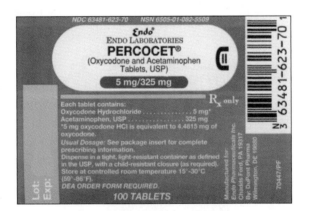

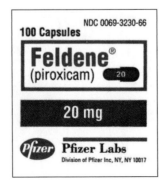

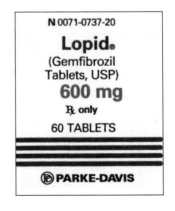

PART V _____

35. cefaclor oral susp. 0.5 g _____

36. spironolactone 0.1 g _____

37. cefpodoxime proxetil 0.2 g _____

38. Augmentin® 0.75 g _____

39. potassium chloride 40 mEq _____

40. penicillin V potassium 600,000 U _____

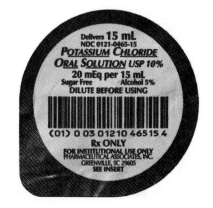

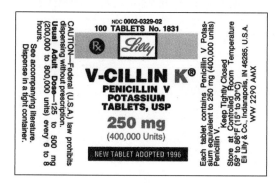

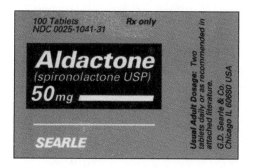

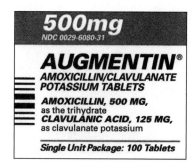

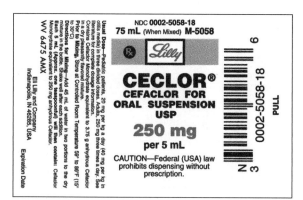

Answers

1. 3 tab	**9.** 3 tab	**18.** 2 cap	**27.** 1 tab	**36.** 2 tab
2. 2 tab	**10.** 2 cap	**19.** 1½ tab	**28.** 1½ tab	**37.** 10 mL
3. 1½ tab	**11.** 2 cap	**20.** 3 tab	**29.** 2 tab	**38.** 1½ tab
4. ½ tab	**12.** 1 cap	**21.** 1 cap	**30.** 10 mL	**39.** 30 mL
5. 1 cap	**13.** 1½ tab	**22.** ½ tab	**31.** 2 tab	**40.** 1½ tab
6. 10 mL	**14.** 2 tab	**23.** 1½ tab	**32.** 1½ tab	
7. 2 tab	**15.** 2 tab	**24.** 1½ tab	**33.** 2 cap	
8. 1 cap	**16.** 3 tab	**25.** 3 cap	**34.** ½ tab	
	17. 2 tab	**26.** 2 tab	**35.** 10 mL	

7

Hypodermic Syringe Measurement

Objectives

The learner will measure parenteral solutions using:

1. a standard 3 mL/cc syringe

2. a tuberculin syringe

3. 5, 6, 10, and 12 mL/cc syringes

4. a 20 cc syringe

A variety of hypodermic syringes are in common clinical use. This chapter focuses most heavily on the frequently used 3 mL/cc syringe. However, larger volume syringes are used on occasion, so it is necessary that you learn the **differences**, as well as the **similarities**, of all syringes in use.

Regardless of a syringe's volume or capacity—0.5, 1, 3, 5, 6, 10, 20, or 50 mL/cc—all except specialized insulin syringes **are calibrated in mL/cc**. However, these various capacity syringes contain **calibrations that differ from each other.** Recognizing the difference in syringe calibrations is the chief safety concern of this chapter.

 The calibrations on different volume syringes differ from each other, requiring particular care in dosage measurement.

STANDARD 3 mL/cc SYRINGE

The most commonly used hypodermic syringe is the 3 mL/cc size illustrated in Figure 7-1. Notice that this syringe contains only one set of calibrations, for the metric mL/cc scale. However, a limited number of 3 mL/cc syringes still contain a second set of smaller calibrations, for the apothecary minim, m, scale. If a syringe you are using contains two calibrated scales be particularly careful not to mistake the minum, m, calibrations for metric mL/cc calibrations. Metric measurements are used almost exclusively in injection dosages.

 If a syringe contains a minim calibration scale, care must be taken not to mistake it for the metric mL/cc scale.

Notice that **longer calibrations** identify zero (0), and each ½ and full mL measure on this 3 mL/cc syringe's calibrated scale. These longer calibrations are numbered: ½, 1, 1½, 2, 2½, and 3.

Next notice the **number of calibrations in each mL**, which is **10**, indicating that on this syringe each mL is **calibrated in tenths**. Tenths of a mL are written as **decimal fractions**, for example 1.2 mL, 2.5 mL, or 0.4 mL. Also notice the arrow on this syringe, which identifies a 0.8 mL dosage.

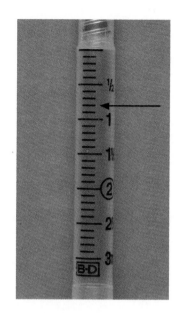

Figure 7-1 A 3 mL Monoject® brand syringe. Manufactured and sold by Kendall (a division of Tyco Healthcare Group, L.P.). Monoject is a proprietary trademark owned by Sherwood Services AG, a Tyco Healthcare Group affiliate.

PROBLEM

Use decimal numbers, for example, 2.2 mL, to identify the measurements indicated by the arrows on the standard 3 mL syringes that follow.

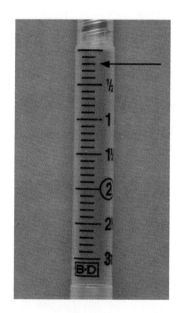

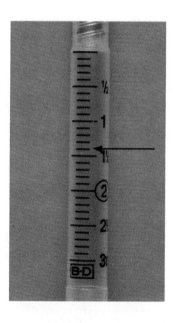

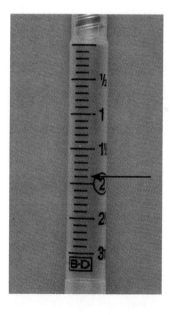

1. _____   2. _____   3. _____

Answers **1.** 0.2 mL **2.** 1.4 mL **3.** 1.9 mL

Did you have difficulty with the 0.2 mL calibration in problem 1? Remember that **the first long calibration on all syringes is zero**. It is slightly longer than the 0.1 cc and subsequent one-tenth calibrations. Be careful not to mistakenly count it as 0.1 cc.

You have just been looking at photos of syringe barrels only. In assembled syringes the colored suction tip of the plunger has two widened areas in contact with the barrel that look like two distinct rings. **Calibrations are read from the front, or top, ring.** Do not become confused by the second, bottom, ring, or by the raised middle section of the suction tip.

PROBLEM

What dosages are measured by the following three assembled syringes?

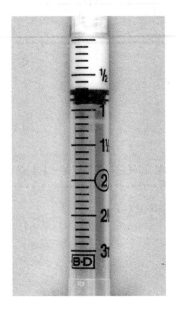 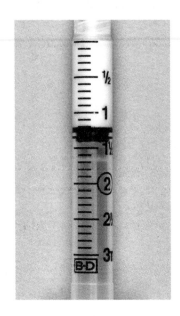 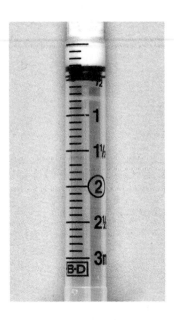

1. _____   2. _____   3. _____

Answers **1.** 0.7 mL **2.** 1.2 mL **3.** 0.3 mL

PROBLEM

Draw an arrow or shade in the following syringe barrels to indicate the required dosages. Have your instructor check your accuracy.

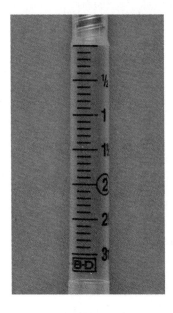 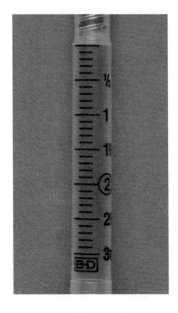 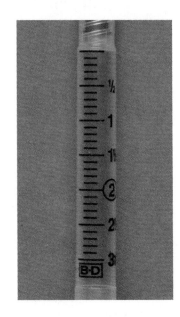

1. 1.3 mL   2. 2.4 mL   3. 0.9 mL

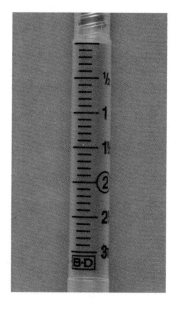

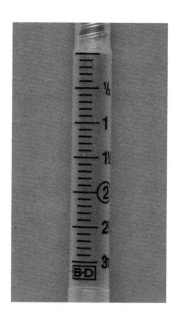

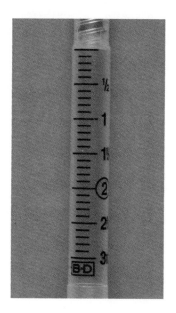

4. 2.5 mL   5. 1.7 mL   6. 2.1 mL

PROBLEM

Identify the dosages measured on the following 3 mL syringes.

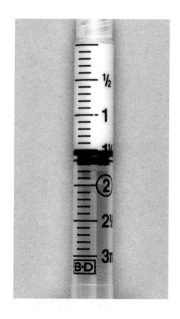

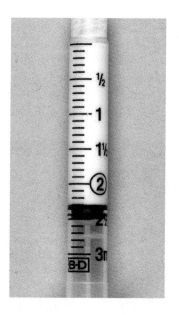

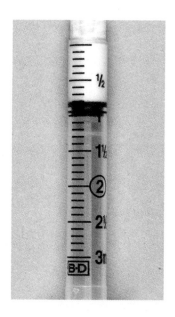

1. _____   2. _____   3. _____

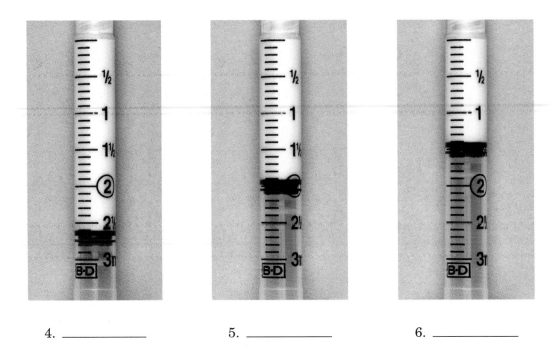

4. _____   5. _____   6. _____

Answers **1.** 1.5 mL **2.** 2.3 mL **3.** 0.8 mL **4.** 2.6 mL **5.** 1.9 mL **6.** 1.4 mL

SAFETY SYRINGES

A number of safety syringes have been developed in recent years to reduce the danger of accidental contaminated needle sticks. Several of these syringes are illustrated in the following photos. Take a few minutes to become familiar with them, as you will in all probability be using them in the clinical setting.

Refer first to the photos in Figure 7-2, which show two B-D SafetyGlide™ syringes. Each of these syringes contains a protective needle guard that can be activated by a single finger to cover and seal the needle after injection.

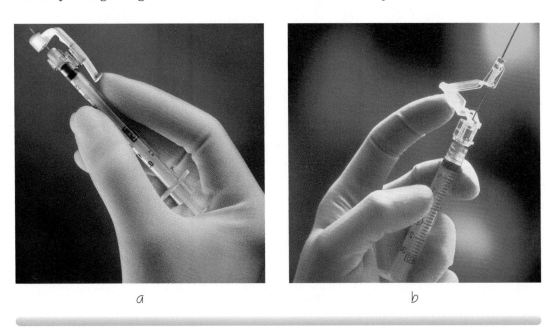

a   b

Figure 7-2a and b   SafetyGlide™ syringes. Product courtesy of BD © 2004 Becton, Dickinson and Company.

The syringe shown in Figure 7-3, the VanishPoint™, has a needle that automatically retracts into the barrel after injection.

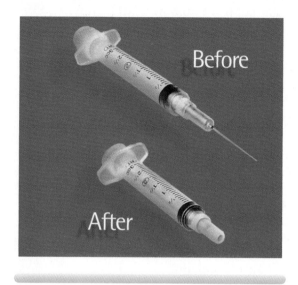

Figure 7-3 Retractable Technologies VanishPoint®

A third type of safety syringe in common use is the Monoject® Safety Syringe (Figure 7-4). This syringe contains a protective sheath that can be used to protect the needle's sterility during transport for injection and be pulled forward and locked into place to provide a permanent needle shield for disposal following injection.

Notice that the Monoject Safety Syringe in Figure 7-4 contains two calibrated scales. The larger is the 3 mL metric scale with which you are already familiar. The smaller scale in the foreground, labeled "30 m," is the apothecary minim scale, which is rarely used by clinicians today.

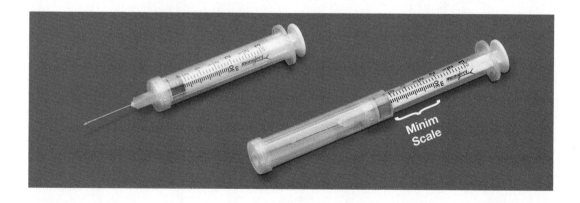

Figure 7-4 Kendall "Monoject® Safety Syringe." Monoject is a proprietary trademark of Sherwood Services AG, a Tyco Healthcare Group affiliate.

The minim scale has been a common source of injection dosage errors. If your clinical facility still uses syringes that contain the minim scale, be extremely careful not to confuse it with the metric calibrations.

TUBERCULIN (TB) SYRINGE

When very small dosages are required they are measured in special tuberculin (TB) **0.5 or 1 mL syringes calibrated in hundredths**. Originally designed for the small dosages required for tuberculin skin testing, these syringes are also widely used in a variety of sensitivity and allergy tests. Pediatric dosages frequently require measurement in hundredths, as does heparin, an anticoagulant drug.

Refer to the 0.5 mL TB syringe in Figure 7-5, and take a careful look at its metric calibrated tenth and hundredth scale. Notice that slightly longer calibrations identify zero, 0.05, 0.1, 0.15, 0.2, and so on through the 0.5 mL measure. Shorter hundredth calibrations lie between these measures. Each tenth mL, .1, .2, .3, .4, and .5 is numbered on this particular TB syringe. Take a moment to study the dosage measured by the arrow in Figure 7-5, which is 0.43 mL.

The closeness and small size of TB syringe calibrations mandate particular care and an unhurried approach in TB syringe dosage measurement

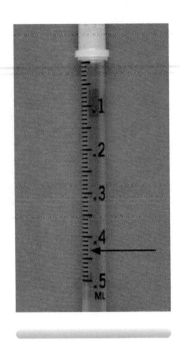

Figure 7-5

PROBLEM

Identify the measurements on the six tuberculin syringes shown below and on the next page.

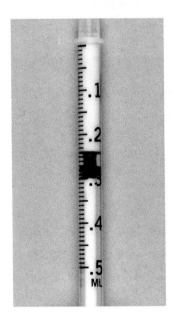

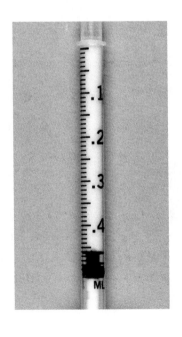

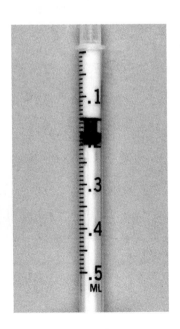

1. _____

2. _____

3. _____

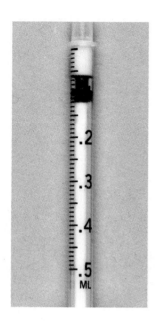

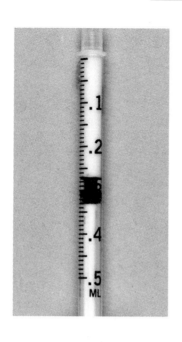

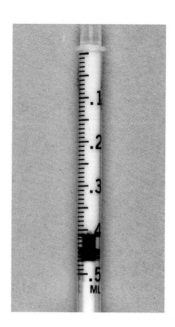

4. _____   5. _____   6. _____

Answers **1.** 0.24 mL **2.** 0.46 mL **3.** 0.15 mL **4.** 0.06 mL **5.** 0.27 mL **6.** 0.41 mL

PROBLEM

Draw an arrow or shade in the barrel to identify the dosages indicated on the following TB syringes. Have your instructor check your answers.

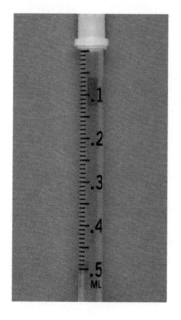

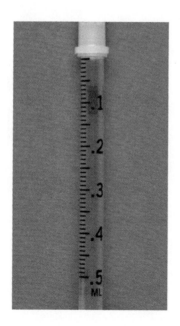

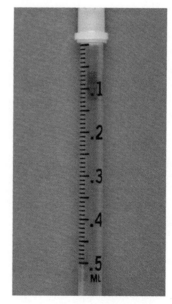

1. 0.28 mL   2. 0.32 mL   3. 0.45 mL

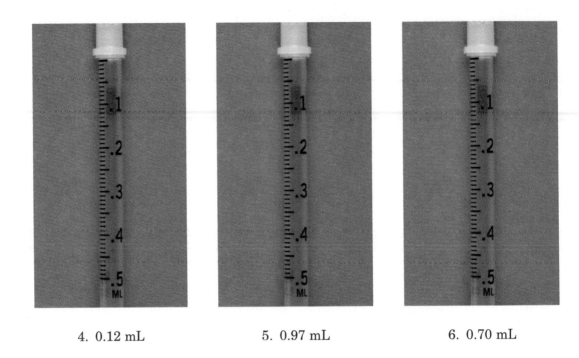

4. 0.12 mL   5. 0.97 mL   6. 0.70 mL

5, 6, 10, AND 12 mL/cc SYRINGES

When volumes larger than 3 mL/cc are required, a 5, 6, 10 or 12 mL/cc syringe may be used. Refer to Figure 7-6 and examine the calibrations between the numbered cc's to determine how these syringes are calibrated.

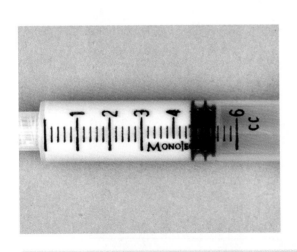
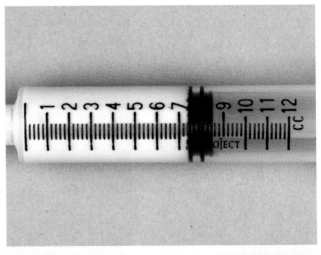

Figure 7-6

As you have discovered, the calibrations divide each cc of these syringes into **five**, so that **each shorter calibration actually measures two-tenths, 0.2 cc**. The 6 cc syringe on the left measures 4.6 cc, and the 12 cc syringe on the right measures 7.4 cc. These syringes are most often used to measure whole rather than fractional cc, but in your practice readings we will include a full range of measurements.

7

PROBLEM

What dosages are measured on the following syringes?

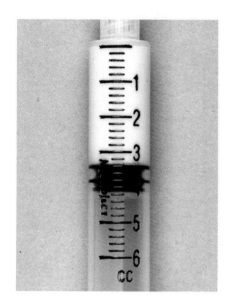

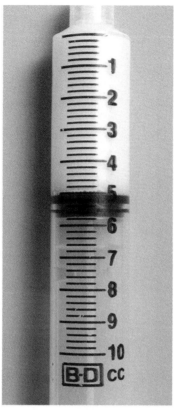

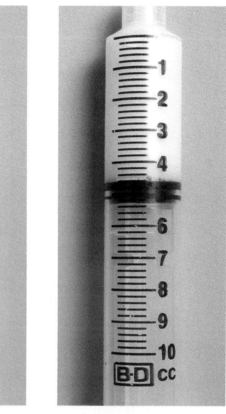

1. _____

2. _____

3. _____

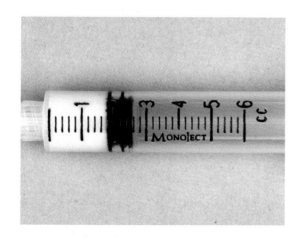

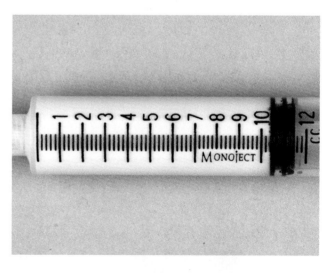

4. _____

5. _____

Answers **1.** 3.4 cc **2.** 5 cc **3.** 4.6 cc **4.** 1.8 cc **5.** 10.4 cc

PROBLEM

Measure the dosages indicated on the six syringes shown below and on the next page. Have an instructor check your accuracy.

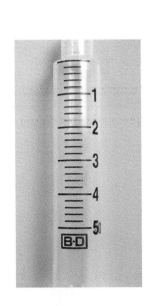

1. 1.4 cc

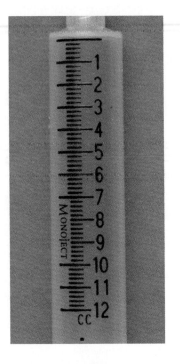

2. 3.2 cc

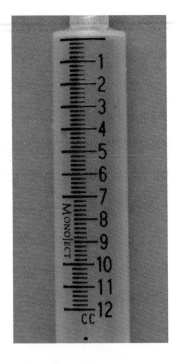

3. 6.8 cc

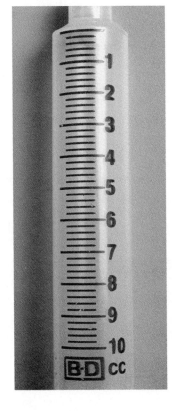

4. 9.4 cc

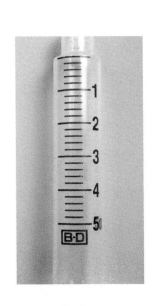

5. 3 cc

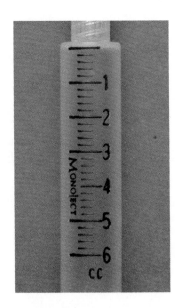

6. 5.6 cc

20 cc AND LARGER SYRINGES

Examine the 20 cc syringe in Figure 7-7 and determine how it is calibrated.

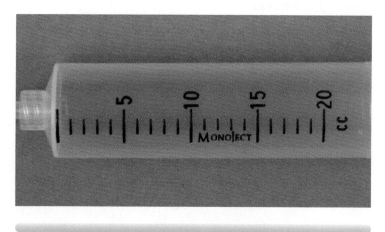

Figure 7-7

As you can see, this syringe is calibrated in **1 cc increments**, with longer calibrations identifying the 0, 5, 10, 15, and 20 cc volumes. Syringes with a 50 cc capacity are also calibrated in full cc measures. These syringes are used only for measurement of large volumes.

PROBLEM

What dosages are measured on the following syringes?

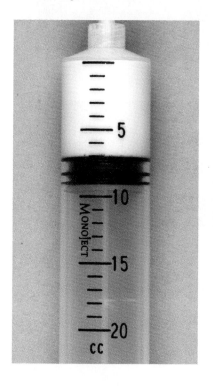

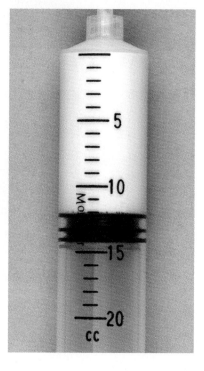

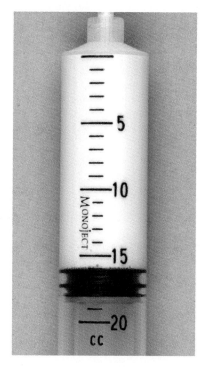

1. _____

2. _____

3. _____

Answers **1.** 7 cc **2.** 12 cc **3.** 16 cc

PROBLEM

Shade in or draw arrows on the three syringe barrels shown below to identify the volumes listed. Have your answers checked by your instructor.

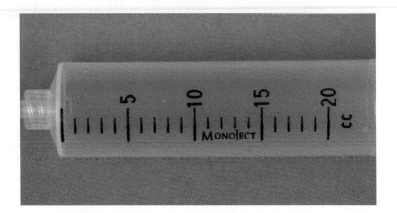

1. 11 cc

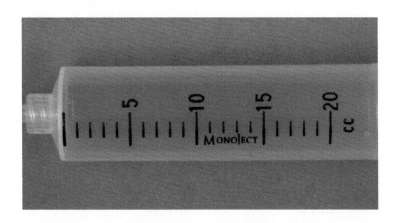

2. 18 cc

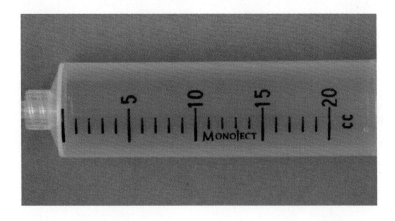

3. 9 cc

Summary

This concludes your introduction to syringe calibrations. The important points to remember from this chapter are:

- 3 mL/cc syringes are calibrated in tenths.

- TB syringes are calibrated in hundredths.

- If a syringe contains the apothecary minim, m, scale, care must be taken not to mistake it for metric, mL, calibrations.

- 5, 6, 10, and 12 mL/cc syringes are calibrated in fifths (two-tenths).

- Syringes larger than 12 mL/cc are calibrated in full mL/cc measures.

- The first long calibration on all syringes indicates zero.

- All syringe calibrations must be read from the top, or front, ring of the plunger's suction tip.

Summary Self-Test

Identify the dosages measured on the following syringes and cartridges.

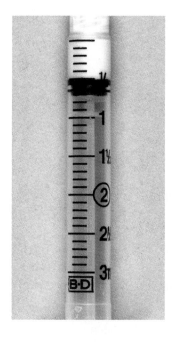

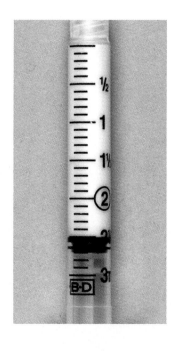

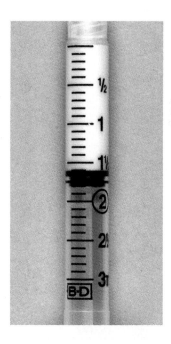

1. _____   2. _____   3. _____

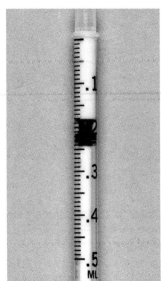

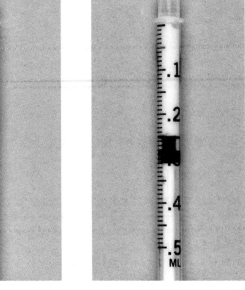

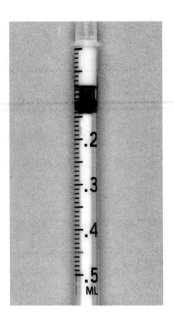

4. _____

5. _____

6. _____

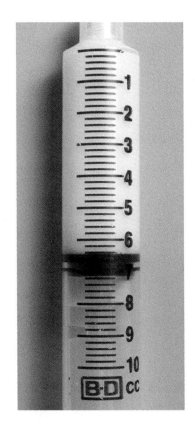

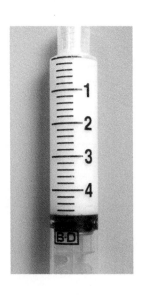

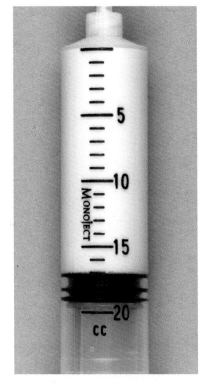

7. _____

8. _____

9. _____

Answers **1.** 0.5 mL **2.** 2.5 mL **3.** 1.6 mL **4.** 0.18 mL **5.** 0.25 mL **6.** 0.08 mL **7.** 6.4 cc **8.** 4.8 cc **9.** 17 cc

Draw arrows or shade the barrels on the following syringes/cartridges to measure the indicated dosages. Have your answers checked by your instructor.

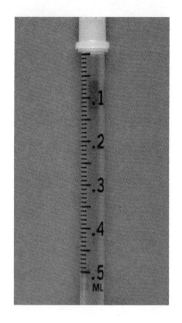

10. 0.52 mL

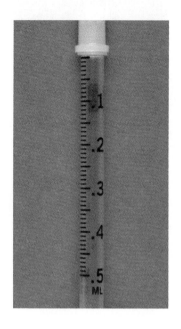

11. 0.31 mL

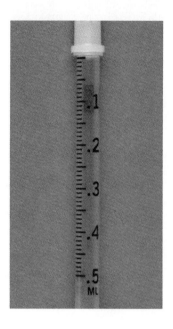

12. 0.94 mL

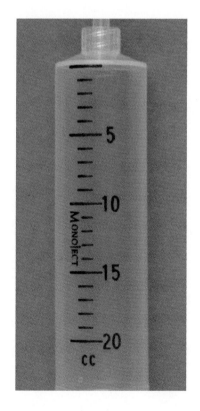

13. 13 cc

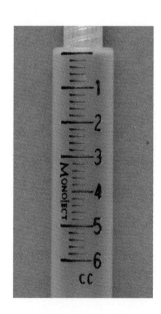

14. 1.2 cc

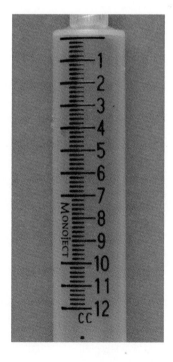

15. 7.6 cc

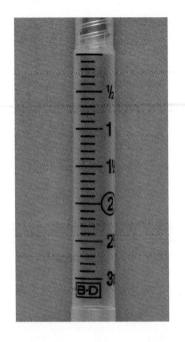 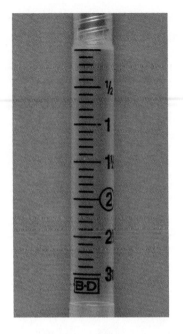 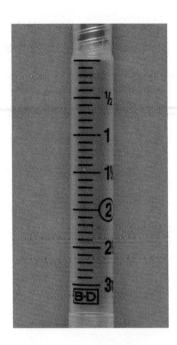

16. 1.7 mL   17. 2.2 mL   18. 0.9 mL

Reading Parenteral Medication Labels

Parenteral medications are administered by injection, the intravenous (IV), intramuscular (IM), and subcutaneous (s.c.) being the most frequently used routes. The labels of oral and parenteral solutions are very similar, but the size of the average parenteral dosage label is much smaller. Intramuscular and subcutaneous solutions in particular are manufactured so that the **average adult dosage will be contained in a volume of between 0.5 mL and 3 mL**. Volumes larger than 3 mL are difficult for a single injection site to absorb. The 0.5–3 mL volume can be used as a guideline for accuracy of calculations in IM and s.c. dosages. Excessively larger or smaller volumes would need to be questioned, and calculations rechecked.

Intravenous medication administration is usually a two-step procedure: the dosage is prepared first, then may be further diluted in IV fluids before administration. In this chapter we will be concerned only with the first step of IV drug preparation, which is accurate measurement of the prescribed dosage.

Parenteral drugs are packaged in a variety of single-use glass ampules, single- and multiple-use rubber-stoppered vials, and in premeasured syringes and cartridges. See Figure 8-1.

Objectives

The learner will:

1. read parenteral solution labels and identify dosage strengths

2. measure parenteral dosages in metric, milliequivalent, unit, percentage, and ratio strengths using 3 mL/cc, TB, 6, 12, and 20 mL/cc syringes

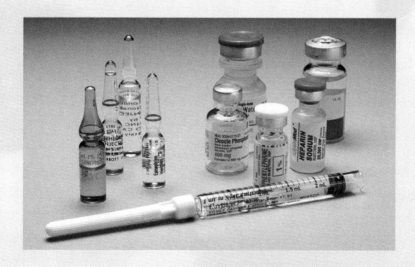

Figure 8-1 Ampules, vials, and a prefilled cartridge

READING METRIC/SI SOLUTION LABELS

We will begin by looking at parenteral solution labels on which the dosages are expressed in metric dosages.

EXAMPLE 1

Refer to the Vistaril® label in Figure 8-2. The immediate difference you will notice between this and oral solution labels is the **size**. Ampules and vials are small and their labels are small, which requires that they be **read with particular care**. The information, however, is similar to oral labels. Vistaril® is the trade name of the drug; hydroxyzine hydrochloride is the generic name. The dosage strength is 50 mg per mL (in the red rectangular area). The total vial contents are 10 mL (in black, upper left). Calculating dosages is not usually complicated. For example, if a dosage of Vistaril 100 mg were ordered you would give 2 mL; if 50 mg are ordered give 1 mL; for 25 mg give 0.5 mL.

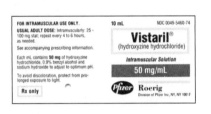

Figure 8-2

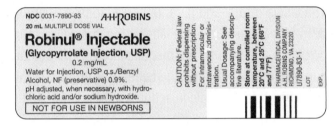

Figure 8-3

EXAMPLE 2

The Robinul® (glycopyrrolate) in Figure 8-3 has a dosage strength of 0.2 mg/mL. To prepare a 0.2 mg dosage you would draw up 1 mL; to prepare a 0.4 mg dosage you would draw up 2 mL; a 0.3 mg dosage would require 1.5 mL.

EXAMPLE 3

The fentanyl citrate solution in Figure 8-4 has a dosage strength of 250 mcg/5 mL. To prepare a 0.25 mg (250 mcg) dosage you will need 5 mL; for a 0.125 mg dosage, 2.5 mL. Once again these simple dosages can be calculated mentally.

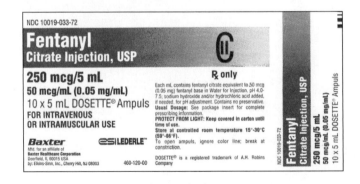

Figure 8-4

PROBLEM

Refer to the gentamicin label in Figure 8-5 and answer the following questions.

1. What is the total volume of this vial? _____

2. What is the dosage strength? _____

3. If gentamicin 80 mg were ordered, how many mL would this be? _____

4. If gentamicin 60 mg were ordered, how many mL would this be? _____

5. How many mL would you need to prepare a 20 mg dosage? _____

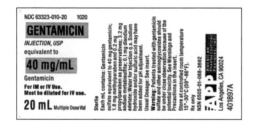

Figure 8-5

Answers **1.** 20 mL **2.** 40 mg/mL **3.** 2 mL **4.** 1.5 mL **5.** 0.5 mL

PERCENT (%) AND RATIO SOLUTION LABELS

Drugs labeled as **percentage solutions** often express the drug strength in **metric measures in addition to percentage strength**. Refer to the lidocaine label in Figure 8-6. Notice that this is a 2% solution, and the vial that contains it has a total volume of 50 mL. Also notice that the dosage strength is listed in metric measures: 20 mg/mL. Lidocaine is most often ordered in mg; for example, 20 mg would require 1 mL, 10 mg would require 0.5 mL, and 30 mg would require 1.5 mL. However, lidocaine is also used as a local anesthetic and a doctor may request, for example, that you prepare 3 mL of 2% lidocaine, which requires no calculation at all, but simply locating the correct percentage strength and drawing up 3 mL.

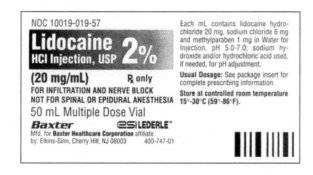

Figure 8-6

PROBLEM

Refer to the lidocaine label in Figure 8-7 and answer the following questions.

1. What is the percentage strength of this solution? _____

2. How many mL does the vial contain? _____

3. If you are asked to prepare 20 mL of solution, how much will you draw up in the syringe? _____

4. The dosage also appears on this label in metric measures. What is the metric dosage strength of this solution? _____

5. If you are asked to prepare 25 mg from this vial, what volume will you draw up? _____

Refer to the calcium gluconate label in Figure 8-8 and answer the following questions.

6. What is the percentage strength of this solution? _____

7. How many mL does this preparation contain? _____

8. What is the mEq dosage strength of this solution? _____

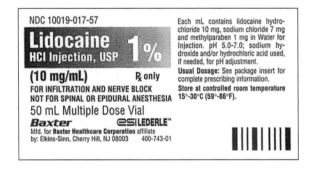

Figure 8-7

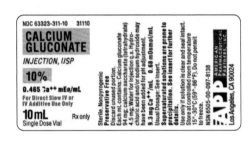

Figure 8-8

Answers **1.** 1% **2.** 50 mL **3.** 20 mL **4.** 10 mg/mL **5.** 2.5 mL **6.** 10% **7.** 10 mL **8.** 0.465 mEq/mL

Parenteral medications expressed in **ratio strengths** are not common, and **when they are ordered it will be by number of mL/cc.** Ratio labels may also contain dosages in metric weights.

PROBLEM

Refer to the epinephrine label in Figure 8-9 and answer the following questions.

1. What is the ratio strength of this solution? _____

2. What volume is this contained in? _____

3. What is the metric dosage strength of this solution? _____

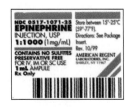

Answers **1.** 1:1000 **2.** 1 mL **3.** 1 mg/mL

Figure 8-9

SOLUTIONS MEASURED IN INTERNATIONAL UNITS (U)

A number of drugs are measured in **International Units**. The next labels will introduce you to several examples.

PROBLEM

Refer to the heparin label in Figure 8-10 and answer the following questions.

1. What is the total volume of this vial?

2. What is the dosage strength?

3. If a volume of 1.5 mL is prepared, how many units will this be?

4. How many mL will you need to prepare a dosage of 5500 U?

5. If 0.25 mL of this medication is prepared, what dosage will this be?

Refer to the oxytocin label in Figure 8-11 and answer the following questions.

6. What is the dosage strength of this solution?

7. If a dosage of 10 U is ordered, what volume will you need?

8. If a dosage of 5 U is ordered, what volume will you prepare?

Refer to the Bicillin® C-R label in Figure 8-12 and answer the following questions.

9. What is the dosage strength of this medication?

10. If 600,000 U was ordered, how many mL would this require?

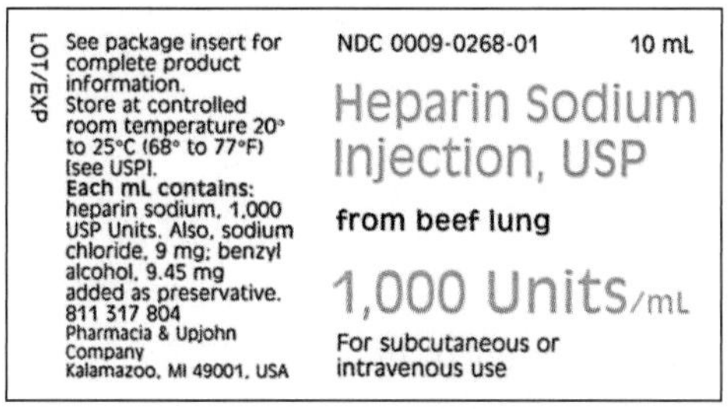

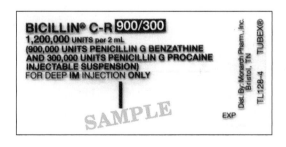

Figure 8-10

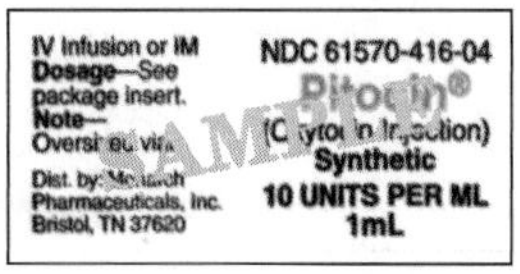

Figure 8-11

Figure 8-12

Answers **1.** 10 mL **2.** 1000 U/mL **3.** 1500 U **4.** 5.5 mL **5.** 250 U **6.** 10 U per mL **7.** 1 mL **8.** 0.5 mL **9.** 1,200,000 U/2 mL
10. 1 mL

SOLUTIONS MEASURED AS MILLIEQUIVALENTS (mEq)

The next four labels will introduce you to milliequivalent (mEq) dosages. Refer to the calcium gluconate label in Figure 8-13 and notice that this solution has a dosage strength of 0.465 mEq/mL. If a dosage of 0.465 mEq were ordered, you would draw up 1 mL in the syringe.

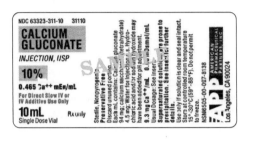

Figure 8-13

PROBLEM

Refer to the potassium chloride label in Figure 8-14 and answer the following questions.

1. What are the total dosage and volume of this vial? _____

2. What is the dosage in mEq per mL? _____

3. If you were asked to prepare 15 mEq for addition to an IV, what volume would you draw up? _____

Refer to the potassium chloride label in Figure 8-15 and answer the following dosage questions.

4. What is the strength of this solution in mEq per mL? _____

5. If you were asked to prepare 40 mEq for addition to an IV solution, what volume would you draw up in the syringe? _____

6. What volume would you need for a dosage of 20 mEq? _____

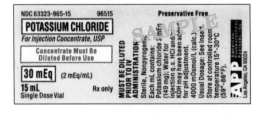

Figure 8-14

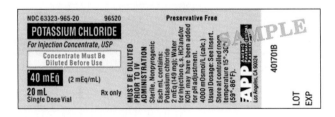

Figure 8-15

Refer to the sodium bicarbonate label in Figure 8-16. Notice that this solution lists the drug strength in mEq, percentage, and mg. Read the label very carefully and locate the answers to the following questions.

7. What is the dosage strength expressed in mEq/mL?   _____

8. What is the total volume of the vial, and how many mEq does this volume contain?   _____

9. What is the strength per mL expressed as mg?   _____

10. If you were asked to prepare 10 mL of an 8.4% sodium bicarbonate solution, what volume would you draw up in a syringe?   _____

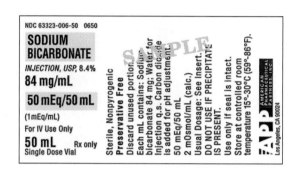

Figure 8-16

Answers   **1.** 30 mEq; 15 mL   **2.** 2 mEq/mL   **3.** 7.5 mL   **4.** 2 mEq/mL   **5.** 20 mL   **6.** 10 mL   **7.** 1 mEq/mL   **8.** 50 mL; 50 mEq
9. 84 mg/mL   **10.** 10 mL

Summary

This concludes the introduction to parenteral solution labels. The important points to remember from this chapter are:

- The most commonly used parenteral administration routes are IV, IM, and s.c.

- The labels of most parenteral solutions are quite small and must be read with particular care.

- The average IM and s.c. dosage will be contained in a volume of between 0.5 mL and 3 mL. This volume can be used as a guideline to accuracy of calculations.

- IV medication preparation is usually a two-step procedure: measurement of the dosage, then dilution according to manufacturers' recommendations or doctor's order.

- Parenteral drugs may be measured in metric, ratio, percentage, unit, or mEq dosages.

- If dosages are ordered by percentage or ratio strength, they are usually specified in mL/cc to be administered.

- Most IM and s.c. dosages are prepared using a 3 mL/cc syringe or 2 mL/cc tuberculin syringe.

Summary Self-Test

Read the parenteral drug labels provided to measure the following dosages. Then indicate on the syringe provided exactly how much solution you will draw up to obtain these dosages. Have your answers checked by your instructor to be sure you have measured the dosages correctly.

Dosage Ordered	mL/cc Needed
1. Depo-Provera® 0.4 g	_____

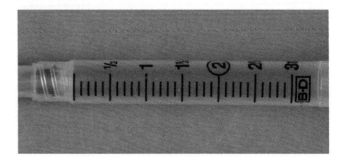

For IM use only.
See package insert for complete product information.
Shake vigorously immediately before each use.
Pharmacia & Upjohn Company
Kalamazoo, MI 49001, USA

NDC 0009-0626-01   2.5 mL Vial
Depo-Provera®
medroxyprogesterone acetate injectable suspension, USP
400 mg /mL

2. furosemide 10 mg   _____

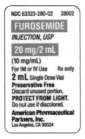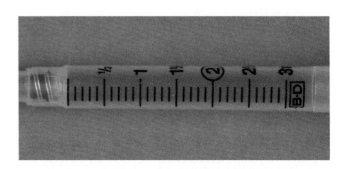

NDC 63323-280-02   28002
FUROSEMIDE
INJECTION, USP
20 mg/2 mL
(10 mg/mL)
For IM or IV Use   Rx only
2 mL Single Dose Vial
Preservative Free
Discard unused portion.
PROTECT FROM LIGHT.
Do not use if discolored.
American Pharmaceutical Partners, Inc.
Los Angeles, CA 90024

3. heparin 2500 U   _____

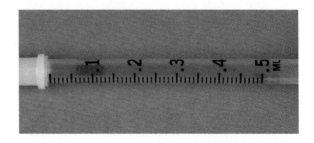

LOT/EXP   811340604

• See package insert for complete product information.
Store at controlled room temperature 20° to 25° C (68° to 77° F)
Isee USPI.
Each mL contains:
Heparin sodium, 5,000 USP Units. Also, sodium chloride, 9 mg; benzyl alcohol, 9.45 mg added as preservative.
Pharmacia & Upjohn Company
Kalamazoo, MI 49001, USA

NDC 0009-0291-01
10 mL
Heparin Sodium Injection, USP
from beef lung
5,000 Units/mL
For subcutaneous or intravenous use

Dosage Ordered	mL/cc Needed

4. Cleocin® 0.9 g   _____

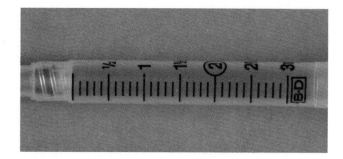

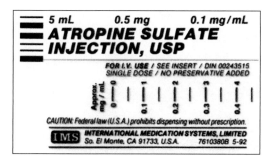

5. atropine 0.2 mg   _____

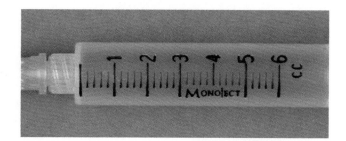

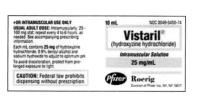

6. hydroxyzine HCl 25 mg   _____

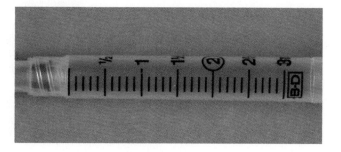

7. Robinul® 100 mcg   _____

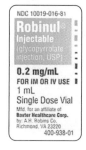

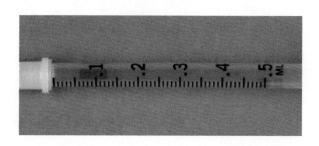

Dosage Ordered	mL/cc Needed
8. Tigan® 0.2 g	_____

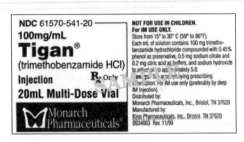

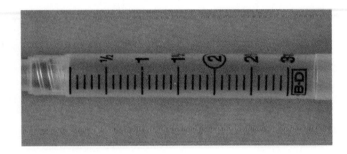

9. methotrexate 0.25 g _____

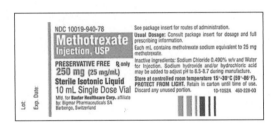

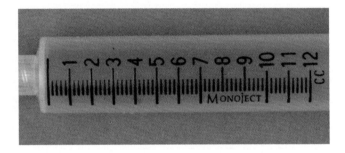

10. cyanocobalamin 0.1 mg _____

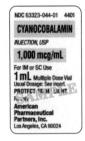

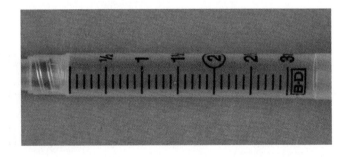

11. tobramycin 120 mg _____

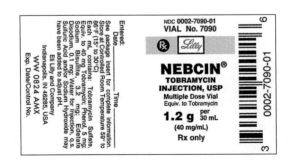

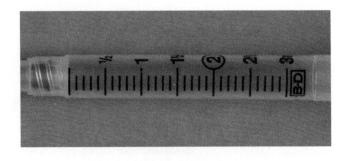

Dosage Ordered	**mL/cc Needed**

12. epinephrine 2 mg   _____

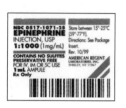

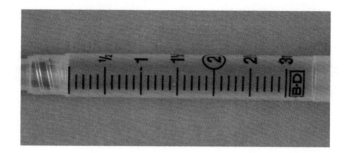

13. Zantac® 25 mg   _____

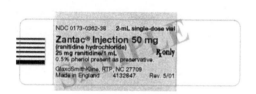

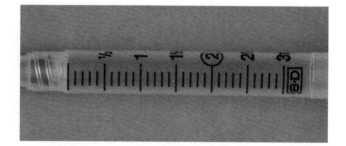

14. calcium gluconate 0.93 mEq   _____

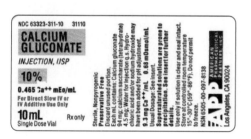

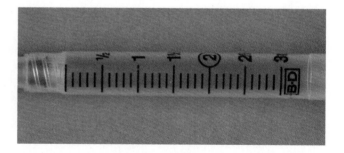

15. Haldol® 7.5 mg   _____

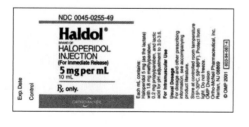

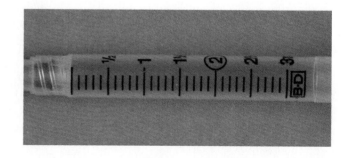

Dosage Ordered	**mL/cc Needed**
16. heparin 500 U	_____

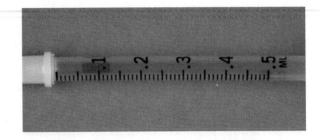

See package insert for complete product information.
Store at controlled room temperature 20° to 25°C (68° to 77°F) [see USP].
Each mL contains: heparin sodium, 1,000 USP Units. Also, sodium chloride, 9 mg; benzyl alcohol, 9.45 mg added as preservative.
811 317 804
Pharmacia & Upjohn Company
Kalamazoo, MI 49001, USA

NDC 0009-0268-01   10 mL

Heparin Sodium Injection, USP

from beef lung

1,000 Units/mL

For subcutaneous or intravenous use

17. benztropine mesylate 500 mcg _____

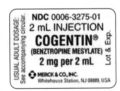

NDC 0006-3275-01
2 mL INJECTION
COGENTIN®
(BENZTROPINE MESYLATE)
2 mg per 2 mL
MERCK & CO., INC.
Whitehouse Station, NJ 08889, USA
USUAL ADULT DOSAGE: See accompanying circular.
Lot & Exp.

18. epinephrine 0.5 mg _____

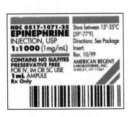

NDC 0517-1071-25
EPINEPHRINE
INJECTION, USP
1:1000 (1mg/mL)
CONTAINS NO SULFITES
PRESERVATIVE FREE
FOR IV, IM OR SC USE
1 mL AMPULE
Rx Only
Store between 15°-25°C (59°-77°F).
Directions: See Package Insert.
Rev. 10/99
AMERICAN REGENT LABORATORIES, INC.
SHIRLEY, NY 11967

19. medroxyprogesterone 1 g _____

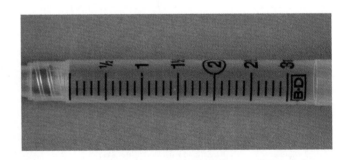

For IM use only.
See package insert for complete product information.
Shake vigorously immediately before each use.
Pharmacia & Upjohn Company
Kalamazoo, MI 49001, USA
812224806
NDC 0009-0626-01   2.5 mL Vial
Depo-Provera®
medroxyprogesterone acetate injectable suspension, USP
400 mg/mL

Dosage Ordered	mL/cc Needed

20. gentamicin 60 mg _____

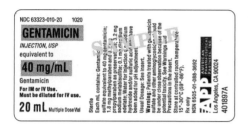 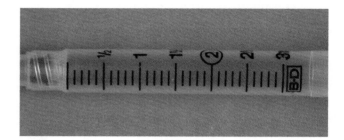

21. lidocaine HCl 50 mg _____

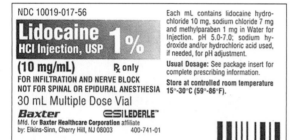 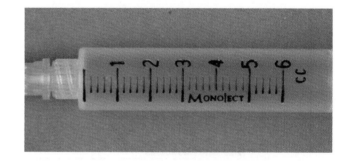

22. sodium chloride 40 mEq _____

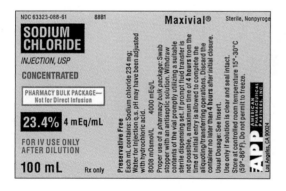 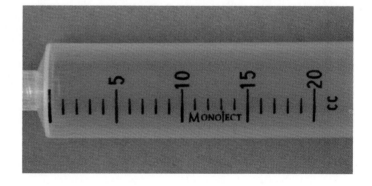

23. atropine 200 mcg _____

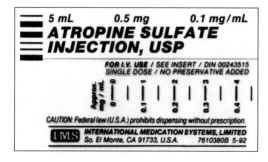 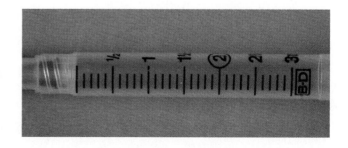

Dosage Ordered **mL/cc Needed**

24. meperidine 50 mg _____

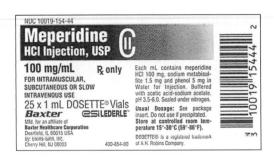

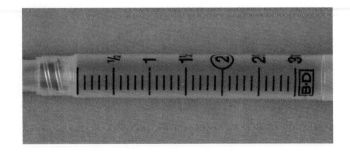

25. Tigan® 0.1 g _____

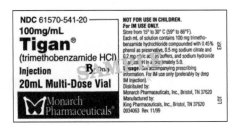

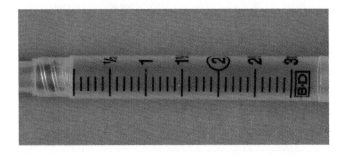

26. clindamycin 0.3 g _____

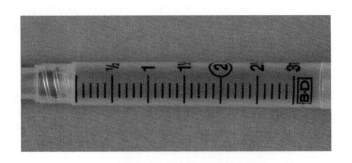

27. morphine sulfate 15 mg _____

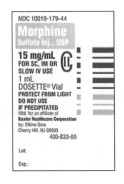

Dosage Ordered   **mL/cc Needed**

28. Terramycin® 0.1 g   _____

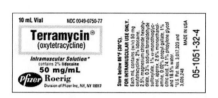

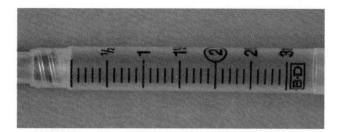

29. Thorazine® 50 mg   _____

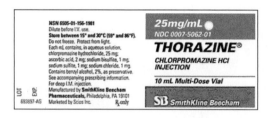

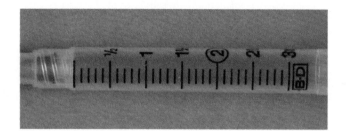

30. sodium chloride 20 mEq   _____

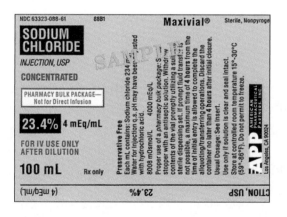

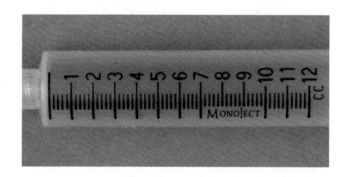

31. meperidine 50 mg   _____

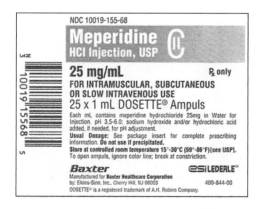

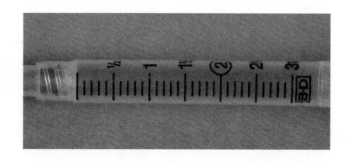

Dosage Ordered	**mL/cc Needed**
32. furosemide 30 mg	_____

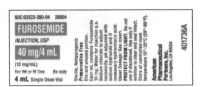

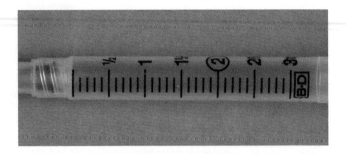

33. gentamicin 60 mg   _____

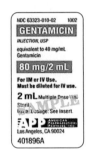

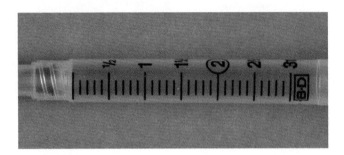

34. chlorpromazine HCl 50 mg   _____

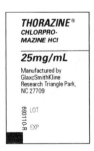

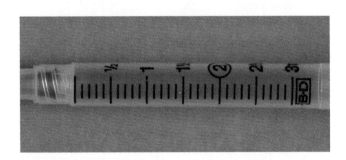

35. dexamethasone 2 mg   _____

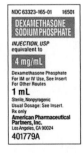

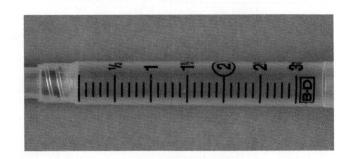

Dosage Ordered	mL/cc Needed

36. chlorpromazine 75 mg _____

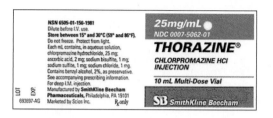

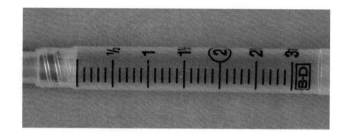

37. fentanyl 0.05 mg _____

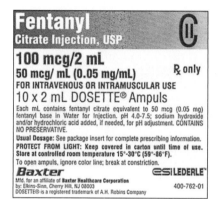

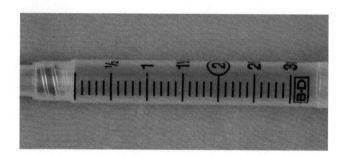

38. enalaprilat 1.25 mg _____

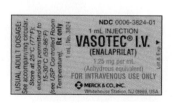

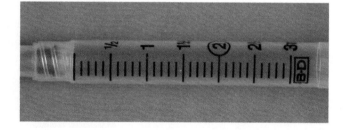

39. morphine 15 mg _____

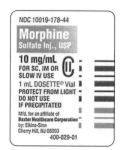

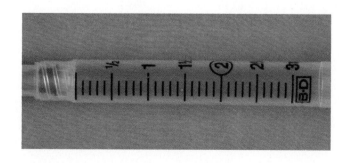

Dosage Ordered	**mL/cc Needed**

40. cyanocobalamin 1 mg　　　　　_____

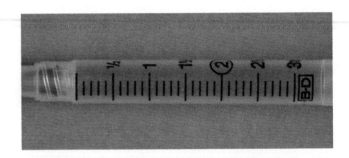

NDC 63323-044-01　4401

CYANOCOBALAMIN

INJECTION, USP

1,000 mcg/mL

For IM or SC Use

1 mL Multiple Dose Vial
Usual Dosage: See insert.
PROTECT FROM LIGHT.
Rx only
**American
Pharmaceutical
Partners, Inc.**
Los Angeles, CA 90024

41. Cogentin® 1000 mcg　　　　　_____

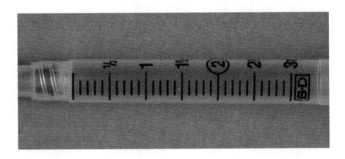

USUAL ADULT DOSAGE:
See accompanying circular.

NDC 0006-3275-01
2 mL INJECTION
COGENTIN®
(BENZTROPINE MESYLATE)
2 mg per 2 mL
♦ MERCK & CO., INC.
Whitehouse Station, NJ 08889, USA
Lot & Exp.

9113908

42. medroxyprogesterone acetate
1000 mg　　　　　_____

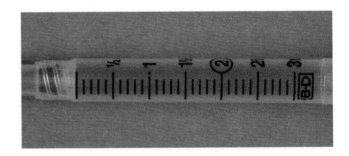

LOT / EXP
812224806

● For IM use only.
See package insert for
complete product
information.
Shake vigorously
immediately before
each use.
Pharmacia & Upjohn Company
Kalamazoo, MI 49001, USA

NDC 0009-0626-01　　2.5 mL Vial
Depo-Provera®
medroxyprogesterone
acetate injectable
suspension, USP
400 mg /mL

Answers

1. 1 mL	**9.** 10 mL	**18.** 0.5 mL	**27.** 1 mL	**36.** 3 mL
2. 1 mL	**10.** 1 mL	**19.** 2.5 mL	**28.** 2 mL	**37.** 1 mL
3. 0.5 mL	**11.** 3 mL	**20.** 1.5 mL	**29.** 2 mL	**38.** 1 mL
4. 6 mL	**12.** 2 mL	**21.** 5 mL	**30.** 5 mL	**39.** 1.5 mL
5. 2 mL	**13.** 1 mL	**22.** 10 mL	**31.** 2 mL	**40.** 1 mL
6. 1 mL	**14.** 2 mL	**23.** 2 mL	**32.** 3 mL	**41.** 1 mL
7. 0.5 mL	**15.** 1.5 mL	**24.** 0.5 mL	**33.** 1.5 mL	**42.** 2.5 mL
8. 2 mL	**16.** 0.5 mL	**25.** 1 mL	**34.** 2 mL	
	17. 0.5 mL	**26.** 2 mL	**35.** 0.5 mL	

Reconstitution of Powdered Drugs

Many drugs are shipped in powdered form because they **retain their potency only a short time in solution**. Reconstitution of these drugs is often the responsibility of hospital pharmacies, but this does not eliminate the need to know how to read and follow reconstitution directions, and how to label drugs with an expiration date and time once they have been reconstituted. The drug label, or instructional package insert, will give specific directions for reconstitution of the drug. Reading these requires care, and this chapter will take you step by step through the entire process.

RECONSTITUTION OF A SINGLE STRENGTH SOLUTION

Let's start with the simplest type of reconstitution instructions for a single strength solution. Examine the label for the oxacillin 2 g vial in Figure 9-1.

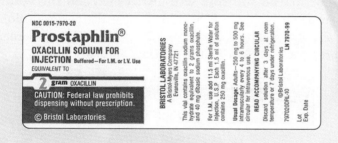

Figure 9-1

The first step in reconstitution is to locate the directions. They are on this oxacillin label at the right side, printed sideways. Notice that the instructions read **"For I.M. use add 11.5 mL Sterile Water for Injection."** Water, or any other solution specified for reconstitution, is called the **diluent**. The **type of diluent** specified will be **different for different drugs**. The **volume of diluent will also vary**. So reading the label carefully to identify both the type and the volume of diluent to be used is mandatory.

Objectives

The learner will:

1. prepare solutions from powdered drugs using directions printed on vial labels

2. prepare solutions from powdered drugs using drug literature or inserts

3. determine expiration dates and times for reconstituted drugs

4. calculate simple dosages from reconstituted drugs

Once the volume and type of diluent are identified, which for this medication is 11.5 mL Sterile Water, the next step is to use a **sterile syringe and aseptic technique** to draw it up. Inject it slowly into the vial **above the medication level**, because air bubbles can distort some drug dosages. If the diluent volume is large, as in this case, be aware that the syringe plunger will be forced out to expel air and re-equalize the internal vial pressure as you inject. Very large volumes of diluent may have to be injected in divided amounts to keep the internal vial pressure equalized. When all the diluent has been injected, the vial must be rotated and upended until all the medication has been dissolved. **Do not shake**, as this also can add air bubbles to the medication.

After reconstitution, locate the information that relates to the **length of time the reconstituted solution may be stored** and **how it must be stored**. The oxacillin label reads "Discard solution after **3 days at room temperature or 7 days under refrigeration**."

 The person who reconstitutes a drug is responsible for labeling it with the date and time of expiration and with her/his name or initials.

Let's assume that this oxacillin solution was **mixed at 2 p.m. on January 3rd**. What expiration information would you print on the vial if it is **stored in the refrigerator**? "**Exp (expires) Jan 10th 2 p.m.**," which is **7 days** from the time mixed. If it is stored at **room temperature**, it must be labeled "**Exp Jan 6th 2 p.m.**," which is **3 days**.

Once the solution is prepared and labeled with your name or initials and the expiration date, you can concentrate on the **dosage strength**. Notice that the label indicates that "**each 1.5 mL of solution contains 250 mg oxacillin.**" There is a total dosage of 2 g in this vial, or eight dosages of 250 mg at 1.5 mL each, for a total volume of 12 mL. You added only 11.5 mL to the vial to reconstitute the drug, and the reason for the increased volume is that the powder itself occupies space. **The total volume of the prepared solution will always exceed the volume of the diluent you add**, because it consists of the diluent plus the powder volume. Refer to the dosage strength again, which is 250 mg per 1.5 mL. If a 250 mg dosage is ordered, you would prepare 1.5 mL; for a 0.5 g dosage, prepare 3 mL.

PROBLEM

Another medication prepared in powdered form is Nebcin® (tobramycin). Refer to the label in Figure 9-2 and answer the following questions about this medication.

1. How much diluent is added to the vial for reconstitution? _____

2. What type of diluent is used? _____

3. What is the dosage strength per mL of the prepared solution? _____

4. If an order is for 80 mg, what volume must you give? _____

5. What is the dosage strength of the total vial? _____

6. How long will the drug retain its potency at room temperature? _____

7. If the drug is reconstituted at 0800 on Oct. 3rd and stored at room temperature, what expiration date will you print on the label? _____

8. How long will the solution retain its potency if refrigerated? _____

9. What expiration date will you print on the label if the solution is reconstituted on June 10th at 9 a.m. and stored under refrigeration? _____

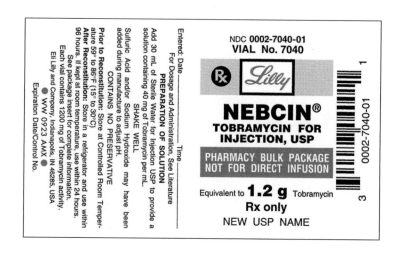

Figure 9-2

PROBLEM

Read the Solu-Medrol® label in Figure 9-3 and answer the following questions.

1. What volume of diluent must be used to reconstitute this vial? _____

2. What kind of diluent is specified? _____

3. How long will the reconstituted solution retain its potency at room temperature? _____

4. If the Solu-Medrol® is reconstituted at 11 a.m. Feb 26th, what expiration date and time will you print on the label? _____

5. What else will you print on the label? _____

6. What will be the dosage strength per mL of this reconstituted solution? _____

7. If a dosage of 125 mg of methylprednisolone is ordered, how much solution will you prepare? _____

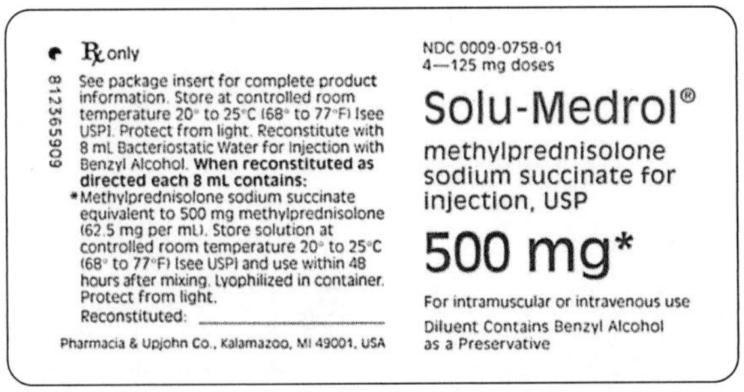

℞ only
See package insert for complete product information. Store at controlled room temperature 20° to 25°C (68° to 77°F) [see USP]. Protect from light. Reconstitute with 8 mL Bacteriostatic Water for Injection with Benzyl Alcohol. **When reconstituted as directed each 8 mL contains:**
*Methylprednisolone sodium succinate equivalent to 500 mg methylprednisolone (62.5 mg per mL). Store solution at controlled room temperature 20° to 25°C (68° to 77°F) [see USP] and use within 48 hours after mixing. Lyophilized in container. Protect from light.
Reconstituted: _____
Pharmacia & Upjohn Co., Kalamazoo, MI 49001, USA

8123565909

NDC 0009-0758-01
4—125 mg doses

Solu-Medrol®
methylprednisolone sodium succinate for injection, USP

500 mg*

For intramuscular or intravenous use
Diluent Contains Benzyl Alcohol as a Preservative

Figure 9-3

Answers   **1.** 8 mL   **2.** Bacteriostatic Water with Benzyl Alcohol   **3.** 48 hours   **4.** Exp 11 a.m. Feb 28th   **5.** your name or initials   **6.** 62.5 mg per mL   **7.** 2 mL

RECONSTITUTION OF MULTIPLE STRENGTH SOLUTIONS

Some powdered drugs offer a choice of dosage strengths. When this is the case you must choose the strength most appropriate for the dosage ordered. For example, refer to the penicillin label in Figure 9-4. The dosage strengths that can be obtained are listed on the right.

Notice that three dosage strengths are listed: 250,000 U, 500,000 U, and 1,000,000 U per mL. If the dosage ordered is 500,000 U, the most appropriate strength to mix would be 500,000 U per mL. Read across from this strength, and determine how much diluent must be added to obtain it. The answer is 33 mL. If the dosage ordered is 1,000,000 U, what would be the most appropriate strength to prepare, and how much diluent would this require? the answer is 1,000,000 U/mL, and 11.5 mL.

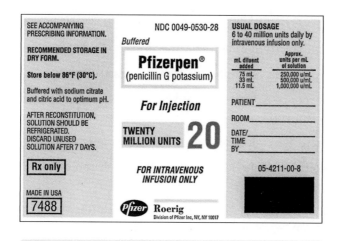

Figure 9-4

Notice that this label does not tell you what type of diluent to use. **When information is missing from the label, look for it on the package information insert that comes with the drug**. Don't start guessing. All the information you need is in print somewhere; just take your time and locate it.

 A multiple strength solution such as this one requires that you add one additional piece of information to the label after you reconstitute it: the dosage strength you have just mixed.

PROBLEM

Refer to the Pfizerpen® label in Figure 9-4 to answer these additional questions.

1. If you add 75 mL of diluent to prepare a solution of penicillin, what dosage strength will you print on the label? _____

2. Does this prepared solution require refrigeration? _____

3. If you reconstitute it on June 1st at 2 p.m., what expiration time and date will you print on the label? _____

4. What is the total dosage strength of this vial? _____

Refer to the Tazicef® label in Figure 9-5 and answer the following questions.

5. What is the total strength of ceftazidime in this vial? _____

6. What kind of diluent is recommended for reconstitution? _____

7. If you wish to prepare a 1 g/10 mL strength, how much diluent will you add to the vial? _____

8. How much diluent will you add for a 1 g/5 mL strength? _____

9. What is the expiration time for this drug if it is stored at room temperature? _____

10. If you reconstitute this drug at 0915 on April 17th and store it under refrigeration, what will you print on the label? _____

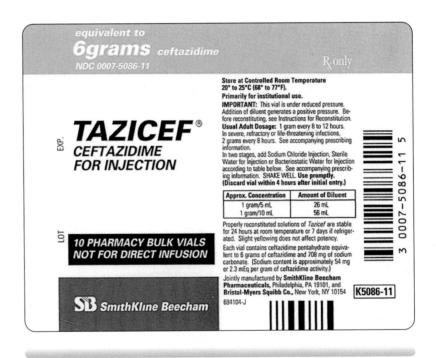

Figure 9-5

RECONSTITUTION FROM PACKAGE INSERT DIRECTIONS

If the label does not contain reconstitution directions, you must obtain these from the information insert that accompanies the vial. The drug Vancocin® HCl falls into this category. Refer to the Vancocin label and its reconstitution directions in Figures 9-6 and 9-7.

PROBLEM

Refer to the Vancocin HCI label and insert in Figures 9-6 and 9-7 and answer the following questions.

1. How much diluent must be added to this 500 mg vial for IV reconstitution?   _____

2. What kind of diluent must be used?   _____

3. If you reconstitute the drug at 3 p.m. on May 4th and the solution is refrigerated, what expiration information will you print on the label?   _____

4. What is the concentration per mL of this solution?   _____

5. What is the total dosage of the vial?   _____

6. What additional minimum dilution will be required for IV administration?   _____

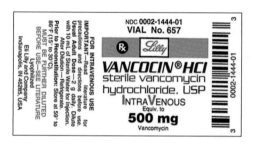

PREPARATION AND STABILITY

At the time of use, reconstitute by adding either 10 mL of Sterile Water for Injection to the 500-mg vial or 20 mL of Sterile Water for Injection to the 1-g vial of dry, sterile vancomycin powder. Vials reconstituted in this manner will give a solution of 50 mg/mL. FURTHER DILUTION IS REQUIRED.

After reconstitution, the vials may be stored in a refrigerator for 14 days without significant loss of potency. Reconstituted solutions containing 500 mg of vancomycin must be diluted with at least 100 mL of diluent. Reconstituted solutions containing 1 g of vancomycin must be diluted with at least 200 mL of diluent. The desired dose, diluted in this manner, should be administered by intermittent intravenous infusion over a period of at least 60 minutes.

Figure 9-6   Figure 9-7

Answers   **1.** 10 mL   **2.** Sterile Water   **3.** Exp 3 p.m. May 28th   **4.** 50 mg/mL   **5.** 500 mg   **6.** 100 mL

Summary

This concludes the chapter on reconstitution of powdered drugs. The important points to remember from this chapter are:

- If the vial label does not contain reconstitution directions, these may be found on the vial package insert.

- The type and amount of diluent to be used for reconstitution must be exactly as specified in the instructions.

- If directions ar given for both IM and IV reconstitution, be careful to read the correct set for the solution you are preparing.

- The person who reconstitutes a powdered drug must initial the vial and print the expiration time and date on the label unless all the drug is used immediately.

- If a multiple strength solution is prepared, the strength of the reconstituted drug also must be printed on the label.

Summary Self-Test

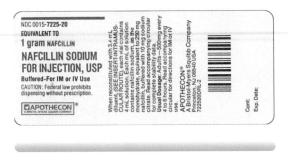

Figure 9-8

Refer to the nafcillin sodium label in Figure 9-8 and answer the following questions about reconstitution.

1. What is the total dosage of this vial? _____

2. What volume of diluent must be used for reconstitution? _____

3. What will be the dosage strength of 1 mL of reconstituted solution? _____

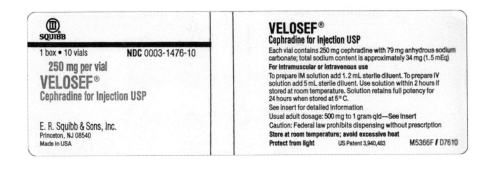

Figure 9-9

Refer to the Velosef® label in Figure 9-9 and answer the following questions.

4. What is the dosage strength of this vial? _____

5. What volume of diluent must you add to prepare the solution for IM use? _____

6. For IV use? _____

7. How long will this reconstituted cephradine retain its potency at room temperature? _____

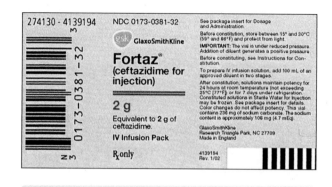

Figure 9-10

Refer to the Fortaz® label in Figure 9-10 and answer the following questions.

8. How much diluent is used to reconstitute this IV solution? _____

9. What is the total strength of the vial? _____

10. How long will the solution retain its potency at room temperature? _____

11. If refrigerated? _____

SQUIBB® MARSAM™

1 box • 10 vials   NDC 0003-0668-05

**5,000,000 units per vial
PENICILLIN G SODIUM
for INJECTION USP**

Caution: Federal law prohibits
dispensing without prescription

PENICILLIN G SODIUM for INJECTION USP

Each vial provides 5,000,000 units penicillin g sodium with approx.
140 mg citrate buffer (composed of sodium citrate and not more than
4.6 mg citric acid). One million units penicillin contains approx. 2.0 mEq
sodium.
Sterile • For intramuscular or intravenous drip use
Usual dosage: See insert
PREPARATION OF SOLUTION: Add 23 mL, 18 mL, 8 mL, or 3 mL diluent to
provide 200,000 u, 250,000 u, 500,000 u, or 1,000,000 u per mL,
respectively.
Sterile solution may be kept in refrigerator 1 week without significant
loss of potency.
Store at room temperature prior to constitution
© 1986 Squibb-Marsam, Inc.
For information contact:
Squibb-Marsam, Inc., Cherry Hill, NJ 08034
Made by Glaxochem, Ltd., Greenford, Middlesex, England.
Filled in Italy by Squibb S.p.A. Dist. by
E. R. Squibb & Sons, Inc., Princeton, NJ 08540   C5277 / 66805

Figure 9-11

Refer to the Penicillin G Sodium label in Figure 9-11 and answer the following questions.

12. How much diluent must be added to obtain a 250,000 U/mL concentration? _____

13. To obtain a 1,000,000 U/mL concentration? _____

14. The type of diluent is not specified. Where would you find this information? _____

15. If this solution is reconstituted at 8:10 p.m. Nov 30th, and stored under refrigeration, what expiration information will you print on the label? _____

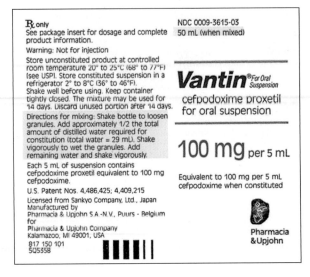

Figure 9-12

Refer to the Vantin® Oral Suspension label in Figure 9-12 and answer the following questions.

16. How much diluent will be required to reconstitute this medication? _____

17. What type of diluent is listed for reconstitution? _____

18. How is this diluent to be added? _____

19. What is the reconstituted dosage strength? _____

20. How long will the reconstituted Vantin solution retain its potency? _____

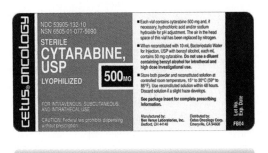

Figure 9-13

Refer to the cytarabine label in Figure 9-13 and answer the following questions.

21. What is the total strength of this medication? _____

22. What diluent must be used for reconstitution? _____

23. How much? _____

24. There is a special precaution on the label about a diluent not to
be used. What is it? _____

25. How long does the reconstituted cytarabine solution retain its potency at room temperature?   _____

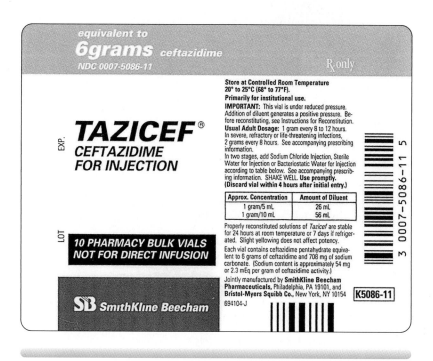

Figure 9-14

Refer to the Tazicef® label in Figure 9-14 and answer the following questions for preparation of a 1 g/5 mL solution.

26. What type of diluent is recommended for IV reconstitution?   _____

27. How much diluent must be added?   _____

28. If this drug is reconstituted at 0200 on March 23rd and stored at room temperature, what expiration information will you print on the label?   _____

29. If it is stored under refrigeration, what date and time will you print?   _____

30. What is the total dosage strength of this vial of ceftazidime?   _____

31. What must you print on the label in addition to the expiration date?   _____

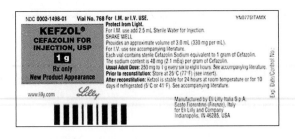

Figure 9-15

Refer to the Kefzol® label in Figure 9-15 and answer the following questions.

32. What is the generic name for Kefzol?

33. What is the total dosage strength of this vial? _____

34. What volume of diluent must be added for IM use? _____

35. What type of diluent is specified? _____

36. What will the reconstituted volume of medication be? _____

37. Why is this volume larger than the amount of diluent added? _____

38. What is the reconstituted dosage strength? _____

39. What volume of solution will be required for a dosage of cefazolin 660 mg? _____

40. How long will Kefzol retain its potency at room temperature? _____

41. If you reconstitute the solution at 2.44 p.m. on Saturday, August 17th and refrigerate it, what must you print on the label? _____

42. What else must you print on the label? _____

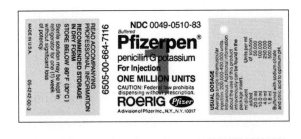

Figure 9-16

Refer to the penicillin G potassium label in Figure 9-16 and answer the following questions.

43. What is the total dosage strength of this vial? _____

44. How much diluent must be added to prepare a 100,000 U/mL strength? _____

45. How much diluent must be added to prepare a 500,000 U/mL strength?   _____

46. How much diluent must be added to prepare a 50,000 U/mL strength?   _____

47. This label has no information on the type of diluent to use. Where will you find this?   _____

48. Penicillin is a suspension that tends to trap air bubbles, which could distort the dosage. List two critical steps in the reconstitution process designed to prevent air bubbles.   _____

49. How must this solution be stored?   _____

50. If reconstituted at 1:10 a.m. on December 18th, what must you print on the label?   _____

51. What else must you print on the label?   _____

52. Why print?   _____

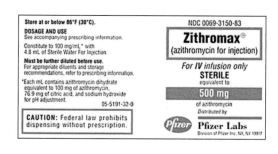

Figure 9-17

Refer to the Zithromax® label in Figure 9-17 and answer the following questions.

53. What is the generic name for Zithromax®?   _____

54. What is the dosage strength of this vial?   _____

55. What diluent is specified for reconstitution?   _____

56. How much diluent is required?   _____

57. What is the reconstituted dosage strength?   _____

Answers
1. 1 g
2. 3.4 mL
3. 250 mg
4. 250 mg
5. 1.2 mL
6. 5 mL
7. 2 hours
8. 100 mL
9. 2 g
10. 24 hours
11. 7 days
12. 18 mL
13. 3 mL
14. package insert information sheet
15. Exp 8:10 p.m. Dec 7th
16. 29 mL
17. distilled water
18. add half and shake, add remainder and shake
19. 100 mg per 5 mL
20. 14 days
21. 500 mg
22. Bacteriostatic Water with benzyl alcohol
23. 10 mL
24. no diluents containing benzyl alcohol if for intrathecal or high investigational use
25. 48 hours
26. Sodium Chloride; Sterile Water; Bacteriostatic Water
27. 26 mL, in 2 stages
28. Exp 0200 March 24th
29. Exp 0200 March 30th
30. 6 grams
31. your name or initials
32. cefazolin
33. 1 g
34. 2.5 mL
35. Sterile Water
36. 3 ml
37. drug also occupies space
38. 330 mg/mL
39. 2 mL
40. 24 hours
41. Exp 2:44 p.m. August 27th
42. your name or initials
43. one million units
44. 10 mL
45. 1.8 mL
46. 20 mL
47. package insert
48. inject diluent above the medication; rotate and upend the vial to mix rather than shake
49. refrigerate
50. Exp 1:10 a.m. December 25th
51. your name or initials
52. handwriting may be difficult to read
53. azithromycin
54. 500 mg
55. Sterile Water for Injection
56. 4.8 mL
57. 100 mg/mL

Measuring Insulin Dosages

Insulin dosages are measured in units (U), with the 100 U per mL/cc (U-100) strength being used almost exclusively. Dosages are measured using **special insulin syringes** that are **calibrated to match the dosage strength of insulin being used**. For example U-100 syringes are used to prepare U-100 strength dosages. This chapter will show you a variety of U-100 syringes to illustrate how to measure dosages. However, let's begin with an introduction to the types of insulin in use.

TYPES OF INSULIN

Insulins are classified by **origin** (animal or human) and by **action** (rapid, intermediate, or long acting). The origin or source of insulins is printed on every label, and it is important to know where to locate this information as physicians may specify origin when writing insulin orders. Notice the small print on the Regular insulin label in Figure 10-1, which identifies its animal (pork) origin, and the Regular insulin label in Figure 10-2, which identifies its human (recombinant DNA) origin. Also notice how similar these labels are, making careful reading of insulin labels essential for correct identification. Insulins prepared in multiple use vials are routinely labeled with each patient's name. However, this does not eliminate the need to read the label

Objectives

The learner will:

1. distinguish between insulins of animal and human origin

2. discuss the difference between rapid-, intermediate-, and long-acting insulins

3. read insulin labels to identify origin and type

4. read calibrations on U-100 insulin syringes

5. measure single insulin dosages

6. measure combined insulin dosages

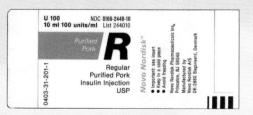

Figure 10-1   Figure 10-2

carefully prior to dosage preparation. Next look at the labels in Figures 10-3 and 10-4. Both of these insulins are of human origin and use the trade name Humulin®. Then notice the initials that follow the trade name: L (Lente®) and U (Ultralente®). These identify the type of insulin by action time. There are three basic action times of insulins. Regular and Semilente® have a rapid action, beginning in ½ hr, peaking in 2½–5 hr, and ending in 8 hr. In the intermediate range are the Lente® and NPH insulins, beginning in 1½–2½ hr, peaking in 4–15 hr, and ending in 16–24 hr. Among the long-acting insulins are the Ultralente®, whose action begins in 4 hr, peaks in 10–30 hr, and ends in 36 hr.

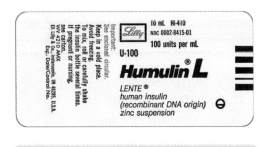

Figure 10-3

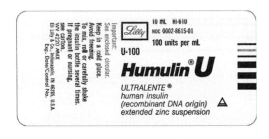

Figure 10-4

Combined rapid and medium action insulins are also in use. Two examples are the 70/30 illustrated in Figure 10-5, and the 50/50 combination illustrated in Figure 10–6.

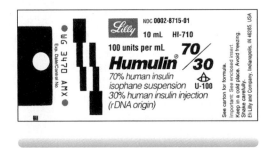

Figure 10-5

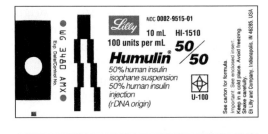

Figure 10-6

PROBLEM

Identify the type and origin of each of the insulins from the following six labels (Figures 10-7 through 10-12).

Type of Insulin	Origin
1. _____	_____
2. _____	_____
3. _____	_____
4. _____	_____
5. _____	_____
6. _____	_____

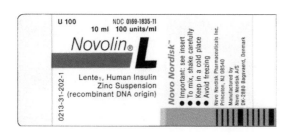

1.   Figure 10-7

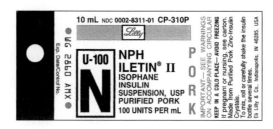

2.   Figure 10-8

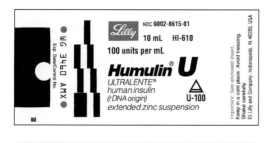

3.   Figure 10-9

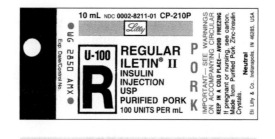

4.   Figure 10-10

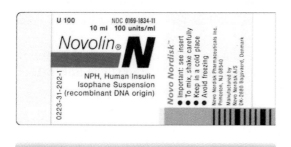

5.   Figure 10-11

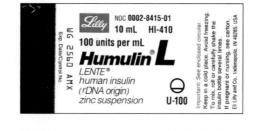

6.   Figure 10-12

Answers   **1.** Lente; human   **2.** NPH; pork   **3.** Ultralente; human   **4.** Regular; pork   **5.** NPH; human   **6.** Lente; human

U-100 INSULIN AND SYRINGES

Refer back to each of the labels you have just read and you will notice that **all have a U-100 strength** (100 U per mL/cc).

 To prepare U-100 insulin dosages you must use a U-100 calibrated syringe.

Refer to the U-100 syringe pictured in Figure 10-13 and you will notice that it is very small. In order to read the calibrations and number of units it is necessary to **rotate insulin syringes from side to side**. To make it possible for you to practice measuring insulin dosages in this chapter, the syringe calibrations have been flattened out. These are the identical calibrations that appear on the syringes, so your dosage practice will be authentic.

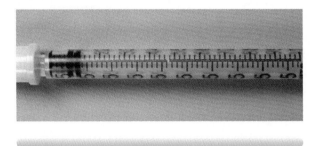

Figure 10-13

The designation U-100 means that the insulin dosage strength is 100 U per mL/cc. Insulin syringes are calibrated to this 100 U/mL/cc dosage, but they do not all have a 1 mL/cc capacity. There are actually several sizes (capacities) of U-100 syringes in use. The easiest of these to read and use are the Lo-Dose® syringes.

LO-DOSE SYRINGES

Lo-Dose® syringes have a capacity of 30 or 50 U. Lo-Dose insulin syringes do exactly what their name implies: they **measure low dosages, but on an enlarged and easier to read scale**. This larger scale is an important safety feature for diabetic patients, who frequently have vision problems, as well as for ease of use by medical personnel.

Refer to the calibrations for 50 U (½ cc) Lo-Dose capacity syringes in the problems that follow. Notice that **each calibration measures 1 U**, and that **each 5 U increment is numbered**.

PROBLEM

Refer to the syringe calibrations for the 50 U Lo-Dose syringes below and identify the dosages indicated by the shaded areas.

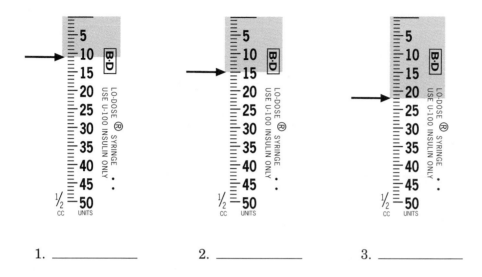

1. _____   2. _____   3. _____

Answers   **1.** 11 U   **2.** 15 U   **3.** 22 U

PROBLEM

Use the U-100 Lo-Dose® calibrations below to shade in the following dosages. Have your instructor check your accuracy.

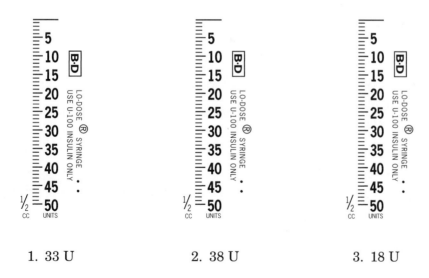

1. 33 U   2. 38 U   3. 18 U

1 cc CAPACITY SYRINGES

There are two 1 mL/cc U-100 insulin syringes in common use. Refer to the first of these syringe calibrations below. Notice the 100 U capacity, and that, in contrast to the Lo-Dose syringes, only **each 10 U increment is numbered**: 10, 20, 30, etc. Next notice the number of calibrations in each 10 U increment, which his five, indicating that **this syringe is calibrated in 2 U increments. Odd numbered units cannot be measured accurately using this syringe**.

PROBLEM

Identify the dosages indicated by the shading on the 1 cc U-100 syringes.

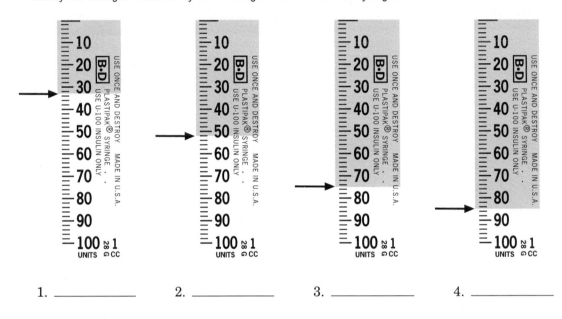

1. _____   2. _____   3. _____   4. _____

Answers   **1.** 32 U   **2.** 52 U   **3.** 74 U   **4.** 84 U

PROBLEM

Shade in the following syringes to measure the dosages indicated. Have your instructor check your accuracy.

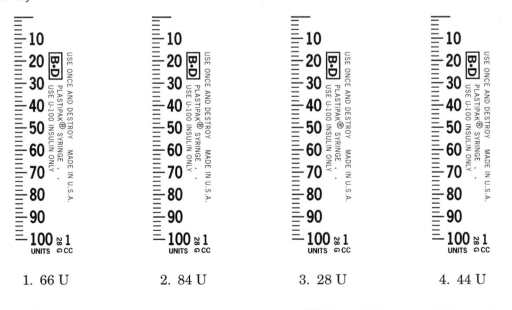

1. 66 U   2. 84 U   3. 28 U   4. 44 U

The second type of 1 mL/cc U-100 syringe is illustrated in Figure 10-14. Notice that this syringe has a **double scale, the odd numbers are on the left, and the even are on the right**. Each 5 U increment is numbered, but on **opposite sides** of the syringe. This syringe does have a calibration for each 1 U increment, but in order to count every one to measure a dosage the syringe would have to be rotated back and forth, which could cause confusion. There is a safer way to read the calibrations. **To measure uneven numbered dosages**, for example, 7, 13, 27, etc., **use the uneven (left) scale only; for even numbered dosages** such as 6, 10, 56, etc., **use the even (right) scale only. Count each calibration (on one side only) as 2 U, because that is what it is measuring.**

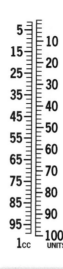

Figure 10-14

EXAMPLE 1

To prepare an 89 U dosage, start at 85 U on the uneven left scale, count the first calibration above this as 87 U, the next as 89 U (**each calibration on the same side measures 2 U**).

EXAMPLE 2

To measure a 26 U dosage, use the even numbered right side calibrations. Start at 20 U, move up one calibration to 22 U, another to 24 U, and one more to 26 U (**each calibration is 2 U**).

PROBLEM

Identify the dosages measured on the 1 cc U-100 syringes provided.

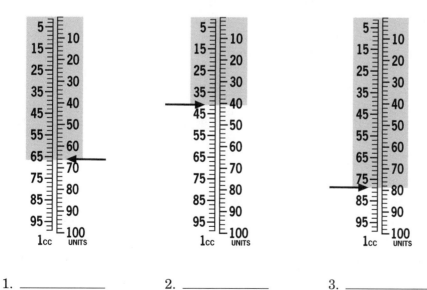

1. _____   2. _____   3. _____

PROBLEM

Shade in each U-100 syringe provided to identify the following dosages.

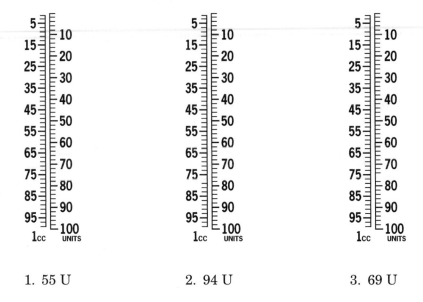

1. 55 U   2. 94 U   3. 69 U

COMBINING INSULIN DOSAGES

Insulin-dependent individuals must have at least one, and, sometimes several, subcutaneous injections of insulin per day. In order to reduce the number of injections as much as possible, it is common to combine two insulins in a single syringe, for example, a short-acting with either an intermediate- or long-acting insulin.

 When two insulins are combined in the same syringe, the regular (shortest acting) insulin is drawn up first.

Both insulins will be withdrawn from sealed 10 mL vials, which requires that an amount of air equal to the insulin to be withdrawn be injected into each vial as a preliminary step. This keeps the pressure inside the vials equalized. An additional step concerns preparation of the insulin itself. Regular insulin does not need to be mixed prior to withdrawal, but intermediate- and long-acting insulins precipitate out. They need to be rotated and mixed immediately before withdrawal from the vial. **The smallest capacity syringe possible should be selected to prepare the dosage**, as the enlarged scale is easier to read and therefore more accurate.

The actual step-by-step procedure for combining insulins is as follows:

EXAMPLE 1

A dosage of 10 U of Regular and 48 U of NPH insulin has been ordered.

STEP 1 | **Locate the correct insulins and rotate and upend the NPH until it is thoroughly mixed.**

STEP 2 | **Use an alcohol wipe to cleanse both vial tops.**

STEP 3 The combined dosage (10 U + 48 U = 58 U) requires the use of a 1 mL/cc U-100 syringe. Draw up 48 U of air and insert the needle into the NPH vial. Keep the needle tip above the insulin and inject the air. Withdraw the needle from the vial.

STEP 4 Draw up 10 U of air and inject this into the Regular insulin vial. Draw up the 10 U of Regular insulin.

STEP 5 Insert the needle back into the NPH vial and draw up 48 U of NPH insulin. This will require that you draw the plunger back until the total insulin in the syringe is 58 U (10 U Regular + 48 U NPH). Withdraw the needle and administer the insulin promptly so that the NPH does not have time to precipitate out.

EXAMPLE 2

The order is to give 16 U of Regular insulin and 33 U of Lente insulin.

STEP 1 Locate the correct insulins and rotate the Lente to mix it.

STEP 2 Cleanse both vial tops.

STEP 3 Use a 50 U capacity syringe (16 U + 22 U = 38 U). Draw up 22 U of air. Insert the needle in the Lente vial. Keep the needle tip above the insulin as you inject the air into the vial. Withdraw the needle.

STEP 4 Draw up 16 U of air and inject it into the Regular insulin vial. Draw up the 16 U of Regular insulin.

STEP 5 Insert the needle back into the Lente vial and draw up Lente insulin until the syringe capacity is 38 U (16 U Regular + 22 U Lente). Administer the dosage promptly.

PROBLEM

For each of the following combined insulin dosages, indicate the total volume of the combined dosage and the smallest capacity syringe you can use to prepare it (30 U, 50 U, and 100 U capacity syringes are available).

	Total Volume	**Syringe Size**
1. 28 U Regular, 64 U NPH	_____	_____
2. 16 U Ultralente, 6 U Regular	_____	_____
3. 33 U Regular, 41 U Lente	_____	_____
4. 21 U Regular, 52 U NPH	_____	_____
5. 13 U Regular, 27 U Ultralente	_____	_____

Answers **1.** 92 U; 100 U **2.** 22 U; 30 U **3.** 74 U; 100 U **4.** 73 U; 100 U **4.** 73 U; 100 U **5.** 40 U; 50 U

Summary

This concludes the chapter on measuring insulin dosages. The important points to remember from this chapter are:

- Insulin labels must be read very carefully because they all look very similar.
- U-100 insulins are measured using U-100 calibrated syringes.
- The smallest capacity syringe possible is used to increase accuracy of dosage preparation.
- Calibrations on 30 U and 50 U syringes are in 1 U increments.
- Calibrations on 100 U syringes may be in 1 U or 2 U increments.
- When insulin dosages are combined, the Regular insulin is drawn up first.
- The intermediate- and long-acting insulins precipitate out and must be thoroughly mixed before measurement and administered promptly after measurement.

Summary Self-Test

Use the syringe calibrations provided to measure the following dosages. For combined insulin dosages, use arrows to indicate the exact calibration to be used for each insulin ordered. Have your instructor check your answers.

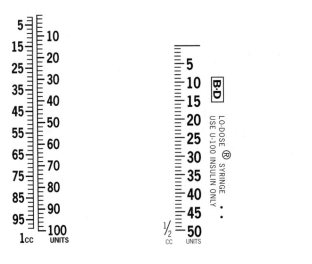

1. 37 U Regular

2. 17 U Regular
   12 U Lente

3. 48 U NPH

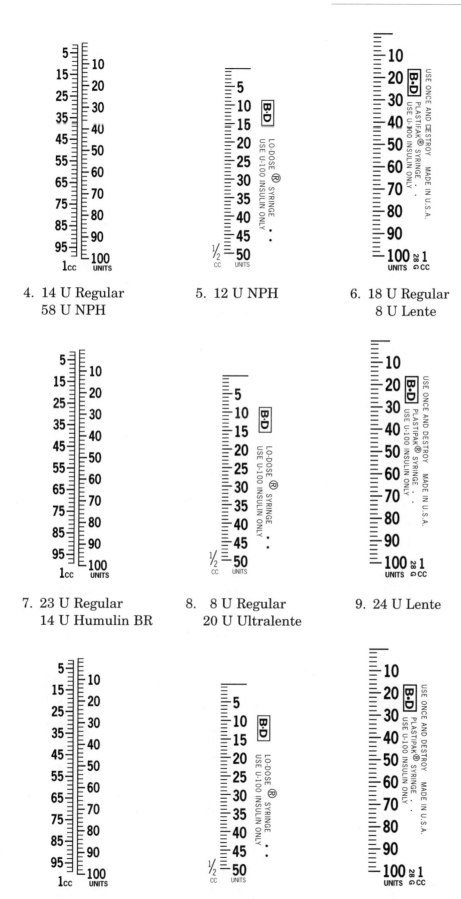

4. 14 U Regular
58 U NPH

5. 12 U NPH

6. 18 U Regular
8 U Lente

7. 23 U Regular
14 U Humulin BR

8. 8 U Regular
20 U Ultralente

9. 24 U Lente

10. 57 U NPH

11. 22 U Regular
U Lente

12. 14 U Regular
44 U NPH

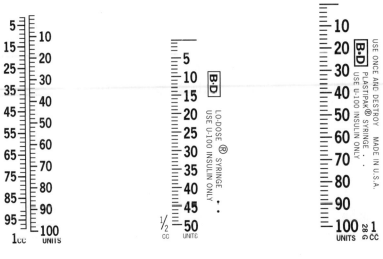

13. 24 U Regular
    27 U Lente

14. 33 U Regular
    10 U Humulin L

15. 56 U Regular

Identify the dosages measured on the following syringes.

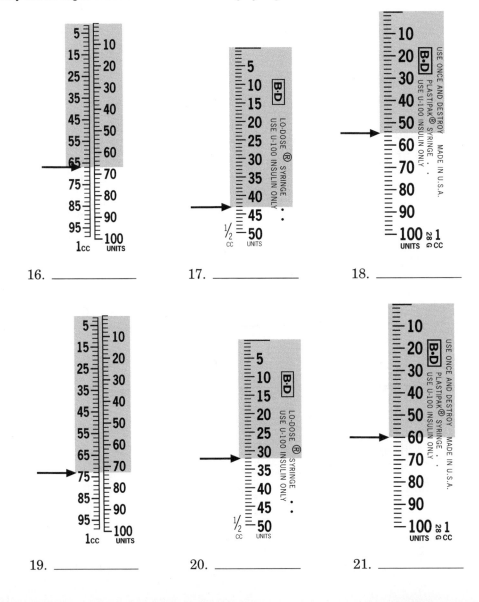

16. _____

17. _____

18. _____

19. _____

20. _____

21. _____

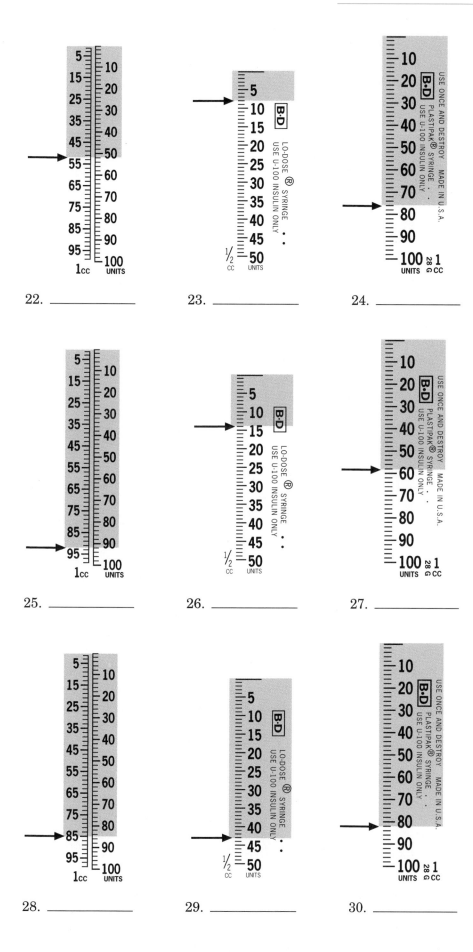

22. _____

23. _____

24. _____

25. _____

26. _____

27. _____

28. _____

29. _____

30. _____

Answers

1–15. See instructor	18.	54 U	22.	52 U	26.	14 U	30.	82 U
16. 67 U	19.	73 U	23.	8 U	27.	58 U		
17. 43 U	20.	32 U	24.	76 U	28.	85 U		
	21.	60 U	25.	92 U	29.	43 U		

SECTION 4

Dosage Calculations

Dosage Calculation Using Ratio and Proportion

Objectives

The learner will:

1. define ratio

2. define proportion

3. solve dosage problems using ratio and proportion

4. assess answers obtained to determine if they are logical

Prerequisites

Chapters 1–8

RATIOS

A **ratio** consists of **two different numbers or quantities that have a significant relationship to each other**. Earlier in the text you learned how to read the dosage on drug labels. Each of these dosages was expressed as a ratio: a certain weight (strength) of drug in a tablet (tab), capsule (cap), or a certain volume of solution, most commonly mL/cc; for example, 50 mg per mL, 100 mcg per tab, 1000 U per mL.

There are **two ways to express (write)** a ratio. The numbers can be **separated by a colon**, or they can be **written as a common fraction**. For example,

Separated by a colon		As a common fraction
50 mg : 1 mL	or	$\dfrac{50 \text{ mg}}{1 \text{ mL}}$
100 mcg : 1 tab	or	$\dfrac{100 \text{ mcg}}{1 \text{ tab}}$
1000 U : 1 mL	or	$\dfrac{1000 \text{ U}}{1 \text{ mL}}$

Although it is more common to see ratios written with the quantity of drug first as in the above examples, it is equally correct to reverse this order and express the quantity or volume first, as follows:

1 mL : 50 mg	or	$\dfrac{1 \text{ mL}}{50 \text{ mg}}$
1 tab : 100 mcg	or	$\dfrac{1 \text{ tab}}{100 \text{ mcg}}$
1 mL : 1000 U	or	$\dfrac{1 \text{ mL}}{1000 \text{ U}}$

A ratio consists of two numbers that have a significant relationship to each other. It can be expressed with the numbers separated by a colon, or as a common fraction.

PROBLEM

Express the following dosages as ratios using whichever form of ratio you prefer, either common fraction, or separated by a colon. Include the units of measure as well as the numerical value when you write the ratios.

1. An injectable solution that contains 100 mg in each 1.5 mL   _____

2. An injectable solution that contains 250 mg in each 0.7 mL   _____

3. A tablet that contains 0.4 mg of drug   _____

4. Two tablets that contain 450 mg of drug   _____

Answers **1.** 1.5 mL : 100 mg; 100 mg : 1.5 mL; $\frac{1.5 \text{ mL}}{100 \text{ mg}}, \frac{100 \text{ mg}}{1.5 \text{ mL}}$ **2.** 250 mg : 0.7 mL; 0.7 mL : 250 mg; $\frac{250 \text{ mg}}{0.7 \text{ mL}}, \frac{0.7 \text{ mL}}{250 \text{ mg}}$

3. 1 tab : 0.4 mg; 0.4 mg : 1 tab; $\frac{1 \text{ tab}}{0.4 \text{ mg}}, \frac{0.4 \text{ mg}}{1 \text{ tab}}$ **4.** 2 tab : 450 mg; 450 mg : 2 tab; $\frac{2 \text{ tab}}{450 \text{ mg}}, \frac{450 \text{ mg}}{2 \text{ tab}}$

Note: If you did not include the units of measure your answers are incorrect.

 To complete the balance of this chapter you will need to choose the style of ratio (and proportion) you prefer to use. If you wish to express ratios as a common fraction, for example, $\frac{1 \text{ mL}}{50 \text{ mg}}$, turn now to page 147 under the heading "Ratio and Proportion (R and P) Expressed Using Common Fractions." If you prefer ratios separated by a colon, continue on this page.

RATIO AND PROPORTION (R and P) EXPRESSED USING COLONS

Whereas a ratio is an expression of a significant relationship between two numbers, **a proportion** takes this one step further, and is used **to show the relationship between two ratios**. In a proportion the ratios may be separated by an **equal** (=) **sign**, or by a **double colon** (::). For example,

$$1 : 50 = 2 : 100 \qquad \text{or} \qquad 1 : 50 :: 2 : 100$$

The equal (=) sign will be used for all examples of proportion in this text, but you may use the double colon (::) if you prefer this alternate format.

 A true proportion contains two ratios that are equal.

The previous example is a true proportion.

$$1 : 50 = 2 : 100$$

This is a simple comparison, and by using our previous drug strength examples we can mentally verify that the ratios are equal, and that the proportion is true.

EXAMPLE 1 | 1 **tab** : 50 mg = 2 **tab** : 100 mg

If 1 tablet contains 50 mg, 2 tablets will contain 100 mg.

EXAMPLE 2 | 1 **mL** : 50 mg = 2 **mL** : 100 mg

If 1 mL contains 50 mg, 2 mL will contain 100 mg.

You can also prove mathematically that these ratios are equal, and that the proportion is true. Look again at example 1.

$$1 \text{ tab} : 50 \text{ mg} = 2 \text{ tab} : 100 \text{ mg}$$

The numbers on the **ends** of the proportion (1, 100) are called the **extremes**, whereas those in the **middle** (50, 2) are called the **means**.

 It is critical in all mathematics involving proportions that the means and extremes not be mixed up, or an incorrect answer will be obtained.

Here is a memory cue that you can use to prevent confusion. Notice that the **means** are in the **middle** of a proportion. Both of these words begin with an "**m**" (means, middle). The **extremes** are on the **ends** of the proportion. Both of these words begin with an "**e**" (extremes, ends). Use these cues as necessary to prevent mix-ups.

 In a true proportion the product of the means equals the product of the extremes.

If you multiply the means then the extremes, their products (answers), will be equal.

EXAMPLE 1 $1 \text{ tab} : 50 \text{ mg} = 2 \text{ tab} : 100 \text{ mg}$

$$\begin{array}{c} \overbrace{\text{extremes}} \\ 1 : 50 = 2 : 100 \\ \underbrace{} \\ \text{means} \end{array}$$

$$50 \times 2 = 100 \times 1$$
$$100 = 100$$

The product of the means, 100, equals the product of the extremes, 100. We have now proved mathematically what we previously proved mentally; the ratios are equal, and the proportion is true.

EXAMPLE 2 $2 \text{ mL} : 500 \text{ mg} = 1 \text{ mL} : 250 \text{ mg}$

$$2 : 500 = 1 : 250$$

$$500 \times 1 = 2 \times 250$$
$$500 = 500$$

The product of the means, 500 equals the product of the extremes, 500. This is a true proportion; the ratios are equal.

EXAMPLE 3 $1 \text{ mL} : 10 \text{ U} = 2 \text{ mL} : 20 \text{ U}$

$$10 \times 2 = 20$$
$$20 = 20$$

This is a true proportion.

PROBLEM

Determine mathematically if the following are true proportions.

1. 34 mg : 2 mL = 51 mg : 3 mL

2. 15 mg : 4 mL = 45 mg : 12 mL

3. 1.3 mL : 46 mg = 0.65 mL : 23 mg

4. 2.3 mL : 150 U = 1.9 mL : 130 U

5. 40 mg : 1.1 mL = 80 mg : 2.2 mL

6. 0.25 mg : 2 mL = 0.5 mg : 4 mL

Answers   **1.** True (2 × 51 = 102 and 34 × 3 = 102)   **2.** True (4 × 45 = 180 and 15 × 12 = 180)   **3.** True (1.3 × 23 = 29.9 and 46 × 0.65 = 29.9)   **4.** Not true (2.3 × 130 = 299 and 150 × 1.9 = 285}   **5.** True (40 × 2.2 = 88 and 1.1 × 80 = 88)   **6.** True (0.25 × 4 = 1 and 2 × 0.5 = 1)

DOSAGE CALCULATION USING *R* AND *P* EXPRESSED WITH COLONS

Ratio and proportion are important in dosage calculations because they can be used when only **one ratio is known**, or **complete**, and **the second is incomplete**. Look carefully at the following examples for parenteral dosages, which is where calculations using *R* and *P* may be required.

EXAMPLE 1 | A solution strength of **8 mg per mL** will be used to prepare a dosage of **10 mg**.

The known ratio is provided by the solution strength available, 8 mg per mL. The incomplete ratio is the dosage to be given, 10 mg, and *X* is used to represent the mL, which will contain 10 mg.

$$8 \text{ mg} : 1 \text{ mL} \quad = \quad 10 \text{ mg} : X \text{ mL}$$

$$\left(\begin{array}{c}\text{complete ratio}\\\text{drug strength}\end{array}\right) \qquad \left(\begin{array}{c}\text{incomplete ratio}\\\text{dosage to give}\end{array}\right)$$

 The ratios in a proportion must be written in the same sequence of measurement units.

In the above example they are: mg : mL = mg : mL.

Next let's look at the math steps used to determine the value of the unknown, *X* mL. The math will be familiar because it was covered earlier in the refresher math section.

$$8 \text{ mg} : 1 \text{ mL} = 10 \text{ mg} : X \text{ mL}$$

check sequence of measurement units; mg : mL = mg : mL

$$8 : 1 = 10 : X$$

drop the measurement units

$$8X = 10$$

multiply the extremes, then the means, keeping X on the left of the equation

$$X = \frac{10}{8}$$

divide 10 by the number in front of X

$$= \frac{\overset{5}{10}}{\underset{4}{8}}$$

reduce the numbers by their highest common denominator, 2. Divide the final fraction. Divide 5 by 4.

$$= \mathbf{1.25 \text{ mL}}$$

the X in the original proportion was **mL**, so the answer is 1.25 **mL**

The ordered dosage of 10 mg is contained in 1.25 mL

It is routine to check your math twice in dosage calculations. However, it is also necessary to **assess each answer to determine if it seems logical**, and here is where the previous review of relative value of numbers is put to use. Consider the answer just obtained in example 1.

$$8 \text{ mg} : 1 \text{ mL} = 10 \text{ mg} : X \text{ mL}$$
$$X = \mathbf{1.25 \text{ mL}}$$

If **1 mL** contains **8 mg**, you will need a **larger** volume than 1 mL to obtain **10 mg**. The answer obtained, 1.25 mL **is** larger; therefore it is logical. This routine check does not guarantee that your math is correct, but it does indicate that you have not mixed up the means and extremes in your calculations.

 Each answer obtained must be assessed to determine if it is logical.

You **can** prove that the proportion is true (and your math correct) by substituting your answer for X in the original proportion.

$$8 \text{ mg} : 1 \text{ mL} = 10 \text{ mg} : \mathbf{X \text{ mL}}$$
$$8 \text{ mg} : 1 \text{ mL} = 10 \text{ mg} : \mathbf{1.25 \text{ mL}}$$
$$10 = 8 \times 1.25$$
$$10 = 10$$

You have now proved mathematically that your answer is correct. **However, in most routine calculations it is neither necessary nor practical to mathematically prove each answer you obtain.** Dosages such as the 1.25 mL in our example are most often rounded to the nearest tenth (1.25 = 1.3 mL). Once this is done, the math proofing the answer may contain small discrepancies that could cause confusion.

EXAMPLE 2 The dosage strength available is **25 mg in 1.5 mL**. A dosage of **20 mg** has been ordered.

$$25 \text{ mg} : 1.5 \text{ mL} = 20 \text{ mg} : X \text{ mL}$$ make sure the units are written in the same sequence: mg : mL = mg : mL

$$25 : 1.5 = 20 : X$$ drop the measurement units

$$25X = 1.5 \times 20$$ multiply the extremes; then the means; keep *X* on the left

$$= \frac{30}{25}$$ divide by the number in front of *X*

$$= \frac{30^{6}}{25_{5}} = 1.2$$ reduce the common denominator by 5, then divide the final fraction, 6 by 5

$$X = \textbf{1.2 mL}$$

The dosage ordered, 20 mg, is a smaller amount of drug than the strength available, 25 mg (in 1.5 mL). So the answer should be smaller than 1.5 mL, and it is, 1.2 mL. This answer is logical.

EXAMPLE 3 A dosage of **200 mg** must be prepared from a solution strength of **80 mg per mL**.

$$80 \text{ mg} : 1 \text{ mL} = 200 \text{ mg} : X \text{ mL}$$

$$80X = 200$$

$$\frac{200^{5}}{80_{2}} = \frac{5}{2} = \textbf{2.5 mL}$$

The original unknown, *X*, was mL, so the answer must be mL. The dosage ordered, 200 mg, is larger than the 80 mg per mL strength being used, so it must be contained in more than 1 mL. The answer, 2.5 mL, is larger. Therefore, it is logical.

As soon as you are comfortable with the math steps in ratio and proportion you can combine several steps at once and work even more efficiently. You may already have been doing this, but here are a few examples to demonstrate the shortcuts.

EXAMPLE 4 A **300 mg in 1.2 mL** solution will be used to prepare a dosage of **120 mg**.

$$300 \text{ mg} : 1.2 \text{ mL} = 120 \text{ mg} : X \text{ mL}$$ set up the proportion with the known ratios written first

$$X = \frac{1.2 \times 120}{300}$$ multiply the means, and **immediately** divide by the number in front of *X*

$$\frac{1.2 \times 120^{2}}{300_{5}} = \frac{2.4}{5} = 0.48 \times \textbf{0.5 mL}$$ reduce by the common denominator 60. Do final division: 2.4 by 5. Round to the nearest tenth.

The required dosage, 120 mg, is smaller than the 300 mg/1.2 mL available strength. Therefore, the smaller 0.5 mL answer is logical.

EXAMPLE 5 | Prepare a **2 mg** dosage using a **1.5 mg in 0.5 mL** solution.

$$1.5 \text{ mg} : 0.5 \text{ mL} = 2 \text{ mg} : X \text{ mL}$$

$$X = \frac{\overset{1}{\cancel{0.5}} \times 2}{\underset{3}{\cancel{1.5}}} = 0.66 = \textbf{0.7 mL}$$

The dosage ordered, 2 mg, is larger than the 1.5 mg/0.5 mL dosage available. The 0.7 mL answer is logical.

EXAMPLE 6 | A **120 mg** dosage is ordered. The solution available is labeled **80 mg/mL**.

$$80 \text{ mg} : 1 \text{ mL} = 120 \text{ mg} : X \text{ mL}$$

$$X = \frac{\overset{3}{\cancel{120}}}{\underset{2}{\cancel{80}}} = \textbf{1.5 mL}$$

The 1.5 mL answer is logical because the 120 mg ordered is larger than the 80 mg/mL dosage strength available.

PROBLEM

Calculate the following dosages. Express your answers to the nearest tenth, including the appropriate unit of measure. Assess your answers to determine if they are logical.

1. A dosage of 24 mg has been ordered. The solution strength available is 12.5 mg in 1.5 mL. _____

2. A 40 mg/2.5 mL solution will be used to prepare a 30 mg dosage. _____

3. Prepare 0.3 mg from a solution strength of 0.6 mg/0.8 mL. _____

4. A 35 mg per 2 mL strength solution is used to prepare 24 mg. _____

5. A dosage of 52 mg is to be prepared from a 78 mg in 0.9 mL solution. _____

6. A dosage of 150 mg has been ordered. The solution strength is 100 mg per mL. _____

7. A strength of 3 mL containing 750 mcg is available to prepare 600 mcg. _____

8. If the strength available is 1.5 g per cc, how many cc will a 4 g dosage require? _____

9. Prepare a 0.25 mg dosage from a 0.5 mg per 1 mL strength solution. _____

10. Prepare a 3 g dosage from a 4 g in 2.7 mL strength solution. _____

Answers: **1.** 2.9 mL **2.** 1.9 mL **3.** 0.4 mL **4.** 1.3 mL **5.** 0.6 mL **6.** 1.5 mL **7.** 2.4 mL **8.** 2.7 cc **9.** 0.5 mL **10.** 2 mL
Note: If you did not include the units of measure, your answers are incorrect.

This completes your introduction to the use of ratio and proportion separated by a colon in solving simple dosage calculations. **Turn now to page 152 "Calculations When Drug Weights Are in Different Units of Measure" to complete the chapter.**

RATIO AND PROPORTION (*R* AND *P*) EXPRESSED USING COMMON FRACTIONS

Whereas a ratio is an expression of a significant relationship between two numbers, **a proportion** takes this one step further, and is used **to show the relationship between two ratios**. In a proportion the ratios may be separated by an **equal (=) sign**, or by a **double colon (::)**. For example,

$$\frac{1}{50} = \frac{2}{100} \qquad \text{or} \qquad \frac{1}{50} :: \frac{2}{100}$$

The equal (=) sign will be used for all examples of proportion in this text, but you may use the double colon (::) if you prefer this alternate format.

 A true proportion contains two ratios that are equal.

The previous example is a true proportion.

$$\frac{1}{50} = \frac{2}{100}$$

This is a simple comparison, and by using our previous drug strength examples we can mentally verify that the ratios are equal, and that the proportion is true.

EXAMPLE 1 | $\dfrac{1\text{ tab}}{50\text{ mg}} = \dfrac{2\text{ tab}}{100\text{ mg}}$

If 1 tablet contains 50 mg, 2 tablets will contain 100 mg.

EXAMPLE 2 | $\dfrac{1\text{ mL}}{50\text{ mg}} = \dfrac{2\text{ mL}}{100\text{ mg}}$

If 1 mL contains 50 mg, 2 mL will contain 100 mg.

You can also prove mathematically that these ratios are equal, and that the proportion is true. Look again at example 1.

$$\frac{1\text{ tab}}{50\text{ mg}} = \frac{2\text{ tab}}{100\text{ mg}}$$

 In a true proportion the products of cross multiplying will be identical.

To prove a proportion is true, cross multiply. The products (answers) you obtain will be identical.

EXAMPLE 1 | $\dfrac{1\text{ tab}}{50\text{ mg}} = \dfrac{2\text{ tab}}{100\text{ mg}}$

$$\frac{1}{50} = \frac{2}{100}$$ drop the measurement units

$$1 \times 100 = 50 \times 2$$ cross multiply

$$100 = 100$$

The products of cross multiplying in this proportion, 100, are the same. We have now proved mathematically what we previously proved mentally; the ratios are equal, and the proportion is true.

EXAMPLE 2 $\quad \dfrac{2 \text{ mL}}{500 \text{ mg}} = \dfrac{1 \text{ mL}}{250 \text{ mg}}$

$$2 \times 250 = 500 \times 1 \qquad \text{drop the measurement units and cross multiply}$$

$$500 = 500$$

The products of cross multiplying, 500, are identical. This is a true proportion; the ratios are equal.

EXAMPLE 3 $\quad \dfrac{1 \text{ mL}}{10 \text{ U}} - \dfrac{2 \text{ mL}}{20 \text{ U}}$

$$1 \times 20 = 10 \times 2$$

$$20 = 20$$

This is a true proportion. The products of cross multiplying, 20, are equal.

It is critical in calculations involving proportions that the numbers multiplied not be mixed up.

If necessary make a habit of drawing an X as in the examples just given to make sure you cross multiply correctly.

PROBLEM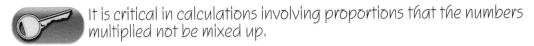

Determine mathematically if the following are true proportions.

1. $\dfrac{34 \text{ mg}}{2 \text{ mL}} = \dfrac{51 \text{ mg}}{3 \text{ mL}}$ _____

2. $\dfrac{15 \text{ mg}}{4 \text{ mL}} = \dfrac{45 \text{ mg}}{12 \text{ mL}}$ _____

3. $\dfrac{1.3 \text{ mL}}{46 \text{ mg}} = \dfrac{0.65 \text{ mL}}{23 \text{ mg}}$ _____

4. $\dfrac{2.3 \text{ mL}}{150 \text{ U}} = \dfrac{1.9 \text{ mL}}{130 \text{ U}}$ _____

5. $\dfrac{40 \text{ mg}}{1.1 \text{ mL}} = \dfrac{80 \text{ mg}}{2.2 \text{ mL}}$ _____

6. $\dfrac{0.25 \text{ mg}}{2 \text{ mL}} = \dfrac{0.5 \text{ mg}}{4 \text{ mL}}$ _____

Answers   **1.** True (2 × 51 = 102 and 34 × 3 = 102)   **2.** True (4 × 45 = 180 and 15 × 12 = 180)
3. True (1.3 × 23 = 29.9 and 46 × 0.65 = 29.9)   **4.** Not true (2.3 × 130 = 299 and 150 × 1.9 = 285}
5. True (40 × 2.2 = 88 and 1.1 × 80 = 88)   **6.** True (0.25 × 4 = 1 and 2 × 0.5 = 1)

DOSAGE CALCULATION USING *R* AND *P* EXPRESSED AS COMMON FRACTIONS

Ratio and proportion are important in dosage calculations because they can be used when only **one ratio is known**, or **complete**, and **the second is incomplete**. Look carefully at the following examples for parenteral dosages, which is where calculations using *R* and *P* may be required.

 A solution strength of **8 mg per mL** will be used to prepare a dosage of **10 mg**.

The known ratio is provided by the solution strength available, 8 mg per mL. The incomplete ratio is the dosage to be given, 10 mg, and *X* is used to represent the mL, which will contain 10 mg.

$$\frac{8 \text{ mg}}{1 \text{ mL}} \quad = \quad \frac{10 \text{ mg}}{X \text{ mL}}$$

$$\left(\begin{array}{c}\text{complete ratio} \\ \text{drug strength}\end{array}\right) \qquad \left(\begin{array}{c}\text{incomplete ratio} \\ \text{dosage to give}\end{array}\right)$$

 The ratios in a proportion must be written in the same sequence of measurement units.

In the above example they are:

$$\frac{\text{mg}}{\text{mL}} = \frac{\text{mg}}{\text{mL}}$$

Both **numerators** are **mg**, both **denominators** are **mL**.

Next let's look at the math steps used to determine the value of the unknown, *X* mL. The math will be familiar because it was covered earlier in the refresher math section.

$$\frac{8 \text{ mg}}{1 \text{ mL}} = \frac{10 \text{ mg}}{X \text{ mL}}$$ set up the proportion to include the measurement units; make sure they are in the same sequence

$$\frac{8 \text{ mg}}{1 \text{ mL}} = \frac{10 \text{ mg}}{X \text{ mL}}$$ drop the measurement units as you cross multiply

$$8X = 10$$ keep *X* on the left of the equation

$$X = \frac{\overset{5}{\cancel{10}}}{\underset{4}{\cancel{8}}}$$ divide 10 by the number in front of *X*; reduce by the highest common denominator (2)

$$= 1.25$$ divide the final fraction to obtain a decimal fraction

$$= 1.25 \text{ mL}$$ the *X* in the original proportion was **mL**, so the answer is 1.25 **mL**

The ordered dosage of 10 mg is contained in 1.25 mL.

It is routine to check your math twice in dosage calculations. However, it is also necessary to **assess each answer to determine if it seems logical**, and here is where the previous review of relative value of numbers is put to use. Consider the answer just obtained in example 1.

$$\frac{8 \text{ mg}}{1 \text{ mL}} = \frac{10 \text{ mg}}{X \text{ mL}}$$

$$X = 1.25 \text{ mL}$$

If **1 mL** contains **8 mg** you will need a **larger** volume than 1 mL to obtain **10 mg**. The answer obtained, 1.25 mL **is** larger, therefore it is logical. This routine check does not guarantee that your math is correct, but it does indicate that you did not mix up the units of measure when you set up the proportion and cross multiplied.

 Each answer obtained must be assessed to determine if it is logical.

You **can** prove that the proportion is true (and your math correct) by substituting your answer for X in the original proportion.

$$\frac{8 \text{ mg}}{1 \text{ mL}} = \frac{10 \text{ mg}}{X \text{ mL}}$$

$$\frac{8 \text{ mg}}{1 \text{ mL}} = \frac{10 \text{ mg}}{1.25 \text{ mL}}$$

$$8 \times 1.25 = 10 \times 1$$

$$10 = 10$$

You have now proved mathematically that your answer is correct. **However, in most routine calculations it is neither necessary nor practical to mathematically prove each answer you obtain.** Dosages such as the 1.25 mL in our example are **most often rounded to the nearest tenth** (1.25 = 1.3 mL). Once this is done, the math proofing the answer may contain small discrepancies, which could cause confusion.

EXAMPLE 2 | The strength available is **25 mg in 1.5 mL**. A dosage of **20 mg** has been ordered.

$$\frac{25 \text{ mg}}{1.5 \text{ mL}} = \frac{20 \text{ mg}}{X \text{ mL}}$$ make sure the units are in the same sequence

$$25X = 1.5 \times 20$$ cross multiply; keep X on the left

$$X = \frac{\cancel{30}^{\;6}}{\cancel{25}_{\;5}}$$ reduce by 5, then divide the final fraction

$$= 1.2 \text{ mL}$$ include the measurement unit in your answer

The dosage ordered, 20 mg, is smaller than the strength available, 25 mg (in 1.5 mL). So the answer should be smaller than 1.5 mL, and it is, 1.2 mL. The answer is logical.

EXAMPLE 3 A dosage of **200 mg** must be prepared from a solution strength of **80 mg per mL**.

$$\frac{80 \text{ mg}}{1 \text{ mL}} = \frac{200 \text{ mg}}{X \text{ mL}}$$

$$80X = 200$$

$$\frac{\overset{5}{\cancel{200}}}{\underset{2}{\cancel{80}}} = \textbf{2.5 mL}$$

The original unknown, X, was mL, so the answer must be mL. The dosage ordered, 200 mg, is larger than the 80 mg per mL strength being used, so it must be contained in more than 1 mL. The answer, 2.5 mL, is larger. Therefore, it is logical.

As soon as you are comfortable with the math steps in ratio and proportion, you can combine several steps at once and work even more efficiently. You may already have been doing this, but here are a few examples to demonstrate the shortcuts.

EXAMPLE 4 A **300 mg in 1.2 mL** solution will be used to prepare a dosage of **120 mg**.

$$\frac{300 \text{ mg}}{1.2 \text{ mL}} = \frac{120 \text{ mg}}{X \text{ mL}}$$

set up the proportion with the known ratio written first

$$X = \frac{1.2 \times 120}{300}$$

cross multiply, and **immediately** divide by the number in front of X

$$\frac{1.2 \times \overset{2}{\cancel{120}}}{\underset{5}{\cancel{300}}} = \frac{2.4}{5} = 0.48 = \textbf{0.5 mL}$$

reduce (by 60); do final division; round to nearest tenth

A dosage of 120 mg will require fewer mL than the 300 mg per 1.2 mL strength available. The smaller 0.5 mL answer is logical.

EXAMPLE 5 Prepare a **2 mg** dosage using a **1.5 mg in 0.5 mL** solution.

$$\frac{1.5 \text{ mg}}{0.5 \text{ mL}} = \frac{2 \text{ mg}}{X \text{ mL}}$$

$$X = \frac{\overset{1}{\cancel{0.5}} \times 2}{\underset{3}{\cancel{1.5}}} = 0.66 = \textbf{0.7 mL}$$

The 0.7 mL answer is a larger volume than the 1.5 mg in 0.5 mL dosage strength available, therefore, it is logical.

EXAMPLE 6 A **120 mg** dosage is ordered. The solution available is labeled **80 mg/mL**.

$$\frac{80 \text{ mg}}{1 \text{ mL}} = \frac{120 \text{ mg}}{X \text{ mL}}$$

$$X = \frac{\overset{3}{\cancel{120}}}{\underset{2}{\cancel{80}}} = \textbf{1.5 mL}$$

The 120 mg dosage ordered will require a volume larger than the 80 mg/mL available dosage strength. The answer, 1.5 mL, is larger, therefore it is logical.

PROBLEM

Calculate the following dosages. Express your answers to the nearest tenth. Include the appropriate unit of measure in your answer. Assess your answers to determine if they are logical.

1. A dosage of 24 mg has been ordered. The solution strength available is 12.5 mg in 1.5 mL. _____

2. A 40 mg/2.5 mL solution will be used to prepare a 30 mg dosage. _____

3. Prepare 0.3 mg from a solution strength of 0.6 mg/0.8 mL. _____

4. A 36 mg per 2 mL strength solution is used to prepare 24 mg. _____

5. A dosage of 52 mg is to be prepared from a 78 mg in 0.9 mL solution. _____

6. A dosage of 150 mg has been ordered. The solution strength is 100 mg per mL. _____

7. A strength of 3 mL containing 750 mcg is available to prepare 600 mcg. _____

8. If the strength available is 1.5 g per cc, how many cc will a 4 g dosage require? _____

9. Prepare a 0.25 mg dosage from a 0.5 mg per 1 mL strength solution. _____

10. Prepare a 3 g dosage from a 4 g in 2.7 mL strength solution. _____

Answers: **1.** 2.9 mL **2.** 1.9 mL **3.** 0.4 mL **4.** 1.3 mL **5.** 0.6 mL **6.** 1.5 mL **7.** 2.4 mL **8.** 2.7 cc **9.** 0.5 mL **10.** 2 mL
Note: If you did not include the units of measure, your answers are incorrect.

CALCULATIONS WHEN DRUG WEIGHTS ARE IN DIFFERENT UNITS OF MEASURE

Consider the following dosage calculations. Follow the examples that use the ratio and proportion method you chose earlier in the chapter.

 EXAMPLE 1 | The order is to give **0.15 g** of medication. The dosage strength available is **200 mg/mL**.

This problem cannot be solved as it is now written because **the drug weights are in different units of measure:** g and mg. In a previous chapter you learned that it may be safer to convert down the scale, higher units to lower, to eliminate or avoid decimals. **Convert the g to mg**.

$$200 \text{ mg} : 1 \text{ mL} = \textbf{0.15 g} : X \text{ mL} \qquad \textbf{or} \qquad \frac{200 \text{ mg}}{1 \text{ mL}} = \frac{\textbf{0.15 g}}{X \text{ mL}}$$

$$200 \text{ mg} : 1 \text{ mL} = \textbf{150 mg} : X \text{ mL} \qquad \textbf{or} \qquad \frac{200 \text{ mg}}{1 \text{ mL}} = \frac{\textbf{150 mg}}{X \text{ mL}}$$

$$200X = 1 \times 150 \qquad\qquad\qquad 200X = 1 \times 150$$

$$X = \frac{150}{200} = 0.75 \qquad\qquad\qquad X = \frac{150}{200} = 0.75$$

$$= \textbf{0.8 mL} \qquad\qquad\qquad\qquad = \textbf{0.8 mL}$$

150 mg is a smaller dosage than 200 mg so it must be contained in a smaller volume than 1 mL. The answer, 0.8 mL, is logical.

EXAMPLE 2   You have a dosage strength of **200 mcg/ml**. The order is to give **0.5 mg**.

$$200 \text{ mcg} : 1 \text{ mL} = \textbf{0.5 mg} : X \text{ mL} \qquad \textbf{or} \qquad \frac{200 \text{ mcg}}{1 \text{ mL}} = \frac{\textbf{0.5 mg}}{X \text{ mL}}$$

$$200 \text{ mcg} : 1 \text{ mL} = \textbf{500 mcg} : X \text{ mL} \qquad \textbf{or} \qquad \frac{200 \text{ mcg}}{1 \text{ mL}} = \frac{\textbf{500 mcg}}{X \text{ mL}}$$

$$200X = 500 \qquad\qquad\qquad\qquad 200X = 500$$

$$X = \textbf{2.5 mL} \qquad\qquad\qquad\qquad X = \textbf{2.5 mL}$$

500 mg is a larger quantity than 200 mcg so it must be contained in a larger quantity than 1 mL. The answer, 2.5 mL, is logical.

Ratio and proportion are also used to solve dosage calculations for **International Units and mEq dosages**.

EXAMPLE 3   The order is to give **1200 U**. The available dosage strength is **1000 U per 1.5 mL**.

$$1000 \text{ U} : 1.5 \text{ mL} = 1200 \text{ U} : X \text{ mL} \qquad \textbf{or} \qquad \frac{1000 \text{ U}}{1.5 \text{ mL}} = \frac{1200 \text{ U}}{X \text{ mL}}$$

$$1000X = 1.5 \times 1200 \qquad\qquad\qquad 1000X = 1.5 \times 1200$$

$$X = \frac{1.5 \times 1200}{1000} \qquad\qquad\qquad X = \frac{1.5 \times 1200}{1000}$$

$$= \textbf{1.8 mL} \qquad\qquad\qquad\qquad = \textbf{1.8 mL}$$

1200 U is a larger dosage than 1000 U so the answer in mL should be larger, which it is.

EXAMPLE 4   A drug has a dosage strength of **2 mEq/mL**. You are to give **10 mEq**.

$$2 \text{ mEq} : 1 \text{ mL} = 10 \text{ mEq} : X \text{ mL} \qquad \textbf{or} \qquad \frac{2 \text{ mEq}}{1 \text{ mL}} = \frac{10 \text{ mEq}}{X \text{ mL}}$$

$$2X = 10 \qquad\qquad\qquad\qquad 2X = 10$$

$$X = \textbf{5 mL} \qquad\qquad\qquad\qquad X = \textbf{5 mL}$$

10 mEq is considerably larger than 2 mEq, so the answer should also be significantly larger, and it is.

PROBLEM

Solve the following dosage problems using your preferred *R* and *P* method. Express your answers to the nearest tenth.

1. The drug label reads 1000 mcg in 2 mL. The order is 0.4 mg. _____

2. The ordered dosage is 275 mg. The available drug is labeled 0.5 g per 2 mL. _____

3. A dosage strength of 0.2 mg in 1.5 mL is available. Give 0.15 mg. _____

4. The strength available is 1 g in 3.6 mL. Prepare a 600 mg dosage. _____

5. A 10,000 U dosage has been ordered. The dosage strength available is 8000 U in 1 mL. _____

6. The dosage available is 20 mEq per 20 mL. You are to prepare 15 mEq. _____

7. The order is for 200,000 U. The strength available is 150,000 U per 2 mL. _____

Answers   **1.** 0.8 mL   **2.** 1.1 mL   **3.** 1.1 mL   **4.** 2.2 mL   **5.** 1.3 mL   **6.** 15 mL   **7.** 2.7 mL

Summary

This concludes the introductory chapter on ratio and proportion and their uses in dosage calculations. The important points to remember from this chapter are:

- A ratio is composed of two numbers that have a significant relationship to each other.

- In medication dosages, ratios can be used to express the amount of drug contained in a tablet or capsule or in a certain volume of solution.

- A true proportion consists of two ratios that are equal to each other.

- If one number of a proportion is missing, it can be determined mathematically by solving an equation to determine the value of *X*.

- The available dosage strength provides the complete or known ratio for calculations.

- The dosage to be given provides the incomplete or unknown ratio.

- The ratios in a proportion must be set up in the same sequence of measurement units, for example, mg : mL = mg : mL.

- If the measurement units in a calculation are different, for example, mg and g, one of these must be converted before the problem can be solved.

- The math of calculations must always be double-checked, and the answer must be assessed logically to determine if *X* is appropriately larger or smaller than the strength available.

- If you have any doubt of your accuracy in calculations seek help.

Summary Self-Test

Use the ratio and proportion method you have chosen to calculate the following parenteral dosages. Express mL answers to the nearest tenth (or hundredth, where indicated). Use the drug labels provided, and assess each answer you obtain to determine if it is logical. Finally, measure the dosages you calculated on the syringes provided, and have your answers checked by your instructor to be sure you have calculated and measured them correctly.

Dosage Ordered   **mL/cc Needed**

1. Depo-Provera® 0.3 g   _____

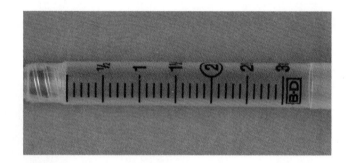

For IM use only.
See package insert for complete product information.
Shake vigorously immediately before each use.
Pharmacia & Upjohn Company
Kalamazoo, MI 49001, USA
NDC 0009-0626-01   2.5 mL Vial
Depo-Provera®
medroxyprogesterone
acetate injectable
suspension, USP
400 mg/mL

2. furosemide 15 mg   _____

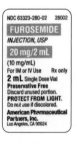

NDC 63323-280-02   28002
FUROSEMIDE
INJECTION, USP
20 mg/2 mL
(10 mg/mL)
For IM or IV Use   Rx only
2 mL Single Dose Vial
Preservative Free
Discard unused portion.
PROTECT FROM LIGHT.
Do not use if discolored.
American Pharmaceutical Partners, Inc.
Los Angeles, CA 90024

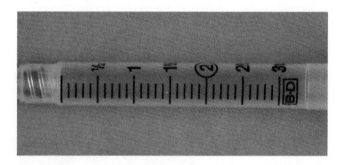

3. heparin 2000 U   _____

LOT/EXP
8113540604
See package insert for complete product information.
Store at controlled room temperature 20°
to 25° C (68° to 77° F)
(see USP).
Each mL contains:
Heparin sodium, 5,000 USP Units. Also,
sodium chloride, 9 mg;
benzyl alcohol,
9.45 mg added as preservative.
Pharmacia & Upjohn Company
Kalamazoo, MI 49001, USA
NDC 0009-0291-01
10 mL
Heparin Sodium
Injection, USP
from beef lung
5,000 Units/mL
For subcutaneous or intravenous use

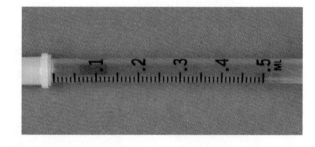

Dosage Ordered	mL/cc Needed

4. Cleocin® 0.75 g
   for an IV additive

_____

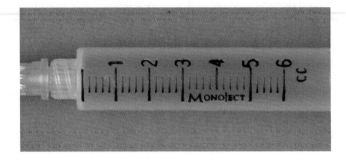

Single Dose Container.
See package insert for complete product information.
Store at controlled room temperature 20° to 25°C (68° to 77°F).
Do not refrigerate.
812 823 707
Pharmacia & Upjohn Company
Kalamazoo, MI 49001. USA

NDC 0009-0902-11   6 mL Vial
Cleocin Phosphate®
clindamycin injection, USP
900 mg
Equivalent to
900 mg clindamycin

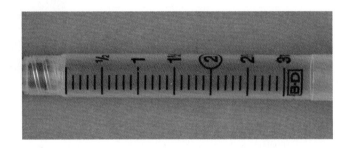

5. naloxone 350 mcg

_____

NDC 63481-358-01
NARCAN®
(Naloxone HCl
Injection, USP)
0.4 mg/mL
1 mL AMPUL
FOR IM, SC OR IV USE
Manufactured for:
Endo Pharmaceuticals Inc.
Chadds Ford, PA 19317

Lot:

Exp:

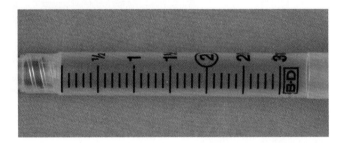

6. clindamycin 225 mg

_____

℞ only
Not for direct infusion. For intramuscular or intravenous use. See package insert.
Warning—if given intravenously, dilute before use. Swab vial closure with an antiseptic solution. Dispense aliquots from the vial via a suitable dispensing device into infusion fluids under a laminar flow hood using aseptic technique. DISCARD VIAL WITHIN 24 HOURS AFTER INITIAL ENTRY.
Store at controlled room temperature 20° to 25° C (68° to 77° F) (see USP). Do not refrigerate.
Each mL contains: clindamycin phosphate equivalent to clindamycin 150 mg; also disodium edetate, 0.5 mg; benzyl alcohol 9.45 mg added as preservative. When necessary, pH was adjusted with sodium hydroxide and/or hydrochloric acid.
DATE/TIME ENTERED
Pharmacia & Upjohn Company

NDC 0009-0728-05
6505-01-246-8718
60 mL Pharmacy Bulk Package

**Cleocin
Phosphate®**
clindamycin
injection, USP

Equivalent to clindamycin

150 mg/mL

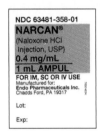

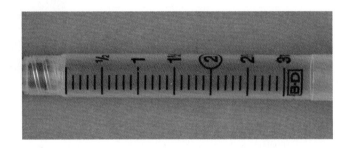

7. Robinul® 75 mcg
   (calculate to the nearest
   hundredth)

_____

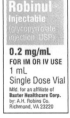

Robinul
Injectable
(glycopyrrolate
injection, USP)
0.2 mg/mL
FOR IM OR IV USE
1 mL
Single Dose Vial
Mfd. for an affiliate of
Baxter Healthcare Corp.
by: A.H. Robins Co.
Richmond, VA 23220

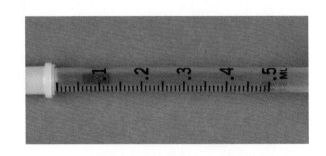

Dosage Ordered   **mL/cc Needed**

8. Tigan® 0.3 g   _____

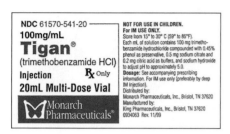

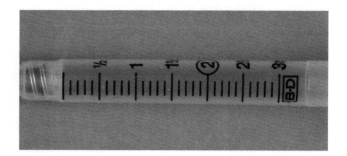

9. benztropine mesylate 2.4 mg   _____

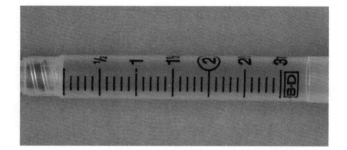

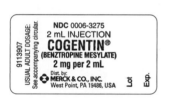

10. cyanocobalamin 800 mcg   _____

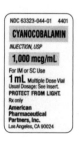

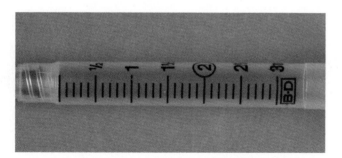

11. tobramycin 65 mg   _____

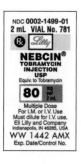

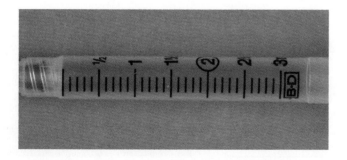

Dosage Ordered	mL/cc Needed

12. amikacin sulfate 0.12 g   _____

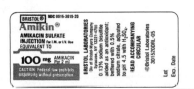

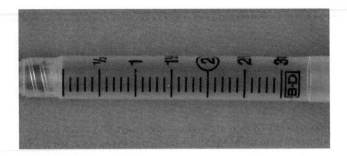

13. Zantac® 70 mg   _____

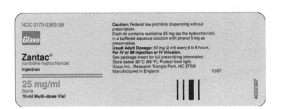

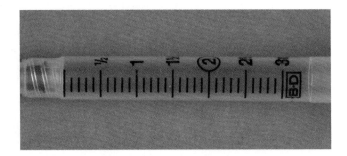

14. calcium gluconate 0.93 mEq   _____
    for an IV additive

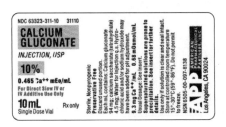

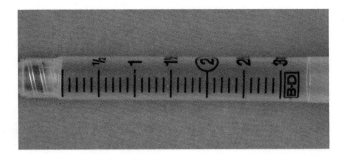

15. morphine sulfate 1.5 mg   _____

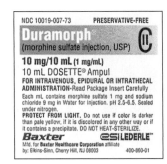

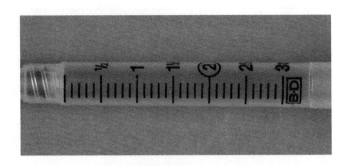

Dosage Ordered	mL/cc Needed

16. heparin 450 U
(calculate to the nearest
hundredth)   _____

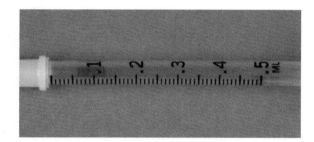

17. perphenazine 3 mg   _____

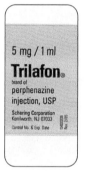 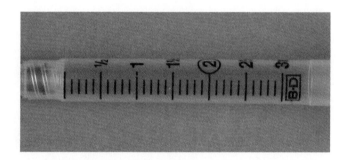

18. Dilantin® 0.1 g   _____

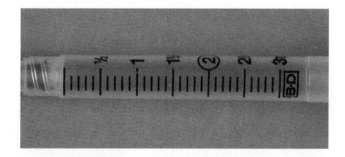

19. medroxyprogesterone 0.9 g   _____

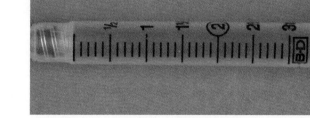

Dosage Ordered	mL/cc Needed

20. gentamicin 70 mg _____

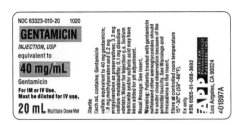

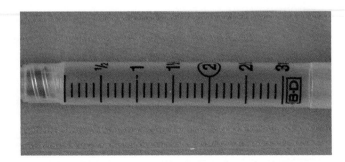

21. Vistaril® 120 mg _____

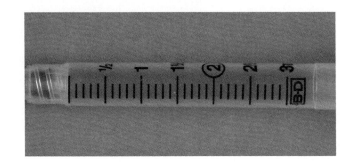

22. sodium chloride 60 mEq for an IV additive _____

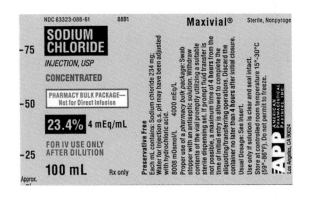

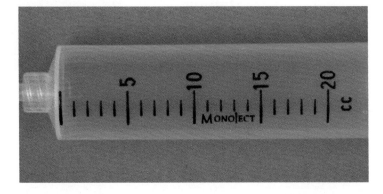

Dosage Ordered   **mL/cc Needed**

23. atropine 150 mcg   _____

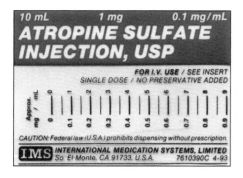

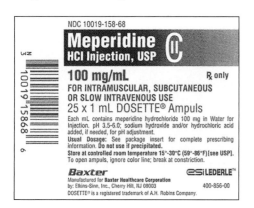

24. meperidine 75 mg   _____

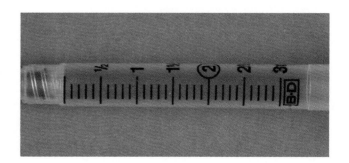

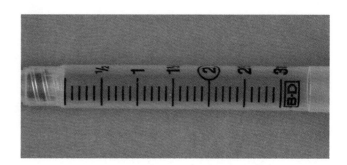

25. fentanyl citrate 80 mcg   _____

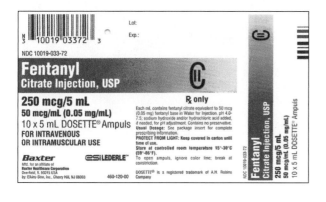

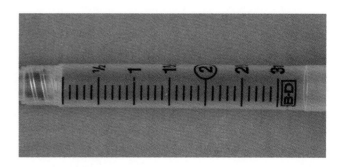

26. clindamycin 0.4 g   _____

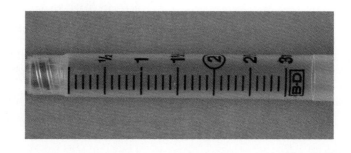

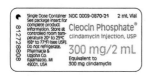

Dosage Ordered	**mL/cc Needed**

27. morphine sulfate 20 mg _____

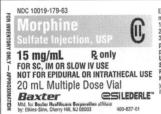

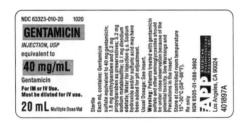

28. gentamycin 0.1 g _____

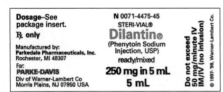

29. Dilantin® 0.15 g _____

30. doxorubicin HCl 16 mg
    for an IV additive _____

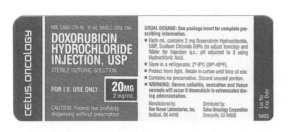

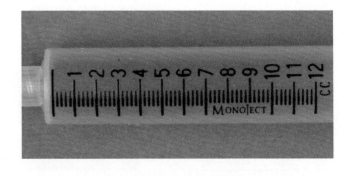

Dosage Ordered	**mL/cc Needed**

31. meperidine HCl 30 mg   _____

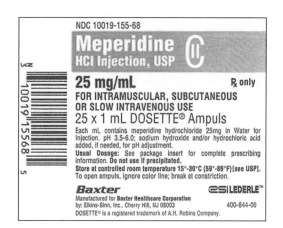
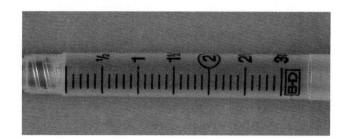

32. methotrexate 40 mg   _____

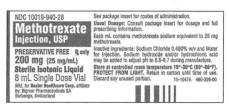
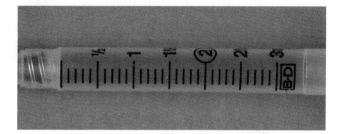

33. Celestone® 12 mg   _____

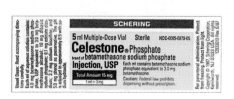
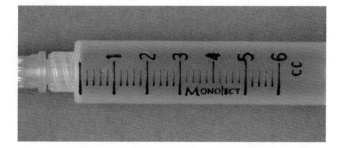

34. haloperidol decanoate 75 mg   _____

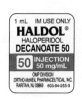
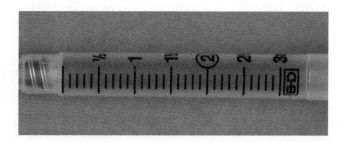

Dosage Ordered	**mL/cc Needed**

35. dexamethasone 5 mg   _____

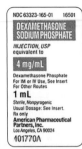

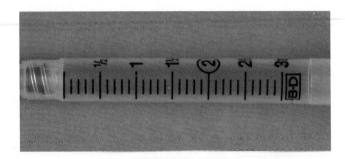

36. chlorpromazine HCl 40 mg   _____

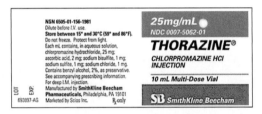

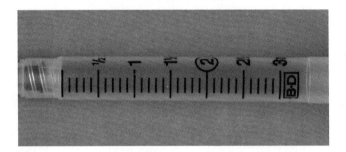

37. Pronestyl® 0.4 g   _____

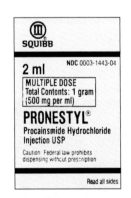

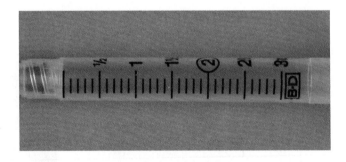

38. nalbuphine HCl 30 mg   _____

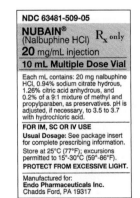

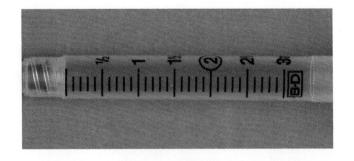

Dosage Ordered   **mL/cc Needed**

39. morphine 15 mg   _____

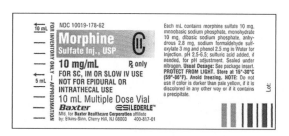

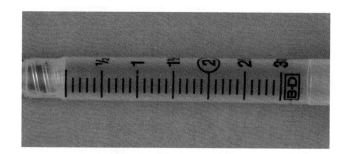

40. cyanocobalamin 750 mg   _____

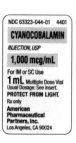

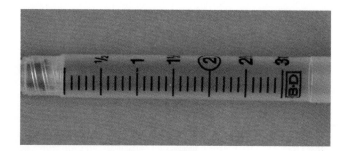

41. tobramycin 70 mg   _____

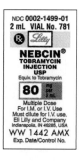

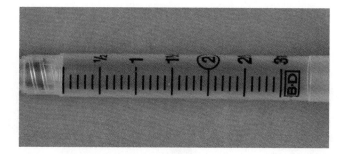

42. aminophylline 0.4 g   _____
    for an IV additive

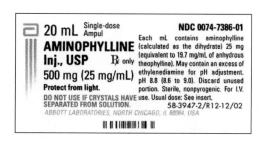

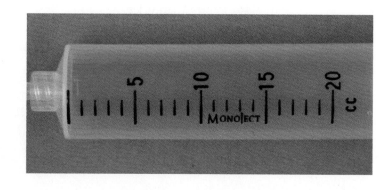

Dosage Ordered	mL/cc Needed

43. naloxone HCl 0.5 mg   _____

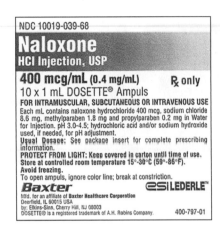

NDC 10019-039-68

Naloxone
HCl Injection, USP

400 mcg/mL (0.4 mg/mL)   R℠ only
10 x 1 mL DOSETTE® Ampuls
FOR INTRAMUSCULAR, SUBCUTANEOUS OR INTRAVENOUS USE
Each mL contains naloxone hydrochloride 400 mcg, sodium chloride
8.6 mg, methylparaben 1.8 mg and propylparaben 0.2 mg in Water
for Injection. pH 3.0-4.5; hydrochloric acid and/or sodium hydroxide
used, if needed, for pH adjustment.
Usual Dosage: See package insert for complete prescribing
information.
PROTECT FROM LIGHT: Keep covered in carton until time of use.
Store at controlled room temperature 15°-30°C (59°-86°F).
Avoid freezing.
To open ampuls, ignore color line; break at constriction.
Baxter   **esi LEDERLE™**
Mfd. for an affiliate of Baxter Healthcare Corporation
Deerfield, IL 60015 USA
by: Elkins-Sinn, Cherry Hill, NJ 08003
DOSETTE® is a registered trademark of A.H. Robins Company.   400-797-01

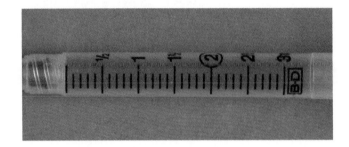

44. Cogentin® 1.5 mg   _____

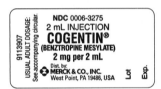

9113907   USUAL ADULT DOSAGE: See accompanying circular.
NDC 0006-3275
2 mL INJECTION
COGENTIN®
(BENZTROPINE MESYLATE)
2 mg per 2 mL.
Dist. by:
MERCK & CO., INC.
West Point, PA 19486, USA   Lot   Exp.

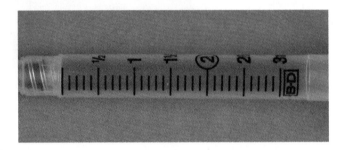

45. chlorpromazine 60 mg   _____

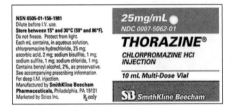

NSN 6505-01-156-1981
Dilute before I.V. use.
Store between 15° and 30°C (59° and 86°F).
Do not freeze. Protect from light.
Each mL contains, in aqueous solution,
chlorpromazine hydrochloride, 25 mg;
ascorbic acid, 2 mg; sodium bisulfite, 1 mg;
sodium sulfite, 1 mg; sodium chloride, 1 mg.
Contains benzyl alcohol, 2%, as preservative.
See accompanying prescribing information.
For deep I.M. injection.
Manufactured by **SmithKline Beecham**
Pharmaceuticals, Philadelphia, PA 19101
Marketed by Scios Inc.   R℠ only

25mg/mL ●
NDC 0007-5062-01
THORAZINE®
CHLORPROMAZINE HCl
INJECTION
10 mL Multi-Dose Vial
SB SmithKline Beecham

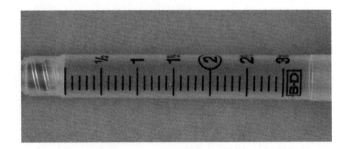

46. gentamicin 0.1 g   _____

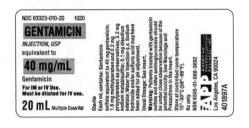

NDC 63323-010-20   1020
GENTAMICIN
INJECTION, USP
equivalent to
40 mg/mL
Gentamicin
For IM or IV Use.
Must be diluted for IV use.
20 mL Multiple Dose Vial

Each mL contains: Gentamicin
sulfate equivalent to 40 mg gentamicin;
1.8 mg methylparaben and 0.2 mg
propylparaben as preservatives; 3.2 mg
sodium metabisulfite; 0.1 mg disodium
edetate; Water for Injection q.s. Sodium
hydroxide and/or sulfuric acid may have
been added for pH adjustment.
Usual Dosage: See insert.
Warning: Patients treated with gentamicin
sulfate and other aminoglycosides should
be under close observation because of the
potential toxicity. See Warnings and
Precautions in the insert.
Store at controlled room temperature
15°-30°C (59°-86°F).
Rx only
NSN 6505-01-088-3692
Los Angeles, CA 90024
401897A

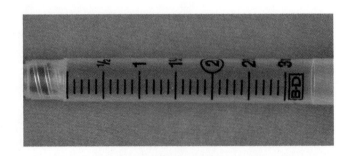

Dosage Ordered   **mL/cc Needed**

47. Robinul® 180 mcg   _____

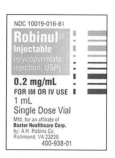
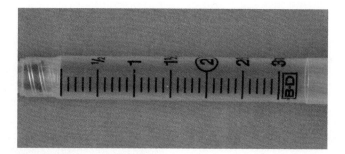

48. hydroxyzine HCl 70 mg   _____

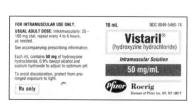
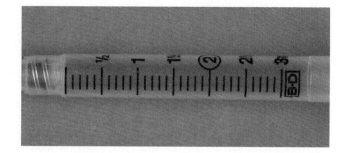

49. Bicillin® C-R 400,000 U   _____

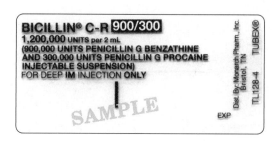
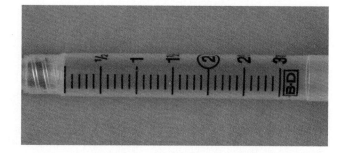

50. heparin sodium 2500 U   _____

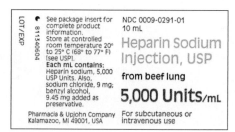
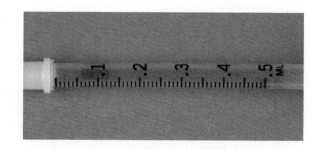

Dosage Ordered   **mL/cc Needed**

51. potassium chloride 20 mEq   _____
    for an IV additive

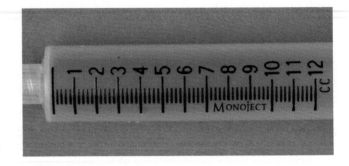

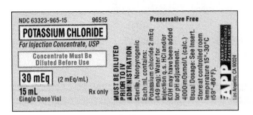

52. oxytocin 25 U   _____

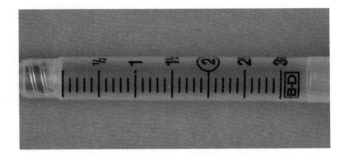

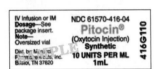

53. epinephrine 1.4 mg   _____

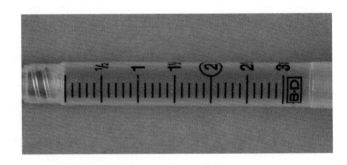

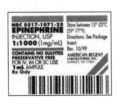

54. heparin Na 4500 U   _____

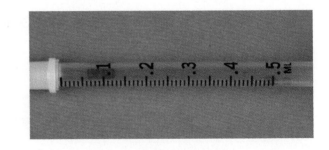

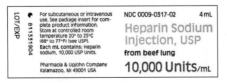

Dosage Ordered   **mL/cc Needed**

55. Depo-Provera® 0.45 g   _____

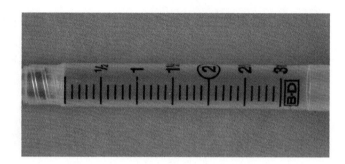

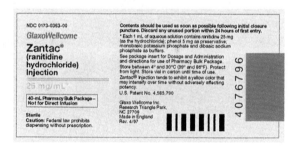

56. ranitidine HCl 35 mg   _____

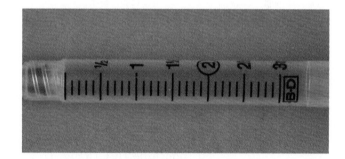

57. furosemide 15 mg   _____

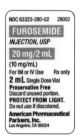
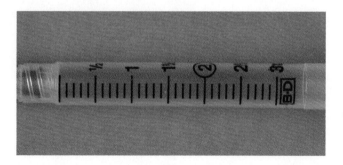

Dosage Ordered	**mL/cc Needed**

58. dexamethasone 6000 mcg   _____

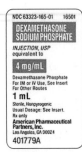

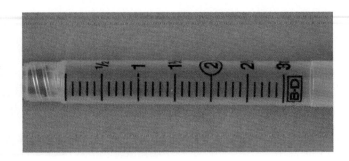

59. phenytoin Na 0.1 g   _____

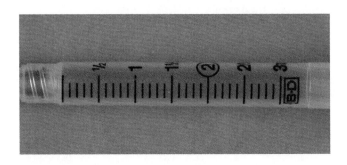

60. lidocaine HCl 15 mg   _____

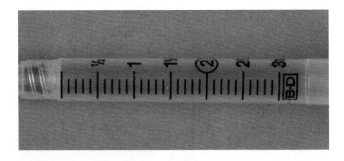

Answers

1. 0.8 mL	**13.** 2.8 mL	**26.** 2.7 mL	**39.** 1.5 mL	**52.** 2.5 mL
2. 1.5 mL	**14.** 2 mL	**27.** 1.3 mL	**40.** 0.8 mL	**53.** 1.4 mL
3. 0.4 mL	**15.** 1.5 mL	**28.** 2.5 mL	**41.** 1.8 mL	**54.** 0.45 mL
4. 5 mL	**16.** 0.45 mL	**29.** 3 mL	**42.** 16 mL	**55.** 1.1 mL
5. 0.9 mL	**17.** 0.6 mL	**30.** 8 mL	**43.** 1.3 mL	**56.** 1.4 mL
6. 1.5 mL	**18.** 2 mL	**31.** 1.2 mL	**44.** 1.5 mL	**57.** 1.5 mL
7. 0.38 mL	**19.** 2.3 mL	**32.** 1.6 mL	**45.** 2.4 mL	**58.** 1.5 mL
8. 3 mL	**20.** 1.8 mL	**33.** 4 mL	**46.** 2.5 mL	**59.** 2 mL
9. 2.4 mL	**21.** 2.4 mL	**34.** 1.5 mL	**47.** 0.9 mL	**60.** 0.8 mL
10. 0.8 mL	**22.** 15 mL	**35.** 1.3 mL	**48.** 1.4 mL	
11. 1.6 mL	**23.** 1.5 mL	**36.** 1.6 mL	**49.** 0.7 mL	
12. 2.4 mL	**24.** 0.8 mL	**37.** 0.8 mL	**50.** 0.5 mL	
	25. 1.6 mL	**38.** 1.5 mL	**51.** 10 mL	

Formula Method

BASIC FORMULA

The formula method may be used for simple one-step dosage calculations. It is really just a variation of ratio and proportion and in other texts has occasionally been presented using different initials. If you are familiar with different initials from those used in this chapter, by all means continue to use them. The important thing is the **answer**, not the means of obtaining it.

The initials most commonly used in the formula method are as follows:

$$\frac{\textbf{D}}{\textbf{H}} \times \textbf{Q} = \textbf{X}$$

Here's what these initials mean.

_D_ = desired	The dosage **ordered**, in mg, g, etc.
_H_ = have	The dosage strength **available**, in mg, g, etc.
_Q_ = quantity	The **volume** the dosage strength **available** is contained in, mL, cc, etc.
_X_ = the unknown	The **volume** the **desired** dosage will be contained in

It is necessary to memorize this formula. Stop and do so now. Print the formula several times to help yourself remember it.

The same three precautions that governed calculations using ratio and proportion also apply to the use of the formula: (1) routinely double-check all math; (2) assess each answer to determine if it is logical; and (3) seek help if you have any doubt of your accuracy. Now let's look at some examples of how the formula is used, so you can begin to be comfortable with it.

 The unknown, **_X_**, will always be expressed in the same units of measure as **_Q_**, the volume the dosage available is contained in.

Objective

The learner will:

1. use the formula method to solve simple dosage problems containing metric, U, and mEq dosages

171

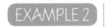 A dosage of **80 mg** is ordered. The dosage strength available is **100 mg in 2 mL**. Calculate the mL necessary to administer this dosage.

The desired dosage (*D*) is 80 mg. You have (*H*) 100 mg in (*Q*) 2 mL available. Remember that *X* will always be expressed in the same units of measure as *Q*, which in this problem is mL. To ensure accuracy **always set up the formula with the units of measure included**.

$$\frac{(D) \quad 80 \text{ mg}}{(H) \quad 100 \text{ mg}} \times (Q) \, 2 \text{ mL} = X \text{ mL}$$

$$\frac{80}{100} \times 2 = X = \textbf{1.6 mL}$$

To give a dosage of 80 mg you must administer 1.6 mL.

After you have double-checked your math, **look at your answer to see if it is logical**. The dosage strength available is 100 mg in 2 mL. **To prepare** 80 mg, which is **a smaller dosage, you will need a smaller volume**. Your answer, 1.6 mL, is smaller; therefore, it is logical.

 The dosage ordered is **0.4 mg**. The strength available is **0.25 mg in 1.2 mL**.

The desired dosage (*D*) is 0.4 mg. You have (*H*) 0.25 mg in (*Q*) 1.2 mL.

$$\frac{0.4 \text{ mg}}{0.25 \text{ mg}} \times 1.2 \text{ mL} = X \text{ mL}$$

$$\frac{0.4}{0.25} \times 1.2 = X = 1.92 = \textbf{1.9 mL}$$

To give a dosage of 0.4 mg you must administer 1.9 mL.

0.4 mg is a larger dosage than 0.25 mg and the volume that contains it must be larger, which it is, 1.9 mL.

 A dosage of **750 mcg** has been ordered. The strength available is **1000 mcg per mL**.

$$\frac{750 \text{ mcg}}{1000 \text{ mcg}} \times 1 \text{ mL} = X \text{ mL}$$

$$\frac{750}{1000} \times 1 = X = 0.75 = \textbf{0.8 mL}$$

To give a dosage of 750 mcg you must administer 0.8 mL.

The answer should be a smaller quantity than 1 mL, and it is, 0.8 mL.

PROBLEM

Determine the volume that will contain the dosage ordered in the following problems. Express your answers as decimal fractions to the nearest tenth.

1. A dosage of 0.8 g has been ordered. The strength available is 1 g in 2.5 mL. _____

2. You have available a dosage strength of 250 mg in 1.5 mL. The order is for 200 mg. _____

3. The strength available is 1 g in 5 mL. The order is for 0.2 g. _____

4. A dosage of 300 mcg has been ordered. The strength available is 500 mcg in 1.2 mL. _____

Answers **1.** 2 mL **2.** 1.2 mL **3.** 1 mL **4.** 0.7 mL

USE WITH METRIC CONVERSIONS

Consider the following problem:

A dosage of 200 mcg is ordered. The strength available is 0.3 mg in 1.5 mL.

This problem cannot be solved as it is now written. The drug strengths, *D* and *H*, are in different units of measure. One of them must be changed before the problem can be solved.

 The drug strengths, D and H, must be expressed in the same units of measure.

 EXAMPLE 1 A dosage of **200 mcg** is ordered. The strength available is **0.3 mg in 1.5 mL**.

• **Convert mg to mcg.**

0.3 mg = 300 mcg

• **Use the formula for the calculation.**

$$\frac{200 \text{ mcg}}{300 \text{ mcg}} \times 1.5 \text{ mL} = X \text{ mL}$$

$$\frac{200}{300} \times 1.5 \text{ mL} = \textbf{1 mL}$$

To give 200 mcg you must administer 1 mL.

Your answer must be a smaller quantity than 1.5 mL, and it is, 1 mL. Therefore, it is logical.

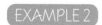 **EXAMPLE 2** A dosage of **0.7 g** has been ordered. Available is a strength of **1000 mg in 1.5 mL**.

• **Convert g to mg.**

0.7 g = 700 mg

• **Use the formula for the calculation.**

$$\frac{700 \text{ mg}}{1000 \text{ mg}} \times 1.5 \text{ mL} = X \text{ mL}$$

$$\frac{700}{1000} \times 1.5 \text{ mL} = 1.05 = \textbf{1.1 mL}$$

To give 0.7 g you must administer 1.1 mL.

The answer should be less than 1.5 mL, which it is, 1.1 mL.

PROBLEM

Determine the volume that will be required to prepare the following dosages. Express your answers to the nearest tenth.

1. The dosage ordered is 780 mcg. The strength available is 1 mg per mL. _____

2. The available dosage strength is 0.1 g per mL. The dosage ordered is 250 mg. _____

3. Prepare a dosage of 0.6 mg from an available strength of 1000 mcg per 2 mL. _____

4. A dosage of 0.4 g has been ordered. The strength available is 500 mg per 1.3 mL. _____

Answers   **1.** 0.8 mL   **2.** 2.5 mL   **3.** 1.2 mL   **4.** 1 mL

USE WITH U AND mEq CALCULATIONS

Dosages expressed in U or mEq are handled in exactly the same way.

 A dosage of **7500 U** is ordered. The available strength is **10,000 U per mL**.

$$\frac{7500 \text{ U}}{10,000 \text{ U}} \times 1 \text{ mL} = X \text{ mL}$$

$$\frac{7500}{10,000} \times 1 = 0.75 = \textbf{0.8 mL}$$

To give 7500 U administer 0.8 mL.

The dosage ordered is less than the strength available and must be contained in a smaller volume of solution than 1 mL, which it is, 0.8 mL.

 A dosage strength of **40 mEq in 5 mL** is available. You are to prepare **30 mEq**.

$$\frac{30 \text{ mEq}}{40 \text{ mEq}} \times 5 \text{ mL} = X \text{ mL}$$

$$\frac{30}{40} \times 5 = 3.75 = \textbf{3.8 mL}$$

A volume of 3.8 mL is necessary to prepare a 30 mEq dosage.

The dosage ordered, 30 mEq, is less than the dosage strength of the solution available. It must be contained in a smaller volume than 5 mL, and the answer, 3.8 mL, indicates that it is.

PROBLEM

Determine the volume that will contain the following dosages. Express your answers to the nearest tenth.

1. A dosage strength of 1000 U per 1.5 mL is available. Prepare a 1250 U dosage. _____

2. A dosage of 45 U has been ordered. The strength available is 80 U per mL. _____

3. The IV solution available has a strength of 200 mEq per 20 mL. You are to prepare a 50 mEq dosage. _____

4. The strength available is 80 mEq per 5 mL. Prepare 30 mEq. _____

Answers **1.** 1.9 mL **2.** 0.6 mL **3.** 5 mL **4.** 1.9 mL

Summary

This concludes the chapter on using the formula method to solve simple dosage calculations. The important points to remember from this chapter are:

- The formula method can be used to solve problems expressed in metric, U, and mEq dosages.

- When the formula method is used, D and H, the dosage strengths, must be expressed in the same units of measure.

- The answer obtained, X, will always be in the same unit of measure as Q, the quantity.

- The math of all calculations is routinely double-checked.

- A logical assessment of the answer you obtain is a routine step in calculations.

Summary Self-Test

Calculate the volume of medication in mL necessary to administer the dosages ordered in the following problems. Express your answers as decimal fractions to the nearest tenth.

1. A 50 mg dosage has been ordered. The strength available is 60 mg in 1.5 mL. _____

2. Prepare a 300 mcg dosage. The dosage available is 0.4 mg/mL. _____

3. Prepare 0.45 g. The strength available is 300 mg/mL. _____

4. The medication is labeled 5 mg/mL. An 8 mg dosage has been ordered. _____

5. Prepare a 70 mg dosage from a solution labeled 250 mg in 5 mL. _____

6. The drug is labeled 25 mg per mL; 30 mg has been ordered. _____

7. The label reads 50 mg/mL. Prepare a 60 mg dosage. _____

8. The order is for 12 mg. The vial is labeled 5 mg per mL. _____

9. A dosage of 7 mg has been ordered. The vial labels reads 10 mg per mL. _____

10. The dosage strength is 10 mg/1 mL; 8 mg has been ordered. _____

11. Prepare a 0.3 g dosage from a medication labeled 900 mg per 6 mL. _____

12. Prepare a 300 mg IV dosage from a vial labeled 0.5 g/20 mL. _____

13. The vial is labeled 0.5 g per 2 mL. A dosage of 750 mg has been ordered. _____

14. Prepare a dosage of 0.2 mg from an available dosage of 250 mcg/5 mL. _____

15. The order is for 130 mg and the single-use ampule is labeled 0.1 g per 2 mL. _____

16. Draw up a 12 mg dosage from a vial labeled 15 mg in 5 mL. _____

17. The ampule is labeled 20 mg/2 mL. Prepare 14 mg. _____

18. The medication is labeled 1.2 g per 30 mL. Draw up an 800 mg dosage for IV administration. _____

19. Prepare an 80 mg dosage of a medication labeled 100 mg in 2 mL. _____

20. The solution strength is 0.4 mg per mL. A dosage of 300 mcg has been ordered. _____

21. Prepare a 600 mg dosage from an available dosage strength of 0.4 g/mL. _____

22. Draw up a 60 mEq dosage for addition to an IV from a solution labeled 40 mEq per 20 mL. _____

23. The label reads 400 mcg/mL; 0.6 mg has been ordered. _____

24. Prepare a 60 mg dosage from a 75 mg/mL strength. _____

25. Prepare a 0.1 g dosage from a vial labeled 40 mg/mL. _____

26. The drug is labeled 50 mg/10 mL. The order is for 8 mg. _____

27. Measure a 0.8 mg dosage from an available strength of 1000 mcg/cc. _____

28. Prepare 40 mg from a vial labeled 25 mg per mL. _____

29. A dosage of 10 mg has been ordered. You have available a strength of 4000 mcg per mL. _____

30. Prepare 200 mg for IV use of a medication labeled 0.25 g per 25 mL. _____

31. The dosage strength available is 15 mg in 1 mL; 10 mg has been ordered. _____

32. Prepare a 4 mg dosage from a strength available of 5 mg/mL. _____

33. A dosage of 75 U has been ordered from an available strength of 90 U in 1.5 mL. _____

34. You are to prepare 100 mEq for addition to an IV solution. The solution available is labeled 80 mEq per 20 mL. _____

35. Prepare a dosage of 180 mg from a 0.15 g in 1 mL solution. _____

36. Prepare a 750 U dosage from an available strength of 1000 U/mL. _____

37. Draw up a 60 mEq dosage for addition to IV solution from a vial labeled 40 mEq/20 mL. _____

38. 400,000 U have been ordered and you have available 300,000 U in 1 mL. _____

39. A dosage of 0.2 mg per 2 mL is available. Prepare a 250 mcg dosage. _____

40. A dosage of 35 mEq has been ordered for addition to an IV solution. The solution is labeled 50 mEq per 50 mL. _____

Answers
1. 1.3 mL
2. 0.8 mL
3. 1.5 mL
4. 1.6 mL
5. 1.4 mL
6. 1.2 mL
7. 1.2 mL
8. 2.4 mL
9. 0.7 mL
10. 0.8 mL
11. 2 mL
12. 12 mL
13. 3 mL
14. 4 mL
15. 2.6 mL
16. 4 mL
17. 1.4 mL
18. 20 mL
19. 1.6 mL
20. 0.8 mL
21. 1.5 mL
22. 30 mL
23. 1.5 mL
24. 0.8 mL
25. 2.5 mL
26. 1.6 mL
27. 0.8 cc
28. 1.6 mL
29. 2.5 mL
30. 20 mL
31. 0.7 mL
32. 0.8 mL
33. 1.3 mL
34. 25 mL
35. 1.2 mL
36. 0.8 mL
37. 30 mL
38. 1.3 mL
39. 2.5 mL
40. 35 mL

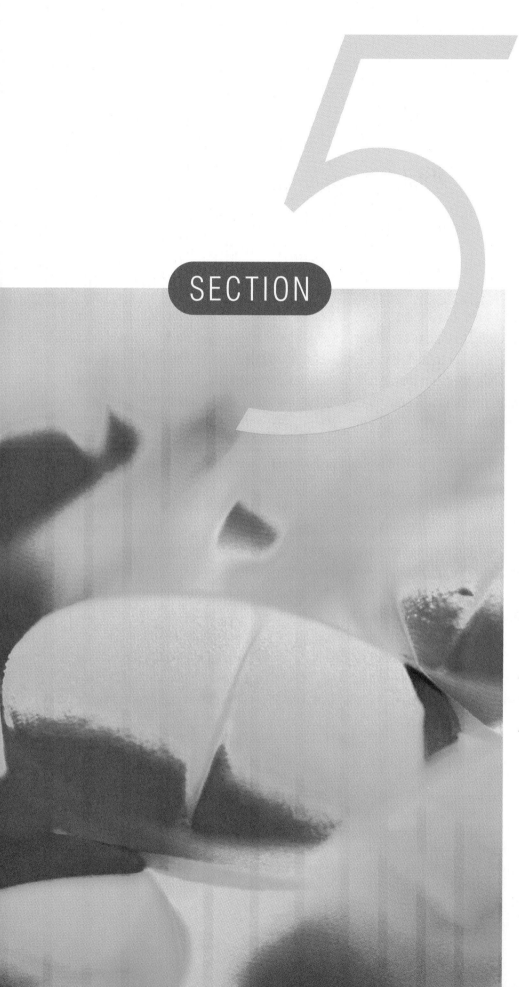

SECTION 5

Dosage Calculation from Body Weight and Body Surface Area

13

Adult and Pediatric Dosages Based on Body Weight

Objectives

The learner will:

1. convert body weight from lb to kg

2. convert body weight from kg to lb

3. calculate dosages using mg/kg, mcg/kg, mg/lb

4. determine if dosages ordered are within the normal range

Body weight is a major factor in calculating drug dosages for both adults and children. It is the most important determiner of dosages for infants and neonates, whose ability to metabolize drugs is not fully developed. The dosage that will produce optimum therapeutic results for any particular individual, either child or adult, depends not only on dosage but on individual variables, including drug sensitivities and tolerance, age, weight, sex, and metabolic, pathologic, or psychologic conditions.

The doctor will, of course, order the drug and dosage. However, it is a nursing responsibility to check each dosage to be sure the order is correct. Each drug label or drug package insert provides specific dosage details, but more complete information is readily available in drug formularies, the *PDR*, and other nursing and medical references. The hospital pharmacist is an excellent resource person who can also supply additional information.

Individualized dosages may be calculated in terms of mcg or mg per kg or lb, per day. The total daily dosage may be administered in divided (more than one) dosages, for example, q.6.h. (four doses), or t.i.d. (three doses).

Because body weight is critical in calculating infant and neonatal dosages, measurement is done using a scale calibrated in kg. Adult weights may be recorded in either kg or lb, and, occasionally, conversions between these two measures are necessary.

CONVERTING lb TO kg

If body weight is recorded in lb, but the drug literature lists dosage per kg, a conversion from lb to kg will be necessary. There are 2.2 lb in 1 kg. This means that kg body weights are smaller than lb weights, so **the conversion from lb to kg is made by dividing body weight by 2.2**. For ease of calculation, fractional lb may be converted to the nearest quarter lb, and written as decimal fractions instead of oz: ¼ lb (4 oz) as 0.25, ½ lb (8 oz) as 0.5, and ¾ lb (12 oz) as 0.75.

EXAMPLE 1 | A child weighs 41 lb 12 oz. Convert to kg.

41 lb 12 oz = 41.75 ÷ 2.2 = 18.97 = **19 kg**

The kg weight should be a smaller number than 41.75 because you are dividing, and it is, 19 kg.

EXAMPLE 2 | Convert the weight of a 144½ lb adult to kg.

144½ = 144.5 ÷ 2.2 = 65.68 = **65.7 kg**

EXAMPLE 3 | Convert the weight of a 27¼ lb child to kg.

27¼ lb = 27.25 ÷ 2.2 = 12.38 = **12.4 kg**

PROBLEM

Convert the following body weights from lb to kg. Round weights to the nearest tenth kg.

1. 58¾ lb	= _____ kg		6. 134½	= _____ kg
2. 63½ lb	= _____ kg		7. 112¾	= _____ kg
3. 163¼	= _____ kg		8. 73¼	= _____ kg
4. 39¾	= _____ kg		9. 121½	= _____ kg
5. 100¼	= _____ kg		10. 92¾	= _____ kg

Answers **1.** 26.7 kg **2.** 28.9 kg **3.** 74.2 kg **4.** 18.1 kg **5.** 45.6 kg **6.** 61.1 kg **7.** 51.3 kg **8.** 33.3 kg **9.** 55.2 kg **10.** 42.2 kg

CONVERTING kg TO lb

There are 2.2 lb in 1 kg. To convert from kg to lb, **multiply by 2.2**. Because you are multiplying, the answer, in lb, will be **larger** than the kg you started with. Express weight to the nearest tenth lb.

EXAMPLE 1 | A child weighs 23.3 kg. Convert to lb.

23.3 kg = 23.2 × 2.2 = 51.26 = **51.3 lb**

The answer must be larger because you are multiplying, and it is.

EXAMPLE 2 | Convert an adult weight of 73.4 kg to lb.

73.4 kg = 73.4 × 2.2 = 161.48 = **161.5 lb**

EXAMPLE 3 | Convert the weight of a 14.2 kg child to lb.

14.2 kg = 14.2 × 2.2 = 31.24 = **31.2 lb**

PROBLEM

Convert the following body weights from kg to lb. Round weights to the nearest tenth lb.

1. 21.3 kg   = _____ lb   6. 43.7 kg   = _____ lb

2. 99.2 kg   = _____ lb   7. 63.8 kg   = _____ lb

3. 28.7 kg   = _____ lb   8. 57.1 kg   = _____ lb

4. 71.4 kg   = _____ lb   9. 84.2 kg   = _____ lb

5. 30.8 kg   = _____ lb   10. 34.9 kg   = _____ lb

Answers   **1.** 46.9 lb   **2.** 218.2 lb   **3.** 63.1 lb   **4.** 157.1 lb   **5.** 67.8 lb   **6.** 96.1 lb   **7.** 140.4 lb   **8.** 125.6 lb   **9.** 185.2 lb
10. 76.8 lb

CALCULATING DOSAGES FROM DRUG LABEL INFORMATION

Information you will need to calculate dosages from body weight may be on the actual drug label, which is common for pediatric oral liquid medications.

Calculating the dosage is a two-step procedure. First the **total daily dosage** is calculated, then it is **divided by the number of doses per day** to obtain the actual dose administered at one time.

Let's start by looking at some pediatric oral antibiotic labels that contain the mg/kg/day dosage guidelines.

EXAMPLE 1 | Refer to the information written sideways on the left of the Polymox® label in Figure 13-1 for children's dosages. Notice that the average dosage range is 20–40 mg/kg/day. This dosage is to be given in divided doses every 8 hours, or a total of 3 doses (24 hr ÷ 8 hr).

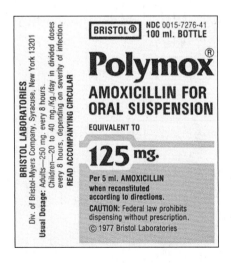

Figure 13-1

Once you have located the dosage information, you can move ahead and calculate the dosage. Let's assume you are checking the dosage ordered for an 18.2 kg child. Start by calculating the **recommended daily dosage range**.

Lower daily dosage = 20 mg/kg

20 mg × 18.2 kg (weight of child) = 364 mg/day

Upper daily dosage = 40 mg/kg

40 mg × 18.2 kg = 728 mg/day

The recommended range for this 18.2 kg child is **364–728 mg/day**.

The drug is to be given in three divided doses.

Lower dosage 364 mg ÷ 3 = **121 mg per dose**

Upper dosage 728 mg ÷ 3 = **243 mg per dose**

The per dose dosage range is **121 mg to 243 mg per dose q.8.h.**

Now that you have the dosage range for this child, you are able to assess the accuracy of physician orders. Let's look at some orders and see how you can use the dosage range you just calculated.

1. **If the order is to give 125 mg q.8.h., is this within the recommended dosage range?**
   Yes, 125 mg q.8.h. is within the average range of 121–243 mg per dose.

2. **If the order is to give 375 mg q.8.h., is this within the recommended dosage range?**
   No, this is an overdosage. The maximum recommended dosage is 243 mg per dose. The 375 mg dose should not be given; the doctor must be called and the order questioned.

3. **If the order is for 75 mg q.8.h., is this an accurate dosage?**
   The recommended lower limit for an 18.2 kg child is 121 mg. Although 75 mg might be safe, it will probably be ineffective. Notify the doctor that the dosage appears to be too low.

4. **If the order is for 250 mg q.8.h., is this accurate?**
   Because 243 mg per dose is the recommended upper limit, 250 mg q.8.h. is essentially within normal range. The drug strength is 125 mg per 5 mL, and a 250 mg dosage is 10 mL. The doctor has probably ordered this dosage based on the available dosage strength and for ease of preparation.

 Discrepancies in dosages are much more significant if the number of mg ordered is small.

For example, the difference between 4 mg and 6 mg is much more critical than the difference between 243 mg and 250 mg, because the drug potency is obviously greater. Additional factors that must be considered are age, weight, and medical condition. Although these factors cannot be dealt with at length, keep in mind that **the younger, the older, or more compromised by illness the patient is, the more critical a discrepancy is likely to be.**

5. **If the dosage ordered is 125 mg q.4.h., is this an accurate dosage?**
   In this order the frequency of administration, q.4.h., does not match the recommended q.8.h. The total daily dosage of 750 mg (125 mg × 6 doses = 750 mg) is slightly, but not significantly, higher than the 728 mg maximum. There may be a reason the doctor ordered the q.4.h. dosage, but call to verify the order.

 To determine the safety of an ordered dosage, use the patient's weight to calculate the dosage range ordered, and compare this with the recommended dosage range in mg/kg/day (or mg/lb/day). Assessment must also include the frequency of dosage ordered.

PROBLEM

Refer to the cloxacillin (Tegopen®) label in Figure 13-2 and answer the following questions.

1. What is the average children's dosage?   _____

2. How is this dosage to be administered?   _____

3. How many divided doses will this be in 24 hours?   _____

4. What will the total daily dose be for a child weighing 10.4 kg?   _____

5. The dosage strength of this oral cloxacillin solution is 125 mg per 5 mL, and the doctor has ordered 125 mg q.6.h for this 10.4 kg child. Is there any need to question this order?   _____

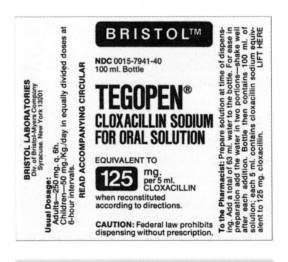

Figure 13-2

Answers **1.** 50 mg/kg/day **2.** Equal doses q.6.h. **3.** 4 doses in 24 hr. **4.** 520 mg **5.** No

PROBLEM

Refer to the ampicillin (Principen®) label in Figure 13-3. Answer the following questions for a 20 lb child.

1. What is the child's body weight in kg to the nearest tenth kg? _____

2. What is the recommended dosage in mg per day for this child? _____

3. How many doses will this be divided into? _____

4. How many mg will this be per dose? _____

5. The order is to give 250 mg q.6.h. Is this dosage accurate? _____

6. How many mL would you need to administer a 250 mg dosage? _____

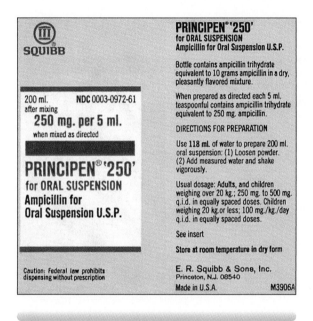

Figure 13-3

Answers **1.** 9.1 kg **2.** 910 mg/day **3.** 4 doses **4.** 227.5 mg/dose **5.** Yes **6.** 5 mL

CALCULATING DOSAGES FROM DRUG LITERATURE

The labels you have just been reading were from oral syrups and suspensions, but the same calculation steps are necessary for dosages to be administered by the IV or IM route. Parenteral labels are much smaller in size and usually do not include dosage recommendations. To obtain these, you will have to refer to the drug package inserts, the *PDR*, or similar references. These references will contain extensive details about each drug's chemistry, actions, adverse reactions, recommended administration, and so on, so it will be necessary for you to search for and select the information you need under the heading "Dosage and Administration." In the following exercises the searching has been done for you, and only those excerpts necessary for your calculations are shown.

PROBLEM

Refer to the cefazolin (Kefzol®) insert in Figure 13-4 and locate the following information for pediatric dosages.

1. What is the dosage range in mg/kg/day for mild to moderate infections? _____

2. What is the dosage range for mild to moderate infections in mg/lb/day? _____

3. The total dosage will be divided into how many doses per day? _____

4. In severe infections, what is the maximum daily dosage recommended in mg/kg? _____

   in mg/lb? _____

KEFZOL®, STERILE CEFAZOLIN SODIUM, USP

ADMINISTRATION AND DOSAGE

In children, a total daily dosage of 25 to 50 mg/kg (approximately 10 to 20 mg/lb) of body weight, divided into 3 or 4 equal doses, is effective for most mild to moderately severe infections (Table 5). Total daily dosage may be increased to 100 mg/kg (45 mg/lb) of body weight for severe infections.

TABLE 5. PEDIATRIC DOSAGE GUIDE

Weight		25 mg/kg/Day Divided into 3 Doses		25 mg/kg/Day Divided into 4 Doses	
lb	kg	Approximate Single Dose (mg q8h)	Vol (mL) Needed with Dilution of 125 mg/mL	Approximate Single Dose (mg q6h)	Vol (mL) Needed with Dilution of 125 mg/mL
10	4.5	40 mg	0.35 mL	30 mg	0.25 mL
20	9	75 mg	0.6 mL	55 mg	0.45 mL
30	13.6	115 mg	0.9 mL	85 mg	0.7 mL
40	18.1	150 mg	1.2 mL	115 mg	0.9 mL
50	22.7	190 mg	1.5 mL	140 mg	1.1 mL

Weight		50 mg/kg/Day Divided into 3 Doses		50 mg/kg/Day Divided into 4 Doses	
lb	kg	Approximate Single Dose (mg q8h)	Vol (mL) Needed with Dilution of 225 mg/mL	Approximate Single Dose (mg q6h)	Vol (mL) Needed with Dilution of 225 mg/mL
10	4.5	75 mg	0.35 mL	55 mg	0.25 mL
20	9	150 mg	0.7 mL	110 mg	0.5 mL
30	13.6	225 mg	1 mL	170 mg	0.75 mL
40	18.1	300 mg	1.35 mL	225 mg	1 mL
50	22.7	375 mg	1.7 mL	285 mg	1.25 mL

Figure 13-4

Answers **1.** 25 mg–50 mg **2.** 10 mg–20 mg **3.** 3–4 doses per day **4.** 100 mg/kg; 45 mg/lb

Notice that in this table sample dosages are provided for several kg and lb weights, for both the 25 mg and 50 mg dosage, and for both 3 and 4 doses per day. Tables of this sort may be helpful or harmful. They are helpful if they are easy to understand and the child whose dosage you are calculating fits exactly one of the weights listed; they are harmful if they tend to confuse, which could happen.

PROBLEM

Use the information you just obtained for Kefzol to do the following calculations for a child who weighs 35 lb and has a moderately severe infection.

1. What is the lower daily dosage range? _____

2. What is the upper daily dosage range? _____

3. If the medication is given in four divided dosages, what will the per dosage range be? _____

4. If a dosage of 125 mg q.6.h. is ordered, will you need to question it? _____

Answers **1.** 350 mg/day **2.** 700 mg/day **3.** 87.5 mg to 175 mg per dose **4.** No; within normal range

PROBLEM

Refer to the dosage information on Mezlin® in Figure 13-5 and answer the following questions about adult IV dosages.

1. What is the recommended daily dosage range for serious infections? _____

2. How many divided doses and at what intervals should this dosage be given? _____

3. What is the maximum daily dosage? _____

4. Calculate the daily dosage range in g for a 176 lb adult. _____

5. If this dosage is to be given q.6.h., what will the individual dosage range be? _____

6. If a dosage of 2 g is ordered, what initial assessment would you make about it? _____

7. If a dosage of 10 g q.6.h. is ordered, what assessment would you make? _____

DOSAGE AND ADMINISTRATION
MEZLIN® (sterile mezlocillin sodium) may be administered intravenously or intramuscularly. For serious infections, the intravenous route of administration should be used. Intramuscular doses should not exceed 2g per injection.
The recommended adult dosage for serious infections is 200-300 mg/kg per day given in 4 to 6 divided doses. The usual dose is 3g given every 4 hours (18g/day) or 4g given every 6 hours (16g/day). For life-threatening infections, up to 350 mg/kg per day may be administered, but the total daily dosage should ordinarily not exceed 24g.
[See table below.]
For patients with life-threatening infections, 4g may be administered every 4 hours (24g/day).

Figure 13-5

Answers **1.** 200 mg/kg to 300 mg/kg **2.** 4 to 6 doses; q.6.h. or q.4.h. **3.** 24 g **4.** 16 g–24 g **5.** 4 g–6 g **6.** The dosage is too low
7. The dosage is too high

PROBLEM

Refer to the dosage recommendations for Mithracin® in Figure 13-6 and answer the following questions for treatment of testicular tumors in a patient weighing 240 lb.

1. What is the recommended daily dosage range in mcg/kg? _____

2. How often is this dosage to be given and for how long?

   _____   _____

3. What is the daily dosage range in mcg for this patient? in mg? (Calculate kg weight to the nearest tenth.) _____   _____

4. If a dosage of 3 mg IV q.a.m. is ordered, does this need to be questioned? _____

Answers **1.** 25–30 mcg/kg **2.** 1× day; 8–10 days **3.** 2728–3273 mcg/day; 2.7–3.3 mg/day **4.** No; within normal range

MITHRACIN® ℞
(plicamycin)
FOR INTRAVENOUS USE

DOSAGE
The daily dose of Mithracin is based on the patient's body weight. If a patient has abnormal fluid retention such as edema, hydrothorax or ascites, the patient's ideal weight rather than actual body weight should be used to calculate the dose.
Treatment of Testicular Tumors: In the treatment of patients with testicular tumors the recommended daily dose of Mithracin (plicamycin) is 25 to 30 mcg (0.025–0.030 mg) per kilogram of body weight. Therapy should be continued for a period of 8 to 10 days unless significant side effects or toxicity occur during therapy. A course of therapy consisting of more than 10 daily doses is not recommended. Individual daily doses should not exceed 30 mcg (0.030 mg) per kilogram of body weight.

VELOSEF® for INJECTION
Cephradine for Injection USP

DOSAGE AND ADMINISTRATION

Infants and Children
The usual dosage range of VELOSEF is 50 to 100 mg/kg/day (approximately 23 to 45 mg/lb/day) in equally divided doses four times a day and should be regulated by age, weight of the patient and severity of the infection being treated.

PEDIATRIC DOSAGE GUIDE				
		50 mg/kg/day		100 mg/kg/day	
Weight		Approx. single dose mg q6h	Volume needed @ 208 mg/mL dilution	Approx. single dose mg q6h	Volume needed @ 227 mg/mL dilution
lbs	kg				
10	4.5	56 mg	0.27 mL	112 mg	0.5 mL
20	9.1	114 mg	0.55 mL	227 mg	1 mL
30	13.6	170 mg	0.82 mL	340 mg	1.5 mL
40	18.2	227 mg	1.1 mL	455 mg	2 mL
50	22.7	284 mg	1.4 mL	567 mg	2.5 mL

Figure 13-6

Figure 13-7

PROBLEM

Refer to the cephradine (Velosef®) literature in Figure 13-7 and answer the following questions.

1. What is the daily dosage range in mg/kg/day? _____

2. What is the daily dosage range in mg/lb/day? _____

3. What is the recommended number of dosages per day? _____

4. What will the daily dosage range be for a child weighing 12.6 kg? _____

5. What is the dosage range per dose for this child? _____

6. Is an order for cephradine 250 mg q.6.h. within the dosage range? _____

7. What is the daily dosage range for a child weighing 19½ lb? _____

8. What will the q.6.h. dose be for this child? _____

9. Is 340 mg q.6.h. within the ordered range? _____

Answers **1.** 50–100 mg/kg/day **2.** 23–45 mg/lb/day **3.** 4 doses per day **4.** 630–1260 mg/day **5.** 158–315 mg/dose **6.** Yes
7. 449–876 mg/day **8.** 112–219 mg/dose **9.** No, too high. Check with the physician.

Summary

This concludes the chapter on calculation and assessment of dosages based on body weight. The important points to remember from this chapter are:

- Dosages are frequently ordered on the basis of weight, especially for children.

- Dosages may be recommended based on mcg or mg per kg or lb per day, usually in divided doses.

- Body weight may need to be converted from kg to lb, or lb to kg, to correlate with dosage recommendations.

- To convert lb to kg divide by 2.2; to convert kg to lb multiply by 2.2.

- Calculating dosage is a two-step procedure: first calculate the total daily dosage for the weight; then divide this by the number of doses to be administered.

- To check the accuracy of a doctor's order, calculate the correct dosage and compare it with the dosage ordered.

- Dosage discrepancies are much more critical if the dosage range is low, for example, 2–5 mg, as opposed to high, for example, 250 mg.

- Factors that make discrepancies particularly serious are age, low body weight, and severity of medical condition.

- If the drug label does not contain all the necessary information for safe administration, additional information should be obtained from drug package inserts, the *PDR*, drug formularies, or the hospital pharmacist.

Summary Self-Test

Read the dosage labels and literature provided to indicate if dosages are within normal safety limits. If they are not, give the correct range. Express body weight conversions to the nearest tenth, and dosages to the nearest whole number in your calculations.

1. A 48 lb child has an order for cefaclor 250 mg q.6.h. What is the daily dosage for this child? What is the per dose dosage? Is the ordered dosage for this child correct?

   _____   _____   _____

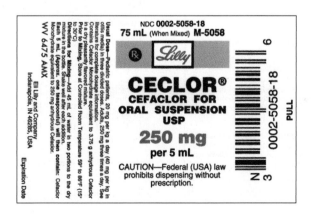

2. Zinacef® (cefuroxime) 375 mg has been ordered IV q.8.h. for a child weighing 20.1 kg. Calculate the per day and q.8.h. per dose dosage ranges. Is the ordered dosage correct?

_____ _____ _____

3. Cefuroxime also has been ordered for a child weighing 84 lb. If this medication is given q.6.h., what will be the dosage range per day, and per dose?

_____ _____

4. Oxacillin 250 mg has been ordered q.6.h. for a 43 lb child. Calculate the per dose dosage, and determine if this order is correct.

_____ _____

5. Prostaphlin® oral solution has been ordered for a 21 lb child. A dosage of 125 mg q.6.h. has been ordered. Calculate the daily and per dose dosage. Is this dosage correct?

_____ _____ _____

6. A 140 lb adult has an order for IV methylprednisolone. Calculate this patient's per dose dosage.

_____

7. A 7.9 kg infant has an order for Veetids® 125 mg q.8.h. Calculate the per dose dosage based on this infant's body weight. Is the dosage ordered correct?

_____ _____

ZINACEF®
[zin 'ah-sef]
(sterile cefuroxime sodium, Glaxo)

DOSAGE AND ADMINISTRATION

Infants and Children Above 3 Months of Age: Administration of 50 to 100 mg/kg/day in equally divided doses every six to eight hours has been successful for most infections susceptible to cefuroxime. The higher dose of 100 mg/kg/day (not to exceed the maximum adult dose) should be used for the more severe or serious infections.
In bone and joint infections, 150 mg/kg/day (not to exceed the maximum adult dose) is recommended in equally divided doses every eight hours. In clinical trials a course of oral antibiotics was administered to children following the completion of parenteral administration of ZINACEF.
In cases of bacterial meningitis, larger doses of ZINACEF are recommended, 200 to 240 mg/kg/day intravenously in divided doses every six to eight hours.
In children with renal insufficiency, the frequency of dosage should be modified consistent with the recommendations for adults.

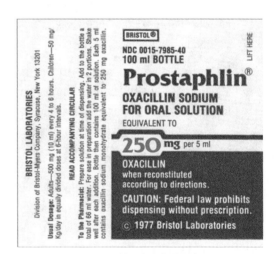

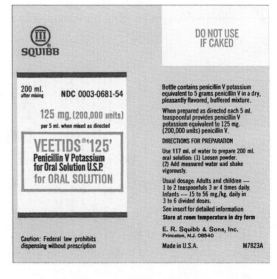

SOLU-MEDROL®
brand of methylprednisolone sodium succinate sterile powder
(methylprednisolone sodium succinate for injection, USP)
For Intravenous or Intramuscular Administration

DOSAGE AND ADMINISTRATION
When high dose therapy is desired, the recommended dose of SOLU-MEDROL Sterile Powder (methylprednisolone sodium succinate) is 30 mg/kg administered intravenously over at least 30 minutes. This dose may be repeated every 4 to 6 hours for 48 hours.

Dosage may be reduced for infants and children but should be governed more by the severity of the condition and response of the patient than by age or size. It should not be less than 0.5 mg per kg every 24 hours.

8. A 130 mg q.8.h. dosage of Vancocin® IV has been ordered for a child weighing 9.7 kg. Calculate the per dose dosage, and determine if this order is correct.   _____   _____

9. Another child weighing 25.1 kg has an IV order for vancomycin. Calculate the per day and q.8.h. per dose dosages.   _____   _____

10. Amoxil® oral suspension 125 mg q.8.h. has been ordered for an infant weighing 6.4 kg. Calculate the per dose dosage range. Is this a correct dosage?   _____   _____

11. Calculate the q.8.h. dosage of amoxicillin suspension for a child weighing 41½ lb who has a severe infection. The Amoxil has a dosage strength of 250 mg/5 mL. What per dose dosage would you expect to be ordered from this available dosage strength?   _____   _____

12. A child weighing 15.9 kg with a diagnosis of bacterial meningitis has an order for cefuroxime sodium 850 mg q.6.h. IV. From the available information, calculate the per dose range and assess the dosage ordered.   _____   _____

VANCOCIN® HCl
[văn ′kō-sĭn ăch ′sē-ĕl]
(vancomycin hydrochloride)
Sterile, USP
IntraVenous

DOSAGE AND ADMINISTRATION

Patients with Normal Renal Function
Adults —The usual daily intravenous dose is 2 g divided either as 500 mg every 6 hours or 1 g every 12 hours. Each dose should be administered over a period of at least 60 minutes. Other patient factors, such as age or obesity, may call for modification of the usual daily dose.
Children —The total daily intravenous dosage of Vancocin® HCl (vancomycin hydrochloride, Lilly), calculated on the basis of 40 mg/kg of body weight, can be divided and incorporated into the child's 24-hour fluid requirement. Each dose should be administered over a period of at least 60 minutes.
Infants and Neonates —In neonates and young infants, the total daily intravenous dosage may be lower. In both neonates and infants, an initial dose of 15 mg/kg is suggested, followed by 10 mg/kg every 12 hours for neonates in the first week of life and every 8 hours thereafter up to the age of 1 month. Close monitoring of serum concentrations of vancomycin may be warranted in these patients.

KEFUROX™
[kĕf ′ōō-rŏcks]
sterile cefuroxime sodium)

DOSAGE AND ADMINISTRATION

Infants and Children Above 3 Months of Age —Administration of 50 to 100 mg/kg/day in equally divided doses every 6 to 8 hours has been successful for most infections susceptible to cefuroxime. The higher dose of 100 mg/kg/day (not to exceed the maximum adult dose) should be used for the more severe or serious infections.
In cases of bacterial meningitis, larger doses of Kefurox are recommended, initially 200 to 240 mg/kg/day intravenously in divided doses every 6 to 8 hours.

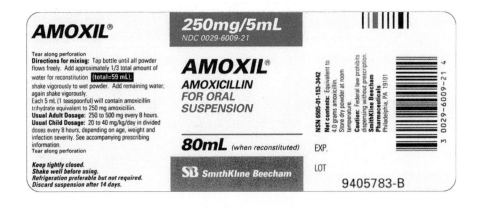

13. A child suffering from a genitourinary tract infection has an order of IV Omnipen®-N 175 mg q.6.h. The child weighs 30¼ lb. What is the recommended per dose dosage? Is the dosage ordered correct?

    _____   _____

14. A 7.7 kg infant has ampicillin 62.5 mg ordered IV q.6.h. for a respiratory infection. Calculate the per dose dosage range, and determine if the dosage ordered is correct.

    _____

15. A dosage of Ancef® 125 mg q.6.h. has been ordered for a child weighing 16 kg. Calculate the per dose dosage range for this child, and decide if it is within the normal range.

    _____

Wyeth®
Omnipen®-N
(ampicillin sodium)
For Parenteral Administration

Dosage (IM or IV)

Infection	Organisms	Adults	Children*
Respiratory tract	streptococci, pneumococci, nonpenicillinase-producing staphylococci, *H. influenzae*	250-500 mg q. 6 h.	25-50 mg/kg/day in equal doses q. 6 h.
Gastrointestinal tract	susceptible pathogens	500 mg q. 6 h.	50 mg/kg/day in equal doses q. 6 h.
Genitourinary tract	susceptible gram-negative or gram-positive pathogens	500 mg q. 6 h.	50 mg/kg/day in equal doses q. 6 h.
Urethritis (acute) in adult males	*N. gonorrhoeae*	500 mg b.i.d. for 1 day (IM)	
	(In complications such as prostatitis and epididymitis, prolonged and intensive therapy is recommended. Gonorrhea cases with suspected primary lesion of syphilis should have dark-field examinations before treatment. In any case suspected of concomitant syphilis, monthly serologic tests for at least 4 months are necessary.)		
Bacterial meningitis	*N. meningitidis,* *H. influenzae*	8-14 gram/day	100-200 mg/kg/ day
	(Initial treatment is usually by IV drip, followed by frequent [q. 3-4 h.] IM injections.) *S. viridans*		

*Children's dosage recommendations are intended for those whose weight will not result in a dosage higher than for the adult.

ANCEF®
brand of
sterile cefazolin sodium
and
cefazolin sodium
injection

Pediatric Dosage
In children, a total daily dosage of 25 to 50 mg per kg (approximately 10 to 20 mg per pound) of body weight, divided into three or four equal doses, is effective for most mild to moderately severe infections. Total daily dosage may be increased to 100 mg per kg (45 mg per pound) of body weight for severe infections. Since safety for use in premature infants and in infants under one month has not been established, the use of Ancef (sterile cefazolin sodium) in these patients is not recommended.

Pediatric Dosage Guide

Weight		25 mg/kg/Day Divided into 3 Doses		25 mg/kg/Day Divided into 4 Doses	
Lbs	Kg	Approximate Single Dose mg/q8h	Vol. (mL) needed with dilution of 125 mg/mL	Approximate Single Dose mg/q6h	Vol. (mL) needed with dilution of 125 mg/mL
10	4.5	40 mg	0.35 mL	30 mg	0.25 mL
20	9.0	75 mg	0.60 mL	55 mg	0.45 mL
30	13.6	115 mg	0.90 mL	85 mg	0.70 mL
40	18.1	150 mg	1.20 mL	115 mg	0.90 mL
50	22.7	190 mg	1.50 mL	140 mg	1.10 mL

Weight		50 mg/kg/Day Divided into 3 Doses		50 mg/kg/Day Divided into 4 Doses	
Lbs	Kg	Approximate Single Dose mg q8h	Vol (mL) needed with dilution of 225 mg/mL	Approximate Single Dose mg/q6h	Vol (mL) needed with dilution of 225 mg/mL
10	4.5	75 mg	0.35 mL	55 mg	0.25 mL
20	9.0	150 mg	0.70 mL	110 mg	0.50 mL
30	13.6	225 mg	1.00 mL	170 mg	0.75 mL
40	18.1	300 mg	1.35 mL	225 mg	1.00 mL
50	22.7	375 mg	1.70 mL	285 mg	1.25 mL

16. A 198 lb adult is to be treated with IV Ticar® for bacterial
     septicemia. What is the daily dosage range in mg for this patient? _____

17. If the drug is administered q.4.h., what will the per dose be in g?   _____

18. Do you need to question a per dose dosage of 4 g for this patient?   _____

TICAR ®

brand of
sterile ticarcillin disodium
for Intramuscular or Intravenous Administration

DOSAGE AND ADMINISTRATION
Clinical experience indicates that in serious urinary tract and systemic infections, intravenous therapy in the higher doses should be used. Intramuscular injections should not exceed 2 grams per injection.
Adults:

Bacterial septicemia	200 to 300 mg/kg/day by I.V. infusion in divided doses every 4 or 6 hours.
Respiratory tract infections	(The usual dose is 3 grams given every 4 hours [18 grams/day] or 4 grams given every 6 hours
Skin and soft-tissue infections	[16 grams/day] depending on weight and the severity of the infection.)
Intra-abdominal infections	
Infections of the female pelvis and genital tract	
Urinary tract infections	
Complicated:	150 to 200 mg/kg/day by I.V. infusion in divided doses every 4 or 6 hours.
	(Usual recommended dosage for average [70 kg] adults: 3 grams q.i.d.)
Uncomplicated:	1 gram I.M. or direct I.V. every 6 hours.

(continues)

19. An adult weighing 77.3 kg with good cardiorenal function who tolerated a test dose of Fungizone® is to receive this drug IV. What will the daily dosage be?

      _____

20. Another patient who weighs 67.4 kg is also to receive amphotericin B for a severe rapidly progressive fungal infection. What will the daily dosage be?

      _____

21. What would be the **maximum** daily Fungizone dosage for an adult weighing 80.3 kg?

      _____

FUNGIZONE® INTRAVENOUS ℞
Amphotericin B For Injection USP

> **WARNING**
> This drug should be used *primarily* for treatment of patients with progressive and potentially life-threatening fungal infections; it should not be used to treat noninvasive forms of fungal disease such as oral thrush, vaginal candidiasis and esophegeal candidiasis in patients with normal neutrophil counts.

DOSAGE AND ADMINISTRATION

CAUTION: Under no circumstances should a total daily dose of 1.5 mg/kg be exceeded. Amphotericin B overdoses can result in cardio-respiratory arrest (see OVERDOSAGE).
FUNGIZONE Intravenous should be administered by *slow* intravenous infusion. Intravenous infusion should be given over a period of approximately 2 to 6 hours (depending on the dose) observing the usual precautions for intravenous therapy (see PRECAUTIONS, General). The recommended concentration for intravenous infusion is 0.1 mg/mL (1 mg/10 mL).
Since patient tolerance varies greatly, the dosage of amphotericin B must be individualized and adjusted according to the patient's clinical status (e.g., site and severity of infection, etiologic agent, cardio-renal function, etc.).
A single intravenous **test dose** (1 mg in 20 mL of 5% dextrose solution) administered over 20–30 minutes may be preferred. The patient's temperature, pulse, respiration, and blood pressure should be recorded every 30 minutes for 2 to 4 hours.
In patients with **good cardi-renal function** and a **well tolerated test dose**, therapy is usually initiated with a daily dose of 0.25 mg/kg of body weight. However, in those patients having **severe and rapidly progressive fungal infection**, therapy may be initiated with a daily dose of 0.3 mg/kg of body weight. In patients with **impaired cardio-renal function** or a **severe reaction to the test dose**, therapy should be initiated with smaller daily doses (i.e., 5 to 10 mg).
Depending on the patient's cardio-renal status (see PRECAUTIONS, Laboratory Tests), doses may gradually be increased by 5 to 10 mg per day to final daily dosage of 0.5 to 0.7 mg/kg.

Answers

1. 436 mg/day; 145 mg/dose. The 250 mg dosage is too high. Also the order is q.6.h., 4 times a day, not the usual q.8.h., which is 3 times a day
2. 1005–2010 mg/day; 335–670 mg/dose; 375 mg dosage ordered is correct
3. 1910–3820 mg/day; 478–955 mg/dose
4. 244 mg/dose; the 250 mg q.6.h. dosage is correct
5. 475 mg/day; 119 mg/dose; the dosage ordered is correct
6. 1908 mg/dose
7. Per dose range is 40–147 mg; the 125 mg order is correct
8. 129 mg/dose; the 130 mg ordered is correct
9. Per day dosage is 1004 mg; per dose dosage is 335 mg
10. Normal dose is 43–85 mg; the dosage ordered is too high
11. Per dose dosage range is 126–252 mg; 250 mg q.8.h. would be ordered
12. The q.6.h. per dosage range is 795–954 mg; the 850 mg dosage ordered is correct
13. 173 mg/dose; the 175 mg dosage ordered is correct
14. The 62.5 mg ordered is within the 48–96 mg per dose range
15. The 125 mg ordered is within the 100–200 mg per dose range
16. 18,000–27,000 mg/day
17. 3–4.5 g/dose
18. No
19. 19 mg/day
20. 20 mg/day
21. 120–121 mg/day

Adult and Pediatric Dosages Based on Body Surface Area

Body surface area (BSA or SA) is a major factor in calculating dosages for a number of drugs, because many of the body's physiologic processes are more closely related to body surface than they are to weight. Body surface is used extensively to calculate dosages of antineoplastic agents for cancer chemo-therapy, and for patients with severe burns. However, an increasing number of other drugs also are calculated using BSA. The nursing responsibility for checking dosages based on BSA varies widely among hospitals; therefore, this chapter covers all three essentials: calculation of BSA, calculation of dosages based on BSA, and assessment of physician orders based on BSA.

Body surface is calculated in **square meters** (m^2) using the patient's **weight and height**, by using a calculator that has square root ($\sqrt{}$) capabilities and a simple formula. Two formulas are used by physicians and pharmacists, one using kg and cm measurements, and another using lb and in (inch) measurements.* We'll look at these separately.

*Taketomo, Carol K. *Pediatric Dosage Handbook*, 10th ed. Hudson/Cleveland/Akron: Lexi-Comp, Inc. 2003.

Objectives

The learner will:

1. calculate BSA using formulas for weight and height

2. use BSA to calculate dosages

3. assess the accuracy of dosages prescribed on the basis of BSA

CALCULATING BSA FROM kg AND cm

The formula used to calculate BSA from kg and cm measurements is very easy to remember.

FORMULA

$$BSA = \sqrt{\frac{wt\ (kg)\ \times\ ht\ (cm)}{3600}}$$

EXAMPLE 1 Calculate the BSA of a man who weighs **104 kg** and whose height is **191 cm**. Express BSA to the nearest hundredth.

$$\sqrt{\frac{104\ (kg)\ \times\ 191\ (cm)}{3600}}$$

$$= \sqrt{5.517}$$

$$= 2.346 = \textbf{2.35 m}^2$$

Calculators may vary in the way square root must be obtained. Here is how the BSA was calculated in this example and throughout the chapter:

$$104. \times 191. \div 3600. = 5.517, \text{ then immediately enter } \sqrt{}$$

Practice with your own calculator to determine how it must be used to calculate a square root. Be careful to **insert periods after all whole numbers**, or you may obtain a wrong answer from pre-set decimal placement.

Only the final m² BSA is rounded to hundredths. Answers may vary slightly depending on how your calculator is set. Consider answers within 2–3 hundredths correct. Fractional weights and heights are also simple to calculate.

EXAMPLE 2 | Calculate the BSA of an adolescent who weighs **59.1 kg** and is **157.5 cm** in height. Express BSA to the nearest hundredth.

$$\sqrt{\frac{59.1 \text{ (kg)} \times 157.5 \text{ (cm)}}{3600}}$$

$$= \sqrt{2.585}$$

$$= 1.607 = \mathbf{1.61 \ m^2}$$

EXAMPLE 3 | A child who is **96.2 cm** tall weighs **15.17 kg**. What is this child's BSA in m² to the nearest hundredth?

$$\sqrt{\frac{15.17 \text{ (kg)} \times 96.2 \text{ (cm)}}{3600}}$$

$$= \sqrt{0.4053}$$

$$= 0.636 = \mathbf{0.63 \ m^2}$$

PROBLEM

Calculate the BSA in m² for the following patients. Express your answers to the nearest hundredth.

1. An adult weighing 59 kg whose height is 160 cm   _____

2. A child whose weight is 35.9 kg and whose height is 63.5 cm   _____

3. A child whose weight is 7.7 kg and whose height is 40 cm   _____

4. An adult whose weight is 92 kg and whose height is 178 cm   _____

5. A child whose weight is 46 kg and whose height is 102 cm   _____

Answers **1.** 1.62 m² **2.** 0.8 m² **3.** 0.29 m² **4.** 2.13 m² **5.** 1.14 m²

CALCULATING BSA FROM lb AND in

The formula for calculating BSA from lb and in measurements is equally easy to use. **The only difference is the denominator, which is 3131.**

FORMULA
$$BSA = \sqrt{\frac{wt\ (lb)\ \times\ ht\ (in)}{3131}}$$

EXAMPLE 1   Calculate BSA to the nearest hundredth of a child who is **24 in** tall weighing **34 lb**.

$$\sqrt{\frac{34\ (lb)\ \times\ 24\ (in)}{3131}}$$

$$= \sqrt{0.260}$$

$$= 0.510 = \textbf{0.51 m}^2$$

EXAMPLE 2   Calculate BSA to the nearest hundredth of an adult who is **61.3 in** tall and weighs **142.7 lb**.

$$\sqrt{\frac{142.7\ (lb)\ \times\ 61.3\ (in)}{3131}}$$

$$= \sqrt{2.793}$$

$$= 1.671 = \textbf{1.67 m}^2$$

EXAMPLE 3   A child weighs **105 lb** and is **51 in** tall. Calculate BSA to the nearest hundredth.

$$\sqrt{\frac{105\ (lb)\ \times\ 51\ (in)}{3131}}$$

$$= \sqrt{1.710}$$

$$= 1.307 = \textbf{1.31 m}^2$$

PROBLEM

Determine the BSA for the following patients. Express your answers to the nearest hundredth.

1. A child weighing 92 lb who measures 35 in   _____

2. An adult who weighs 175 lb and who is 67 in tall   _____

3. An adult who is 70 in tall and weighs 194 lb   _____

4. A child who weighs 72.4 lb and is 40.5 in tall   _____

5. A child who measures 26 in and weighs 36 lb   _____

Answers   **1.** 1.01 m² **2.** 1.94 m² **3.** 2.08 m² **4.** 0.97 m² **5.** 0.55 m²

DOSAGE CALCULATION BASED ON BSA

Once you know the BSA, dosage calculation is simple multiplication.

EXAMPLE 1 | Dosage recommended is **5 mg per m²**. The child has a BSA of **1.1 m²**.

1.1 (m²) × 5 mg = **5.5 mg**

EXAMPLE 2 | The recommended child's dosage is 25–50 mg per m². The child has a BSA of **0.76 m²**.

Lower dosage   0.76 (m²) × 25 mg = 19 mg

Upper dosage   0.76 (m²) × 50 mg = 38 mg

The dosage range is **19–38 mg**.

PROBLEM

Determine the child's dosage for the following drugs. Express your answers to the nearest whole number.

1. The recommended child's dosage is 5–10 mg/m². The BSA is 0.43 m². _____

2. A child with a BSA of 0.81 m² is to receive a drug with a recommended dosage of 40 mg/m². _____

3. Calculate the dosage of a drug with a recommended child's dosage of 20 mg/m² for a child with a BSA of 0.50 m². _____

4. An adult is to receive a drug with a recommended dosage of 20–40 U per m². The BSA is 1.93 m². _____

5. The adult recommended dosage is 3–5 mg per m². Calculate dosage for 2.08 m². _____

Answers   **1.** 2–4 mg   **2.** 32 mg   **3.** 10 mg   **4.** 39–77 U   **5.** 6–10 mg

ASSESSING ORDERS BASED ON BSA

In most situations in which you will have to check a dosage against m² recommendations you will be referring to drug package inserts, medication protocols, or the *PDR* to determine what the dosage should be.

EXAMPLE 1 | Refer to the vinblastine information insert in Figure 14-1 and calculate the first dose for an adult whose BSA is 1.66 m². Calculations are to the nearest whole number.

Recommended first dose = 3.7 mg/m²

1.66 (m²) × 3.7 mg = 6.14 = **6 mg**

EXAMPLE 2 | A child with a BSA of 0.96 m² is to receive her fourth dose of vinblastine.

Recommended fourth dose = 6.25 mg/m²

0.96 (m²) × 6.25 mg = **6 mg**

cetus oncology

STERILE VINBLASTINE SULFATE, USP

DOSAGE AND ADMINISTRATION
Caution: It is extremely important that the needle be properly positioned in the vein before this product is injected.

If leakage into surrounding tissue should occur during intravenous administration of vinblastine sulfate, it may cause considerable irritation. The injection should be discontinued immediately, and any remaining portion of the dose should then be introduced into another vein. Local injection of hyaluronidase and the application of moderate heat to the area of leakage help disperse the drug and are thought to minimize discomfort and the possibility of cellulitis.

There are variations in the depth of the leukopenic response which follows therapy with vinblastine sulfate. For this reason, it is recommended that the drug be given no more frequently than *once every 7 days.* It is wise to initiate therapy for adults by administering a single intravenous dose of 3.7 mg/M² of body surface area (bsa); the initial dose for children should be 2.5 mg/M². Thereafter, white-blood-cell counts should be made to determine the patient's sensitivity to vinblastine sulfate. A reduction of 50% in the dose of vinblastine is recommended for patients having a direct serum bilirubin value above 3 mg/100 mL. Since metabolism and excretion are primarily hepatic, no modification is recommended for patients with impaired renal function.

A simplified and conservative incremental approach to dosage *at weekly intervals* may be outlined as follows:

	Adults	Children
First dose	3.7 mg/M² bsa	2.5 mg/M² bsa
Second dose	5.5 mg/M² bsa	3.75 mg/M² bsa
Third dose	7.4 mg/M² bsa	5 mg/M² bsa
Forth dose	9.25 mg/M² bsa	6.25 mg/M² bsa
Fifth dose	11.1 mg/M² bsa	7.5 mg/M² bsa

The above-mentioned increases may be used until a maximum dose (not exceeding 18.5 mg/M² bsa for adults and 12.5 mg/M² bsa for children) is reached. The dose should not be increased after that dose which reduces the white-cell count to approximately 3000 cells/mm³. In some adults, 3.7 mg/M² bsa may produce this leukopenia; other adults may require more than 11.1mg/M² bsa; and, very rarely, as much as 18.5 mg/M² bsa may be necessary. For most adult patients, however, the weekly dosage will prove to be 5.5 to 7.4 mg/M² bsa.

Figure 14-1

PROBLEM

Calculate the following dosages of vinblastine from the information available in Figure 14-1. Calculate dosages to the nearest whole number.

1. Calculate the dosage for an adult's third dose. The patient's BSA is 1.91 m². _____

2. Calculate the first child's dosage for a patient with a BSA of 1.2 m². _____

3. Calculate the fifth adult dosage. The BSA is 1.53 m². _____

4. Calculate the second child's dosage for a BSA of 1.01 m². _____

5. Calculate the second adult dose for a BSA of 2.12 m². _____

Answers **1.** 14 mg **2.** 3 mg **3.** 17 mg **4.** 4 mg **5.** 12 mg

BiCNU ®
(carmustine for injection)

DOSAGE AND ADMINISTRATION
The recommended dose of BiCNU as a single agent in previously untreated patients is 150 to 200 mg/m^2 intravenously every 6 weeks. This may be given as a single dose or divided into daily injections such as 75 to 100 mg/m^2 on 2 successive days. When BiCNU is used in combination with other myelosuppressive drugs or in patients in whom bone marrow reserve is depleted, the doses should be adjusted accordingly.

Figure 14-2

PROBLEM

Refer to Figure 14-2 for BiCNU® and locate the following information. Express all dosages to the nearest whole number.

1. What is the dosage per m^2 if the drug is to be given in a single dose?   _____

2. If the patient has a BSA of 1.91 m^2, what will the daily dosage range be?   _____

3. If the order for this patient is a single dosage of 325 mg, is there any need to question it?   _____

4. If the dosage ordered is 450 mg, is there any need to question it?   _____

Answers **1.** 150–200 mg/m^2 **2.** 287–382 mg **3.** No **4.** Yes, too high

Summary

This concludes the chapter on dosage calculation based on BSA. The important points to remember from this chapter are:

- BSA is calculated from a patient's weight and height.

- BSA is more important than weight alone in calculating some drug dosages because many physiologic processes are more closely related to surface area than they are to weight.

- BSA is calculated in square meters (m^2) using a formula.

- The formulas for calculation of BSA are:

$$\sqrt{\frac{wt\ (kg)\ \times\ ht\ (cm)}{3600}} \quad and \quad \sqrt{\frac{wt\ (lb)\ \times\ ht\ (in)}{3131}}$$

- Once the BSA has been obtained, it can be used to calculate specific drug dosages and assess accuracy of physician orders.

Summary Self-Test

Use the formula method to calculate the following BSAs. Express the BSA to the nearest hundredth.

1. The weight is 58 lb, and the height is 36 in   _____

2. An adult weighing 74 kg and measuring 160 cm   _____

3. A child who is 14.2 kg and measures 64 cm   _____

4. An adult weighing 69 kg whose height is 170 cm   _____

5. An adolescent who is 55 in and 103 lb   _____

6. A child who is 112 cm and weighs 25.3 kg   _____

7. An adult who weighs 55 kg and measures 157.5 cm   _____

8. An adult who weighs 65.4 kg and is 132 cm in height   _____

9. A child whose height is 58 in and whose weight is 26.5 lb   _____

10. A child whose height and weight are 60 cm and 13.6 kg, respectively _____

Read the drug insert information provided on pages 201–204 and answer the following questions pertaining to it. Calculate dosages to the nearest whole number.

11. Read the information on children's dosage for Periactin® in Figure 14-3 and calculate the daily dosage for a 5-year-old child whose BSA is 0.78 m². _____

12. If a dosage of 4 mg is ordered for this 5-year-old would you question it? _____

13. What would the daily dosage be for a 5-year-old child whose BSA is 0.29 m²? _____

14. What would the daily dosage be for a 5-year-old child with a BSA of 0.51 m²? _____

PERIACTIN®
(CYPROHEPTADINE HCl)
DOSAGE AND ADMINISTRATION

DOSAGE SHOULD BE INDIVIDUALIZED ACCORDING TO THE NEEDS AND THE RESPONSE OF THE PATIENT.

Each PERIACTIN tablet contains 4 mg of cyproheptadine hydrochloride.

Pediatric Patients

Age 2 to 6 years

The total daily dosage for pediatric patients may be calculated on the basis of body weight or body area using approximately 0.25 mg/kg/day or 8 mg per square meter of body surface (8 mg/m²).

The usual dose is 2 mg (½ tablet) two or three times a day, adjusted as necessary to the size and response of the patient. The dose is not to exceed 12 mg a day.

Age 7 to 14 years

The usual dose is 4 mg (1 tablet) two or three times a day, adjusted as necessary to the size and response of the patient. The dose is not to exceed 16 mg a day.

Adults

The total daily dose for adults should not exceed 0.5 mg/kg/day.

The therapeutic range is 4 to 20 mg a day, with the majority of patients requiring 12 to 16 mg a day. An occasional patient may require as much as 32 mg a day for adequate relief. It is suggested that dosage be initiated with 4 mg (1 tablet) three times a day and adjusted according to the size and response of the patient.

Figure 14-3

MUTAMYCIN®   ℞
[*mū″-tĕ-mĭ′-sĭn*]
(mitomycin for injection) USP

DOSAGE AND ADMINISTRATION
Mutamycin should be given intravenously only, using care to avoid extravasation of the compound. If extravasation occurs, cellulitis, ulceration, and slough may result.

Each vial contains either mitomycin 5 mg and mannitol 10 mg, mitomycin 20 mg and mannitol 40 mg, or mitomycin 40 mg and mannitol 80 mg. To administer, add Sterile Water for Injection, 10 mL, 40 mL or 80 mL, respectively. Shake to dissolve. If product does not dissolve immediately, allow to stand at room temperature until solution is obtained.

After full hematological recovery (see guide to dosage adjustment) from any previous chemotherapy, the following dosage schedule may be used at 6- to 8-week intervals:

   20 mg/m² intravenously as a single dose via a functioning intravenous catheter.

Because of cumulative myelosuppression, patients should be fully reevaluated after each course of Mutamycin, and the dose reduced if the patient has experienced any toxicities. Doses greater than 20 mg/m² have not been shown to be more effective, and are more toxic than lower doses.

The following schedule is suggested as a guide to dosage adjustment:

Figure 14-4

PARAPLATIN®   ℞
[*păr-a-plătin*]
(carboplatin for injection)

DOSAGE AND ADMINISTRATION
NOTE: Aluminum reacts with carboplatin causing precipitate formation and loss of potency, therefore, needles or intravenous sets containing aluminum parts that may come in contact with the drug must not be used for the preparation or administration of PARAPLATIN.

PARAPLATIN, as a single agent, has been shown to be effective in patients with recurrent ovarian carcinoma at a dosage of 360 mg/m² IV on day 1 every 4 weeks. In general, however, single intermittent courses of PARAPLATIN should not be repeated until the neutrophil count is at least 2,000 and the platelet count is at least 100,000.

The dose adjustments shown in the table below are modified from a controlled trial in previously treated patients with ovarian carcinoma. Blood counts were done weekly, and the recommendations are based on the lowest posttreatment platelet or neutrophil value.

Figure 14-5

15. A patient is to receive the antineoplastic drug Mutamycin® IV (Figure 14-4). What will the dosage be for this patient, whose BSA is 1.46 m²? _____

16. Another patient with a BSA of 2.12 m² is also to receive Mutamycin. What will the dosage be? _____

17. A patient is to be treated with the drug Paraplatin® for ovarian carcinoma (Figure 14-5). Her BSA is 1.61 m². What will the dosage be? _____

18. Another patient, who weighs 130 lb and measures 62 in, is to receive Paraplatin. What will her dosage be? _____

19. A third patient receiving Paraplatin has a dosage of 637 mg IV ordered. She is 161 cm tall and weighs 70 kg. Assess this dosage. _____

BLENOXANE® ℞
[blĕ-nŏk'sān]
(sterile bleomycin sulfate, USP)
vial, 15 units NSN 6505-01-060-4278(m)

DOSAGE
Because of the possibility of an anaphylactoid reaction, lymphoma patients should be treated with two units or less for the first two doses. If no acute reaction occurs, then the regular dosage schedule may be followed.
The following dose schedule is recommended: Squamous cell carcinoma, lymphosarcoma, reticulum cell sarcoma, testicular carcinoma—0.25 to 0.50 units/kg (10 to 20 units/m²) given intravenously, intramuscularly, or subcutaneously weekly or twice weekly.
Hodgkin's Disease—0.25 to 0.50 units/kg (10 to 20 units/m²) given intravenously, intramuscularly, or subcutaneously weekly or twice weekly. After a 50% response, a maintenance dose of one unit daily or five units weekly intravenously or intramuscularly should be given.
Pulmonary toxicity of Blenoxane appears to be dose related with a striking increase when the total dose is over 400 units. Total doses over 400 units should be given with great caution.

Figure 14-6

PLATINOL® ℞
[plă'tĭ-nŏl"]
(cisplatin for injection, USP)

DOSAGE AND ADMINISTRATION
Note: Needles or intravenous sets containing aluminum parts that may come in contact with PLATINOL® (cisplatin for injection, USP) should not be used for preparation or administration. Aluminum reacts with PLATINOL, causing precipitate formation and a loss of potency.
Metastatic Testicular Tumors—The usual PLATINOL dose for the treatment of testicular cancer in combination with other approved chemotherapeutic agents is 20 mg/m² IV daily for 5 days.
Metastatic Ovarian Tumors—The usual PLATINOL dose for the treatment of metastatic ovarian tumors in combination with Cytoxan or other approved chemotherapeutic agents is 75–100 mg/m² IV once every 4 weeks, (Day 1).[1,2]
The dose of Cytoxan when used in combination with PLATINOL is 600 mg/m² IV once every 4 weeks, (Day 1).[1,2]
For directions for the administration of Cytoxan refer to the Cytoxan package insert.
In combination therapy, PLATINOL and Cytoxan are administered sequentially.
As a single agent, PLATINOL should be administered at a dose of 100 mg/m² IV once every 4 weeks.

Figure 14-7

20. A patient with Hodgkin's disease who weighs 60 kg and is 142 cm tall is to receive Blenoxane® IV (Figure 14-6). What is her BSA? _____

What will her dosage range be? _____

If a dosage of 20 U is ordered must you question it? _____

21. Another patient receiving Blenoxane weighs 91 kg and measures 190 cm. What will his dosage range be? _____

22. Platinol® (Figure 14-7) is being given for metastatic ovarian carcinoma. What is the dosage range of this drug for a patient with a BSA of 1.29 m²? _____

23. Another patient with metastatic testicular carcinoma is to receive Platinol. He weighs 173 lb and is 65 in tall. What is his BSA? _____

What will his dosage be? _____

℞

(Acyclovir Sodium)
FOR INTRAVENOUS INFUSION ONLY

DOSAGE AND ADMINISTRATION
CAUTION— RAPID OR BOLUS INTRAVENOUS AND IN-
TRAMUSCULAR OR SUBCUTANEOUS INJECTION MUST
BE AVOIDED. Therapy should be initiated as early as possible following onset of signs and symptoms. For diagnosis—
see INDICATIONS.
Dosage:
HERPES SIMPLEX INFECTIONS
*MUCOSAL AND CUTANEOUS HERPES SIMPLEX (HSV-1
and HSV-2) INFECTIONS IN IMMUNOCOMPROMISED
PATIENTS* —5 mg/kg infused at a constant rate over 1
hour, every 8 hours (15 mg/kg/day) for 7 days in adult patients with normal renal function. In children under 12
years of age, more accurate dosing can be attained by infusing 250 mg/m^2 at a constant rate over 1 hour, every 8 hours
(750 mg/m^2/day) for 7 days.

*SEVERE INITIAL CLINICAL EPISODES OF HERPES
GENITALIS* —The same dose given above—administered
for 5 days.
HERPES SIMPLEX ENCEPHALITIS —10 mg/kg infused
at a constant rate over at least 1 hour, every 8 hours for 10
days. In children between 6 months and 12 years of age, more
accurate dosing is achieved by infusing 500 mg/m^2, at a constant rate over at least one hour, every 8 hours for 10 days.
VARICELLA ZOSTER INFECTIONS
ZOSTER IN IMMUNOCOMPROMISED PATIENTS —10
mg/kg infused at a constant rate over 1 hour, every 8 hours
for 7 days in adult patients with normal renal function. In
children under 12 years of age, equivalent plasma concentrations are attained by infusing 500 mg/m^2 at a constant rate
over at least 1 hour, every 8 hours for 7 days. Obese patients
should be dosed at 10 mg/kg (Ideal Body Weight). A maximum dose equivalent to 500 mg/m^2 every 8 hours should not
be exceeded for any patient.

Figure 14-8

24. Acylclovir sodium (Figure 14-8) is to be given to a child with
herpes simplex encephalitis. This patient weighs 34 lb and is 24
in tall. What is the BSA?   _____

What will the dosage be?   _____

25. An immunocompromised 10-year-old child with a herpes simplex
infection is to be medicated with acyclovir sodium. Her weight is
72 lb and height 40 in. What is her BSA?   _____

What will the hourly dosage be?   _____

26. Another immunosuppressed child is to receive acyclovir sodium
for a varicella zoster infection. His weight is 43 lb and height
28 in. What is his BSA?   _____

27. What will the dosage be for this patient?   _____

Answers
1. 0.82 m^2
2. 1.81 m^2
3. 0.50 m^2
4. 1.81 m^2
5. 1.35 m^2
6. 0.89 m^2
7. 1.55 m^2
8. 1.55 m^2
9. 0.70 m^2
10. 0.48 m^2
11. 6 mg per day
12. Yes; too low
13. 2 mg per day
14. 4 mg
15. 29 mg
16. 42 mg
17. 580 mg
18. 576 mg
19. Accurate
20. 1.54 m^2;
 15–31 U; No
21. 22–44 U
22. 97–129 mg
23. 1.90 m^2;
 38 mg
24. 0.51 m^2;
 255 mg
25. 0.96 m^2;
 240 mg
26. 0.62 m^2
27. 310 mg

SECTION 6

Intravenous Calculations

15

Introduction to IV Therapy

The calculations associated with IVs will be easier to understand if you have some general understanding of IV therapy. IV fluid and medication administration is one of the most challenging of all nursing responsibilities. There are currently estimated to be over 200 different IV fluids being manufactured, and at least as many additives are used with IV fluids, including medications, electrolytes, and nutrients. In addition there are hundreds of different types of IV administration sets and components, and dozens of different models of electronic infusion devices (EIDs) are used to infuse and monitor IV fluids. This would appear to make the entire subject of IV therapy overwhelming, but it is not. This chapter presents the essentials in understandable segments and gives an excellent base of instruction on which to build. Let's begin by looking at a basic sterile IV setup, which is referred to as a primary line.

PRIMARY LINE

Refer to Figure 15-1, which shows a typical primary IV line connecting an IV fluid bag or bottle to the needle or cannula in a vein. The IV tubing is connected to the IV solution bag (using sterile technique), and the bag is hung on an IV stand.

 Close all roller clamps on the tubing before connecting it to the solution bag. This step prevents air bubbles from forming in the tubing.

The **drip chamber**, A, is then squeezed to **half fill** it with fluid. This level is very important because **IV flow rates are set and monitored by counting the drops falling in this chamber**. If the chamber is too full the drops cannot be counted. On the other hand, if the outlet at the bottom of the chamber is not completely covered, air can enter the tubing during infusions and, subsequently, the vein and circulatory system. So the half full fluid level is extremely important.

 The correct fluid level for IV drip chambers is half full, to allow drops to be counted and prevent air from entering the tubing.

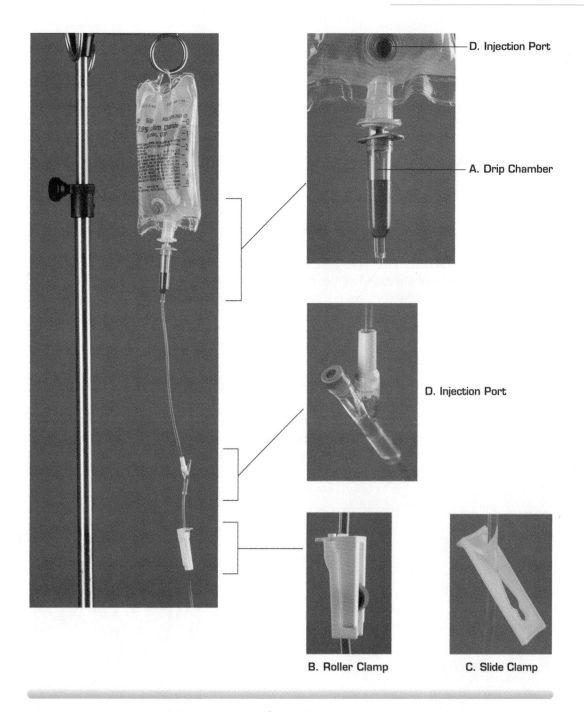

D. Injection Port

A. Drip Chamber

D. Injection Port

B. Roller Clamp

C. Slide Clamp

Figure 15-1

Next notice B, the **roller clamp**. This is adjusted while the drops falling in the drip chamber are counted to set the flow rate. It provides an extremely accurate control of rate. A second type of clamp, C, called a **slide clamp**, is present on tubings. The slide clamp can be used to temporarily stop an IV without disturbing the rate set on the roller clamp.

Next notice D, the **injection port**. Rubber ports are located in several locations on the tubing, typically near the cannula end, drip chamber and middle of the line, and also on most IV solution bags. Ports allow injection of medication directly into the line or bag, or the attachment of secondary IV lines containing compatible IV fluids or medications to the primary line.

Intravenous fluids run by gravity flow. This necessitates that the IV solution bag be hung **above the patient's heart level** to exert sufficient pressure to infuse. Three feet is considered an average height.

 The higher an IV bag is hung, the greater the pressure, and the faster the IV will infuse.

This pressure differential also means that if the flow rate is adjusted while the patient is lying in bed, it will slow down if she/he sits or stands and, in fact, it changes slightly with each turn from side to side. For this reason **monitoring IV flow rate is ongoing**, officially done every hour, but routinely checked after each major position change.

There are two additional terms relating to primary lines that you must know. If an arm or hand (or, less commonly, leg) vein is used for an infusion, it is referred to as a **peripheral line**. This is to distinguish it from a **central line**, which uses a special catheter whose tip is located centrally in a deep chest vein. Central lines may access the chest vein directly through the chest wall, via a neck vein, or through a peripheral vein in the arm or leg.

SECONDARY LINE

Secondary lines attach to the primary line at an injection port. They are used primarily to infuse medications, frequently on an intermittent basis, for example, every 6–8 hours. They may also be used to infuse other compatible IV fluids. Secondary lines are commonly referred to as **IV piggybacks**. They are abbreviated **IVPB**. Refer to Figure 15-2, which illustrates a primary and secondary line setup.

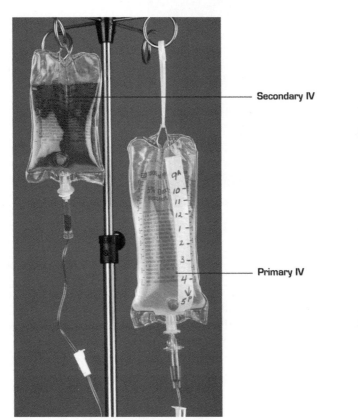

Secondary IV

Primary IV

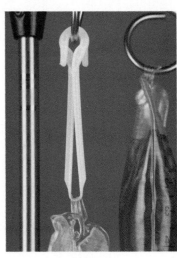

A. Extender

Figure 15-2

15

The IVPB is connected to a port located below the drip chamber on the primary line. Notice that **the IVPB bag is hanging higher than the primary**. This gives it greater pressure and causes it to **infuse first**. Each IVPB set includes a plastic or metal **extender**, A, which is used to lower the primary solution bag to obtain this pressure differential. The flow rate for the IVPB is set by a separate roller clamp located on the secondary line. When the IVPB bag has empties the primary line will automatically resume its flow. Secondary medication bags are usually much smaller than primary bags. Fifty, 100, 150, 200, and 250 mL bags are frequently used.

Another type of secondary medication setup is provided by Abbot Laboratories **ADD-Vantage® system** (Figure 15-3). In this system a specially designed IV fluid bag that contains a **medication vial port** is used. The medication vial containing the ordered drug and dosage is inserted into the port, and the drug (frequently in powdered form) is mixed using IV fluid as the diluent, as illustrated in Figure 15-4. The vial contents are then displaced back into the solution bag and thoroughly mixed in the total solution before infusion. The vial remains in the solution bag port throughout the infusion, making it possible to cross-check the vial label for drug and dosage at any time.

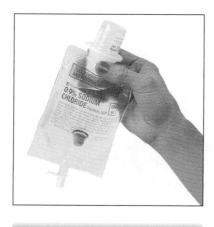

Figure 15-3 ADD-Vantage System®. (Courtesy of Abbott Laboratories)

If a drug is not available in either a prepackaged or ADD-Vantage format, it is often prepared and labeled by the hospital pharmacy. And, finally, an IV medication may be prepared, added to the appropriate IV fluid, thoroughly mixed, labeled and initialed, and administered by the nurse who initiates the infusion.

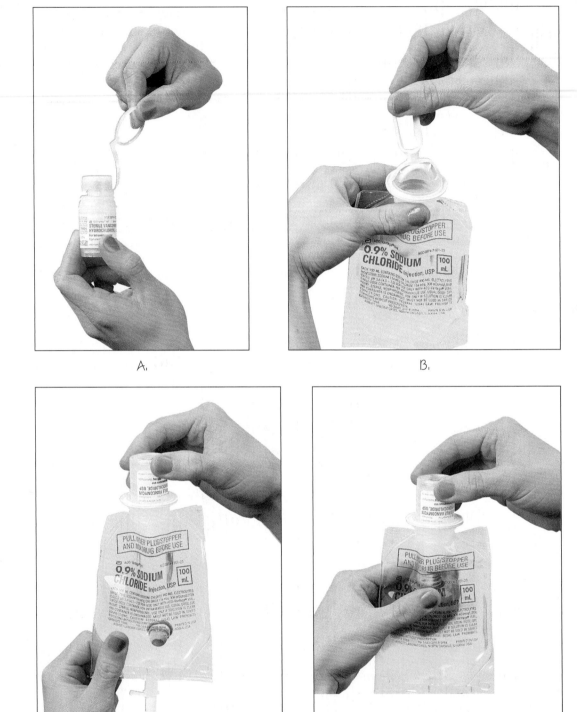

A.

B.

C.

D.

Figure 15-4   ADD-Vantage System® A. The ADD-Vantage medication vial is opened first.
B. The medication vial port on the IV bag is opened.   C. The vial top is inserted into the IV bag
port and twisted to lock tightly in place.   D. The vial stopper is removed "inside" the IV bag, and
the medication and solution are thoroughly mixed before infusion. (Courtesy of Abbott Laboratories)

VOLUME-CONTROLLED BURETTES

For greater accuracy in the measurement of **small volume** IV medications and fluids, a **calibrated burette chamber** such as the one in Figure 15-5 may be used. The total capacity of burettes varies from 100 to 150 mL, calibrated in 1 mL increments. Many burettes are calibrated to deliver very small drops (microdrops), which also contributes to their accuracy. Burettes are most often referred to by their trade names, for example, Buretrols®, Solusets®, or Volutrols®. Burette chambers are often connected to a secondary solution bag and used as a secondary line, but they can also be primary lines. When medication is ordered, it is injected into the burette through its injection port. The exact among of IV fluid is then added as a diluent. After thorough mixing, the flow rate is set using a separate clamp on the burette line. Burettes are extensively used in pediatric and intensive care units, where medication dosages and fluid volumes are critical.

INDWELLING INFUSION PORTS/ INTERMITTENT LOCKS

When a continuous IV is not necessary, but intermittent IV medication administration is, an **infusion port adapter** (Figure 15-6) can be attached to an indwelling cannula in a vein. Infusion ports are frequently referred to as **heplocks** or **saline locks (or ports)**. This terminology evolved because the ports must be irrigated with 1–2 cc of sterile saline every 6–8 hours, or a heparin lock flush solution (100 U/mL) to prevent clotting and blockage. To infuse medication, the port top is cleansed, and the medication line is attached. When the infusion is complete, the line is disconnected until the next dosage is due. Ports are also used for **direct injection of medication using a syringe**, which is called an **IV push**, or **bolus**.

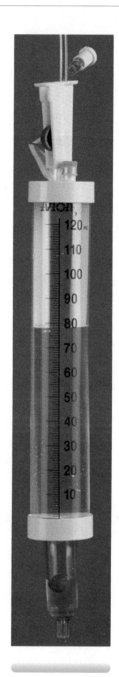

Figure 15-5

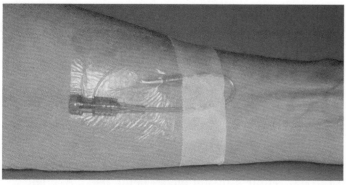

Figure 15-6

PROBLEM

Answer the following questions about IV administration sets as briefly as possible.

1. What is the correct fluid level for an IV drip chamber?

2. Which clamp is used to regulate IV flow rate?

3. When might a slide clamp be used?

4. What is a peripheral line?

5. What is a central line?

6. What is the common abbreviation for an intravenous piggyback?

7. Is this a primary or secondary line?

8. What must the height of a primary solution bag be when a secondary bag is infusing?

9. When is a saline lock used?

Answers **1.** Middle of chamber **2.** Roller clamp **3.** Stop the IV temporarily without disturbing the rate set on the roller clamp **4.** Arm or leg vein **5.** IV catheter inserted into a large chest vein **6.** IVPB **7.** Secondary **8.** Lower than secondary bag **9.** Intermittent infusions when a continuous IV is not necessary

VOLUMETRIC PUMPS

Refer now to Figure 15-7 of the ALARIS Signature Edition® volumetric pump. Notice that the IV tubing with the AccuSlide® flow regulator has been inserted into the channel on the right. On the right is a pumping mechanism that maintains the desired flow rate.

Most of the simpler pumps physically resemble the ALARIS Signature Edition® pump, but the functions of different models vary widely. Some models continue to pump fluids even if an IV infiltrates, whereas others have a built-in pressure sensor that will alarm if a resultant increased infusion resistance pressure occurs. Some models alarm when the solution has completely infused; other models do not.

Because of the wide variation in pump models and their functions, caution is mandatory when they are used. It is estimated that as high as 50% of IV medication errors may result from errors in pump programming.

 Hospital or clinic in-service education is required for the use of all infusion devices.

Infusion devices are now widely used in many households for patient IV medication administration, and the precautions in use apply less to the difficulty of the skill than in becoming familiar with the particular infusion model being used. A single hospital or clinic could realistically have a dozen different models in use, and it is an ongoing nursing responsibility to learn how to use each particular model.

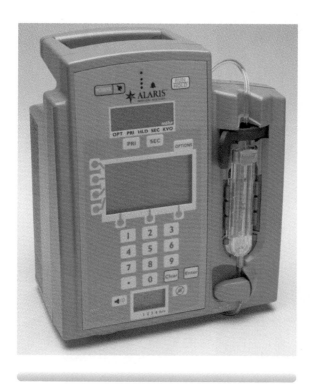

Figure 15-7 ALARIS Signature Edition® Volumetric
Pump. (Courtesy of ALARIS Medical Systems)

 Double-checking of programming is mandatory in the use of infusion devices.

Because errors in infusion device programming are a factor in IV medication errors, it is mandatory that all programming be double-checked. A new generation of sophisticated "smart" pumps that have a built-in library of usual drug dosages and are capable of detecting programming errors are slowly making their appearance. The Outlook™ illustrated in Figure 15-8 is one example. Another dose-specific pump is the ALARIS® *Medley™ Medication Safety System with Guardrails® Safety Software* shown in Figure 15-9, a lightweight, modular platform that integrates infusion, patient monitoring, and clinical best-practice guidelines.

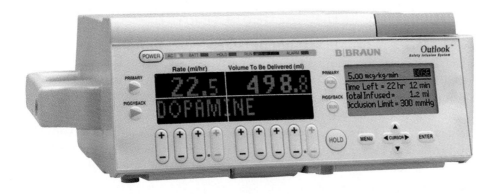

Figure 15-8 The Outlook™. (Courtesy of B. Braun Medical Inc.)

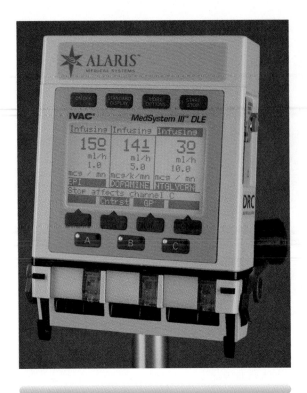

Figure 15-9 ALARIS Medley® Medication Safety System. (Courtesy of ALARIS Medical Systems)

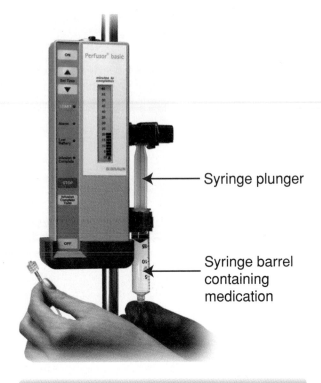

— Syringe plunger

— Syringe barrel containing medication

Figure 15-10 B. Braun Perfusor™ Basic Syringe Pump. (Courtesy of B. Braun Medical Inc.)

SYRINGE PUMPS

Syringe pumps, as their name implies, are devices that use a syringe to administer medications or fluids (Figure 15-10). Syringe pumps are particularly valuable when **drugs that cannot be mixed with other solutions or medications** must be administered at a controlled rate over a short period of time, for example, 5, 10, or 20 minutes. The drug is measured in the syringe, which is inserted into the device, and the medication is infused at the rate set.

PATIENT-CONTROLLED ANALGESIA (PCA) DEVICES

PCA devices allow a patient to **self-administer medication to control pain**. A prefilled syringe or medication bag containing pain medication is inserted into the device (Figure 15-11), and the **dosage and frequency of administration ordered by the doctor are set**. The patient presses the control button, A, as medication is needed, and it is administered and recorded by the PCA.

The device also keeps a record of the number of times a patient **attempts** to use it, and thus provides a record of the effectiveness of the dosage prescribed. If a patient's pain is not being relieved, new orders must be obtained and the PCA reset to administer the new dosage.

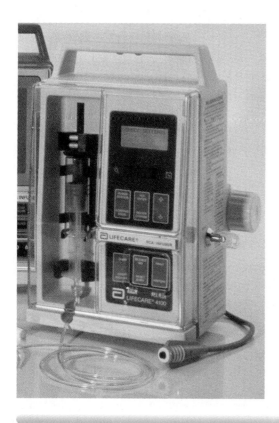
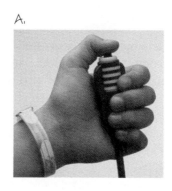

A.

Figure 15-11 Abbott Lifecare® PCA 4100 Infuser. (Courtesy of Abbott Laboratories)

 All electronic devices must be monitored to be sure they are functioning properly.

Is the IV infusing at the rate that was set? Is the patient who activates a PCA getting relief of pain? If not, is it possible the PCA itself is malfunctioning? Electronic devices have been in use for many years and are relatively trouble free, but if the desired goal is not being obtained, in the absence of other obvious reasons, **the possibility of malfunction must always be considered**.

PROBLEM

Answer the following questions about infusion devices as briefly as possible.

1. What is the function of a volumetric pump? _____

2. List two major precautions in their use. _____

3. When might a syringe pump be used? _____

4. What is a PCA? _____

Answers **1.** To administer IVs at a controlled rate **2.** Accurate programming; rate and site monitoring **3.** To infuse small volumes of drugs that are not compatible with other drugs and/or fluids **4.** Patient-controlled analgesia device

INTRODUCTION TO IV FLUIDS

IV fluids are prepared in plastic solution bags or glass bottles in volumes ranging from 50 mL (bags only) to 1000 mL. The 500 and 1000 mL sizes are the most commonly used. IV bags and bottles are labeled with the **complete name** of the fluid they contain, and the fine print under the solution name identifies the exact amount of each component of the fluid. IV **orders and charting**, however, are most often done **using abbreviations**. Some examples of frequently used fluids are: 5% Dextrose in Water, D and 5% Dextrose in Normal Saline.

 In IV fluid abbreviations D always identifies dextrose; W always identifies water; S identifies saline, NS identifies normal saline; and numbers identify percentage (%) strengths.

Solutions may be abbreviated in different ways; for example, D5W, 5%D/W, D5%W, or other combinations. But the **initials and percentage have the identical meaning regardless of the way they are abbreviated**. Normal saline solutions are frequently written with the .9 or % sign included, for example, D5 .9NS, or D5 0.9%S. IV fluids with different percentages of saline are also available: 0.45%, often written as 1/2 (0.45% is half of 0.9%), and 0.225%, sometimes written as 1/4 (¼ of 0.9) are examples. Some typical orders might be abbreviated D5 1/2S, or D5 1/4NS.

Another commonly used solution is **Ringer's lactate**, a balanced electrolyte solution, which is also called Lactated Ringer's Solution. As you would now expect, this solution is abbreviated **RL** or **LR**, and, possibly, RLS. Electrolytes may also be added to the basic fluids (DW and DS) just discussed. One electrolyte so commonly added that it must be mentioned is potassium chloride, which is abbreviated KCl. It is measured in milliequivalents (mEq).

PROBLEM

List as briefly as possible the components and percentage strengths of the following IV solutions.

1. D10 NS _____

2. D5 NS _____

3. D2.5 1/2S _____

4. D5 1/4S _____

5. D20W _____

6. D5NS _____

7. D5NS 20 mEq KCl _____

8. D5RL _____

Answers **1.** 10% Dextrose in 0.9% Saline **2.** 5% Dextrose in Normal (0.9%) Saline **3.** 2.5% Dextrose in 0.45% Saline **4.** 5% Dextrose in 0.225% Saline **5.** 20% Dextrose in Water **6.** 5% Dextrose in Normal (0.9%) Saline **7.** 5% Dextrose in 0.9% Saline with 20 mEq potassium chloride **8.** 5% Dextrose in Ringer's Lactate Solution

PERCENTAGES IN IV FLUIDS

You will recall that **percent means grams of drug per 100 mL of fluid**. This means that a 5% dextrose solution will have 5 g of dextrose in each 100 mL. A 500 mL bag of a 5% solution will contain 5 g $\times$ 5, or 25 g of dextrose, whereas 500 mL of a 10% solution contains 10 g $\times$ 5, or 50 g of dextrose. The fine print on IV labels always lists the name and amount of all ingredients.

The point being made here is that percentages make IV fluids significantly different from each other. As with drugs, reading labels and making sure the IVs administered are what are actually ordered are critically important.

PARENTERAL NUTRITION

One of the options available for providing nutrition when a patient is unable to eat is to administer a nutrient solution via a central vein. This is referred to as parenteral nutrition. The solutions infused are generally high caloric and contain varying percentages of glucose, amino acids, and/or fat emulsions. A number of abbreviations/descriptions are used for parenteral nutrients. Some of the more common are total parenteral nutrition (TPN), partial parenteral nutrition (PPN), and hyperalimentation (nutrition in excess of maintenance needs). There is a noticeable difference in fluids that contain lipids (fat, intralipids) in that they are opaque-white in appearance, not unlike nonfat milk. These fluids are normally infused slowly, but not usually in excess of 24 hours, because they can spoil and support bacterial growth. All precautions applicable to IVs in general apply equally to parenteral nutrients, with more care necessary for the IV site to prevent infection. Flow rate and infusion time calculations covered in subsequent chapters are also applicable for parenteral nutrition solutions.

Summary

This concludes your introduction to IV therapy. The important points to remember from this chapter are:

- Sterile technique is used to set up all IV solutions, tubings, and devices.
- The correct fluid level for an IV drip chamber is half full.
- Injection ports on an IV line are used to connect secondary lines and to infuse medications.
- A peripheral line refers to an IV infusing in a hand, arm, or leg vein.
- A central line refers to an IV infusing into a deep chest vein.
- IVs flow by gravity pressure, and the higher the solution bag, the faster the IV will infuse.
- The average height for an IV solution bag above the patient's heart level is 3 feet.
- Secondary solution bags must hang higher than the primary bag to infuse first.
- Volume-controlled burettes are used for very exact measurements of IV medications and fluids.
- Intermittent infusion locks or ports are used to infuse IV medications or fluids on an intermittent basis when a continuous IV is not necessary.

● Volumetric pumps are electronic devices that force fluids into a vein under pressure and control infusion rates.

● Syringe pumps are used to infuse medications that cannot be mixed with other fluids or medications.

● Patient-controlled analgesia (PCA) devices allow a patient to self-administer pain medication.

● In IV fluid abbreviations, D identifies Dextrose, W identifies Water, S identifies Saline, NS identifies Normal Saline, RL and LR identify Lactated Ringer's Solution, and numbers identify percentage (%) strengths.

Summary Self-Test

You are to assist with some IV procedures. Answer the following situational questions concerning these.

1. A patient is admitted and an IV of 1000 mL D5RL is started. These initials identify what type of solution? _____

   This is referred to as what type of line? _____

2. All roller clamps on the IV tubing are closed before connection to the solution bag. Why? _____

3. The IV is started in the back of the patient's left hand. This makes it what type of line? _____

4. You are asked to check the fluid level in the drip chamber, and you observe that it is correct, which is . . . _____

5. You are then asked to adjust the flow rate. You will use what type of clamp to do this? _____

6. It is decided to use an electronic infusion control device to administer this IV. The device used is a . . . _____

7. An IV antibiotic is ordered for the patient. This is sent from the pharmacy already prepared in a small-volume IV solution bag. The setup used to infuse this medication is referred to as an IV . . . _____

8. This is abbreviated how? _____

9. In order for the antibiotic to infuse first, how must it be hung in relation to the original solution bag? _____

10. Some days later the patient's IV is to be discontinued, but he is to continue to receive IV antibiotics. What is the site used for this intermittent administration called? _____

11. The patient had a PCA in use for one day. What do these initials mean? _____

    What does this device control? _____

Answer the following questions as briefly as possible.

12. A small-volume IV medication is to be diluted in 20 mL and infused. This can be
    most accurately measured using a _____   _____ .

13. These devices are calibrated in _____ increments.

14. When an IV medication is injected directly into the vein via a port, it is called
    an IV _____ or _____ .

15. Ports may be irrigated with _____ mL of _____
    to prevent blockage every _____ hr.

16. In IV fluid abbreviations, D5NS identifies what IV fluid? _____

IV Flow Rate Calculation

There are a number of ways to calculate IV flow rates, and this chapter presents three: ratio and proportion, a formula method, and the division factor method. Use whichever method you are most comfortable with.

Large volumes of intravenous fluids are most often ordered on the basis of **mL/hr** to be administered, for example 125 mL/hr. With the widespread use of electronic infusion devices that can be **set to deliver a mL/hr rate**, simply setting the rate ordered on the device and making sure it is working properly is all that is required for most infusions. Some infusion devices can also be set at a **gtt/min** (drop per minute) rate, which is much less frequently ordered than the mL/hr rate.

The most common calculation, which is necessary **when an infusion device is not being used**, involves **converting an IV order to the gtt/min rate necessary to infuse it**. This calculation may be required for **large-volume orders** written designating a **mL/hr** rate, for example, **1000 mL to infuse at 125 mL/hr**; for infusions of **mL per multiple hours**, for example, **3000 mL/24 hr**; or for **small-volume orders**, usually involving medication administration, for example, **100 mL/40 min**.

IV TUBING CALIBRATION

The size of IV drops is regulated by the type of IV set being used, which is **calibrated in number of gtt/mL**. Unfortunately, not all sets (and their drop size) are the same. Each hospital uses at least two sizes of infusion sets, the standard, or **macrodrip set, calibrated at 10, 15, or 20 gtt/mL**, which is used for routine adult IV administrations; and a **mini, or microdrip set, calibrated at 60 gtt/mL**, which is used when more exact measurements are needed, for example, to infuse medications, or in critical care and pediatric infusions.

 IV administration sets are calibrated in gtt/mL.

The **gtt/mL calibration of each IV set is clearly printed on each package**, and the first step in calculating flow rates is to identify the gtt/mL calibration of the set to be used for infusion.

PROBLEM

Refer to the IV set packages provided in Figures 16-1 and 16-2 and identify the calibration in gtt/mL of each.

1. _____

2. _____

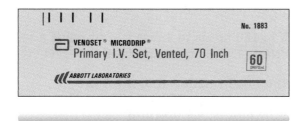

Figure 16-1

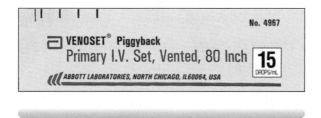

Figure 16-2

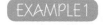Answers **1.** 60 gtt/mL **2.** 15 gtt/mL

CALCULATING LARGE VOLUME gtt/min RATES FROM mL/hr ORDERED

Usually only one **macrodrip** calibrated set of either **10, 15, or 20 gtt/mL** is used in most hospital or clinical settings, and a **mL/hr to gtt/min conversion chart** may be available. If one is not available, the following method is one of the safest and most logical to use to **convert the mL/hr ordered to a gtt/min flow rate**. It can be used if the rate ordered is mL/hr, for example, 125 mL/hr, or mL per multiple hr, for example, 3000 mL/24 hr. Let's now look at some calculations that involve both of these types of orders.

EXAMPLE 1 | An IV is ordered to infuse at a rate of **125 mL/hr** using a set calibrated at **10 gtt/mL**. Calculate the **gtt/min** flow rate.

You are calculating **gtt/min**, so start by determining how many **mL/min** this order represents. This is done by **dividing the 125 mL/hr rate by 60 min**.

- **Change the mL/hr ordered to mL/min.**

  125 mL ÷ 60 min = **2 mL/min**

- **Calculate the gtt/min rate for the 2 mL/min obtained.** To establish consistency in calculations, you may wish to **enter the set calibration as the first ratio in the proportion**.

$$10 \text{ gtt} : 1 \text{ mL} = X \text{ gtt} : 2 \text{ mL} \quad \text{or} \quad \frac{10 \text{ gtt}}{1 \text{ mL}} = \frac{X \text{ gtt}}{2 \text{ mL}} = \textbf{20 gtt}$$
$$X = \textbf{20 gtt}$$

To infuse an IV at 125 mL/hr using a set calibrated at 10 gtt/mL, set the manual drip rate at 20 gtt/min.

 | An IV of **150 mL** is to infuse in **1 hr** using a set calibrated at **15 gtt/mL**. Calculate the **gtt/min** flow rate.

- **Change the mL/hr ordered to mL/min.**

  150 mL ÷ 60 min = **2.5 mL/min**

- **Calculate the gtt/min rate.**

$$15 \text{ gtt} : 1 \text{ mL} = X \text{ gtt} : 2.5 \text{ mL} \quad \text{or} \quad \frac{15 \text{ gtt}}{1 \text{ mL}} = \frac{X \text{ gtt}}{2.5 \text{ mL}} = 37.5 = \textbf{38 gtt}$$
$$X = 37.5 = \textbf{38 gtt}$$

To infuse 150 mL/hr using a set calibrated at 15 gtt/mL, set the manual drip rate at 38 gtt/min.

 Flow rates are routinely rounded to the nearest whole number.

Let's now look at some IVs ordered to infuse in more than 1 hour.

 | An IV of **2500 mL** is to infuse in **24 hr** using a **20 gtt/mL** calibrated set. Calculate the **gtt/min** flow rate.

- **Calculate the mL/hr to infuse.**

  2500 mL ÷ 24 hr = 104.1 = **104 mL/hr**

- **Calculate the mL/min to infuse.**

  104 mL ÷ 60 min = **1.7 mL/min**

- **Calculate the gtt/min rate.**

$$20 \text{ gtt} : 1 \text{ mL} = X \text{ gtt} : 1.7 \text{ mL} \quad \text{or} \quad \frac{20 \text{ gtt}}{1 \text{ mL}} = \frac{X \text{ gtt}}{1.7 \text{ mL}} = \textbf{34 gtt}$$
$$X = \textbf{34 gtt}$$

To infuse an IV of 2500 mL in 24 hr using an IV set calibrated at 20 gtt/mL, set the manual flow rate at 34 gtt/min.

16

EXAMPLE 4 | An IV of **1000 mL** is ordered to infuse in **5 hr** using a set calibrated at **15 gtt/mL**.

- **Calculate the mL/hr to infuse.**

  1000 mL ÷ 5 hr = **200 mL/hr**

- **Calculate the mL/min to infuse.**

  200 mL ÷ 60 min = **3.3 mL/min**

- **Calculate the gtt/min rate.**

  15 gtt : 1 mL = X gtt : 3.3 mL   or $\dfrac{15 \text{ gtt}}{1 \text{ mL}} = \dfrac{X \text{ gtt}}{3.3 \text{ mL}}$ = 49.5 = **50 gtt**

  X = 49.5 = **50 gtt**

To infuse 1000 mL in 5 hr using a set calibrated at 15 gtt/mL, set the rate at 50 gtt/min.

Flow rate answers may vary by 1–2 gtt/min depending on how the numbers are rounded in calculations, or due to calculator setting.

A 1–2 gtt/min variation is considered insignificant for most infusions, because flow rates fluctuate as the patient bends the infusion arm, changes position in bed, or ambulates. Thus, manually set rates are approximate.

PROBLEM

Calculate the gtt/min manual IV flow rates for the following infusions. Round rates to the nearest whole number.

1. An IV of 2000 mL is to infuse over 12 hr using a 10 gtt/mL set.   _____

2. 3500 mL are ordered to infuse in 24 hr using a set calibrated at 20 gtt/mL.   _____

3. Infuse 500 mL in 3 hr using a 15 gtt/mL set.   _____

4. A volume of 1500 mL is to infuse in 5 hr using a 15 gtt/mL set.   _____

5. 1750 mL are ordered to infuse in 9 hr using a 20 gtt/mL set.   _____

6. An IV of 2500 mL is to infuse in 18 hr on a set calibrated at 10 gtt/mL.   _____

7. A 3000 mL volume is to infuse in 24 hr on a set calibrated at 20 gtt/mL.   _____

8. A volume of 2750 mL is to infuse in 22 hr on a 15 gtt/mL set.   _____

9. An IV of 750 mL is ordered to infuse in 8 hr on a 10 gtt/mL set.   _____

10. A volume of 1250 mL is to infuse in 12 hr using a 15 gtt/mL set.   _____

Answers **1.** 28 gtt/min **2.** 49 gtt/min **3.** 42 gtt/min **4.** 75 gtt/min **5.** 65 gtt/min **6.** 23 gtt/min **7.** 41 gtt/min **8.** 31 gtt/min **9.** 16 gtt/min **10.** 26 gtt/min **Note:** Answers that vary by 1–2 gtt/min may be considered correct.

CALCULATING SMALL-VOLUME gtt/min RATES FROM mL/min ORDERED

Small-volume IV solutions are most frequently ordered to administer medications. Because of the immediacy of IV medication action, each dosage is routinely double-checked for accuracy before administration. A small-volume flush of IV solution is usually ordered to follow the administration to ensure that all the medication has cleared the line. The flush volume may vary from 2 to 15 mL depending on the length of the IV tubing used.

There are three common administrative techniques used for small-volume infusions. **Very small volumes** are most often administered by **syringe**, either **manually** or **via syringe pump**. If a syringe pump (see Chapter 15, page 214) is used, the primary responsibilities are to make sure the rate is set correctly on the device **and** that it is working properly.

The two other methods of small-volume administration are via **burettes** calibrated in 1–2 mL increments, with a capacity of 100–150 mL (Chapter 21, page 296), or via **commercial or pharmacy prepared IV bags containing medication** in a volume of 50–250 mL (Chapter 15, page 209).

It is when a **burette** or **small-volume IV solution bag** is to be infused **without the use of an electronic device** that a gtt/min flow rate will need to be calculated. With regard to burettes one precaution must be particularly stressed: **although most are calibrated in 60 gtt/mL microdrips, this calibration cannot be taken for granted**. Some burettes are specifically manufactured for use with electronic volumetric pumps and may have, for example, a 20 gtt/mL calibration. When pumps are used with their companion tubings their setting accommodates for the gtt size, and the main administrative precaution becomes **matching the correct tubing to its pump**, setting the rate correctly, and, as always, making sure the device is working properly.

Let's now look at calculation of small-volume flow rates when no infusion device is used.

 An IV medication of **100 mL** is to be infused in **40 min** using a set calibrated at **15 gtt/mL**. Calculate the **gtt/min** flow rate.

- **Calculate the mL/min to be administered.**

$$100 \text{ mL} : 40 \text{ min} = X \text{ mL} : 1 \text{ min} \quad \text{or} \quad \frac{100 \text{ mL}}{40 \text{ min}} = \frac{X \text{ mL}}{1 \text{ min}} = \textbf{2.5 mL/min}$$
$$X = \textbf{2.5 mL/min}$$

- **Calculate the gtt/min rate.**

$$15 \text{ gtt} : 1 \text{ mL} = X \text{ gtt} : 2.5 \text{ mL} \quad \text{or} \quad \frac{15 \text{ gtt}}{1 \text{ mL}} = \frac{X \text{ gtt}}{2.5 \text{ mL}} = 37.5 = \textbf{38 gtt}$$
$$X = 37.5 = \textbf{38 gtt}$$

To administer an infusion of 100 mL in 40 min using a 15 gtt/mL calibrated set, the flow rate must be 38 gtt/min.

EXAMPLE 2 | An IV medication of **60 mL** is ordered to infuse in **30 min**. The set calibration is **20 gtt/mL**. Calculate the **gtt/min** flow rate.

• **Calculate the mL/min to be administered.**

$$60 \text{ mL} : 30 \text{ min} = X \text{ mL} : 1 \text{ min} \quad \text{or} \quad \frac{60 \text{ mL}}{30 \text{ min}} = \frac{X \text{ mL}}{1 \text{ min}} = \textbf{2 mL/min}$$
$$X = \textbf{2 mL/min}$$

• **Calculate the gtt/min rate.**

$$20 \text{ gtt} : 1 \text{ mL} = X \text{ gtt} : 2 \text{ mL} \quad \text{or} \quad \frac{20 \text{ gtt}}{1 \text{ mL}} = \frac{X \text{ gtt}}{2 \text{ mL}} = \textbf{40 gtt}$$
$$X = \textbf{40 gtt}$$

To administer an infusion of 60 mL in 30 min using a set calibrated at 20 gtt/mL, set the flow rate at 40 gtt/min.

EXAMPLE 3 | A volume of **50 mL** is ordered to infuse in **20 min** using a **10 gtt/mL** calibrated set. Calculate the **gtt/min** flow rate.

• **Calculate the mL/min to be administered.**

$$50 \text{ mL} : 20 \text{ min} = X \text{ mL} : 1 \text{ min} \quad \text{or} \quad \frac{50 \text{ mL}}{20 \text{ min}} = \frac{X \text{ mL}}{1 \text{ min}} = \textbf{2.5 mL/min}$$
$$X = \textbf{2.5 mL/min}$$

• **Calculate the gtt/min rate.**

$$10 \text{ gtt} : 1 \text{ mL} = X \text{ gtt} : 2.5 \text{ mL} \quad \text{or} \quad \frac{10 \text{ gtt}}{1 \text{ mL}} = \frac{X \text{ gtt}}{2.5 \text{ mL}} = \textbf{25 gtt}$$
$$X = \textbf{25 gtt}$$

To infuse a volume of 50 mL in 20 min using a set calibrated at 10 gtt/mL, set the flow rate at 25 gtt/min.

PROBLEM

Calculate the flow rates in gtt/min for the following small-volume infusions. Round rates to the nearest whole gtt.

1. A medication of 75 mL is to be administered in 50 min using a set calibrated at 10 gtt/mL. _____

2. A set calibrated at 15 gtt/mL is to be used to infuse 80 mL in 50 min. _____

3. A volume of 40 mL is to be infused in 20 min using a set calibrated at 20 gtt/mL. _____

4. A 10 gtt/mL set is being used to administer 20 mL in 20 min. _____

5. A 70 mL volume is to infuse in 40 min using a 15 gtt/mL set. _____

Answers **1.** 15 gtt/min **2.** 24 gtt/min **3.** 40 gtt/min **4.** 10 gtt/min **5.** 26 gtt/min **Note:** Answers that vary by 1–2 gtt/min may be considered correct.

FORMULA METHOD OF FLOW RATE CALCULATION

The flow rate can also be determined by using the following formula, which is **useful when the rate can be expressed as mL/60 min or less**.

$$\text{Flow Rate} = \frac{\text{Volume} \times \text{Set Calibration}}{\text{Time (in min)}}$$

EXAMPLE 1   An IV is ordered to infuse at **125 mL/hr**. Calculate the **gtt/min** rate for a set calibrated at **10 gtt/mL**.

• **Convert the hr to min.**

$$\frac{125\ (\text{mL}) \times 10\ (\text{gtt/mL})}{60\ (\text{min})}$$

• **Calculate the gtt/min rate.**

$$\frac{125 \times 10}{60} = 20.8 = \mathbf{21\ gtt/min}$$

EXAMPLE 2   Administer an IV medication of **100 mL** in **40 min** using a set calibrated at **15 gtt/mL**.

$$\frac{100 \times 15}{40} = 37.5 = \mathbf{38\ gtt/min}$$

EXAMPLE 3   A **75 mL** volume of IV medication is ordered to infuse in **45 min**. The set is calibrated at **20 gtt/mL**.

$$\frac{75 \times 20}{45} = 33.3 = \mathbf{33\ gtt/min}$$

PROBLEM

Calculate the flow rate in gtt/min for the following infusions using the formula method.

1. Administer an IV of 110 mL/hr using a set calibrated at 20 gtt/mL.   _____

2. An IV solution is ordered at 200 mL/hr using a set calibrated at 15 gtt/mL.   _____

3. A volume of 80 mL is to be infused in 20 min using a 10 gtt/mL set.   _____

4. An IV is ordered to infuse at 150 mL/hr using a 10 gtt/mL calibrated set.   _____

5. An IV rate of 90 mL/hr is ordered using a 15 gtt/mL calibrated set.   _____

Answers   **1.** 37 gtt/min   **2.** 50 gtt/min   **3.** 40 gtt/min   **4.** 25 gtt/min   **5.** 23 gtt/min   **Note:** Consider answers within 1 gtt/min correct.

When an IV is ordered to infuse in **more than 1 hour**, the formula method can still be used. However, to keep the numbers you are working with as small as possible, it is best to add a preliminary step and determine the **mL/hr** the ordered volume will represent.

EXAMPLE 1

Calculate the gtt/min flow rate for an IV of **1000 mL** to infuse in **8 hr** on a set calibrated at **20 gtt/mL**.

- **Calculate the mL/hr.**

    1000 mL/8 hr $=$ 1000 $\div$ 8 $=$ **125 mL/hr**

- **Calculate the gtt/min flow rate.**

    $$\frac{125 \text{ (mL)} \times 20 \text{ (gtt/mL)}}{60 \text{ (min)}} = 41.6 = \textbf{42 gtt/min}$$

EXAMPLE 2

Calculate the gtt/min flow rate for a volume of **2500 mL** to infuse in **24 hr** on a set calibrated at **10 gtt/mL**.

- **Calculate the mL/hr.**

    2500 mL/24 hr $=$ 2500 $\div$ 24 $=$ **104 mL/hr**

- **Calculate the gtt/min flow rate.**

    $$\frac{104 \times 10}{60} = 17.3 = \textbf{17 gtt/min}$$

EXAMPLE 3

An IV of **1200 mL** is to infuse in **16 hr** on a set calibrated at **15 gtt/mL**.

1200 mL/16 hr $=$ 1200 $\div$ 16 $=$ **75 mL/hr**

$$\frac{75 \times 15}{60} = 18.7 = \textbf{19 gtt/min}$$

PROBLEM

Calculate the gtt/min flow rate for the following infusions using the formula method.

1. A volume of 2000 mL to infuse in 24 hr on a set calibrated at 15 gtt/mL _____

2. A volume of 300 mL to infuse in 6 hr on a 60 gtt/mL microdrip set _____

3. A volume of 500 mL to infuse in 4 hr on a 15 gtt/mL calibrated set _____

4. A 10-hr infusion of 1200 mL using a 20 gtt/mL set _____

5. An infusion of 500 mL in 5 hr on a set calibrated at 10 gtt/mL _____

Answers **1.** 21 gtt/min **2.** 50 gtt/min **3.** 31 gtt/min **4.** 40 gtt/min **5.** 17 gtt/min **Note:** Answers that vary by 1–2 gtt/min may be considered correct.

DIVISION FACTOR METHOD OF CALCULATION

In a clinical setting where all the macrodrip IV sets have the same calibration, either 10,15, or 20 gtt/mL, an alternate "division factor" method can be used to calculate flow rates. However, **this method can only be used if the rate is expressed in mL/hr (mL/60 min)**. Let's start by looking at how the division factor is obtained.

EXAMPLE | Administer an IV at **125 mL/hr**. The set calibration is **10 gtt/mL**. Calculate the gtt/min rate. Express the hr rate as 60 min.

$$\frac{125 \text{ (mL)} \times \overset{1}{\cancel{10}} \text{(gtt/mL)}}{\underset{6}{\cancel{60}} \text{ (min)}} = 20.8 = \textbf{21 gtt/min}$$

Look at the completed equation, and noted that because you are restricting the time to 60 min, the set calibration (10) will be divided into 60 (min) to obtain a constant number (6). This constant (6) is the division factor for a 10 gtt/mL calibrated set.

 The division factor can be obtained for any IV set by dividing 60 by the calibration of the set.

PROBLEM

Determine the division factor for the following IV sets.

1. 20 gtt/mL   _____

2. 15 gtt/mL   _____

3. 60 gtt/mL   _____

4. 10 gtt/mL   _____

Answers **1.** 3 **2.** 4 **3.** 1 **4.** 6

Once the division factor is known, the gtt/min rate can be calculated in one step, by dividing the mL/hr rate by the division factor. Look again at the example.

$$\frac{125 \text{ (mL)} \times \overset{1}{\cancel{10}} \text{(gtt/mL)}}{\underset{6}{\cancel{60}} \text{ (min)}} = 20.8 = \textbf{21 gtt/min}$$

or 125 (mL/hr) ÷ 6 = 20.8 = **21 gtt/min**

The 125 mL/hr flow rate divided by the division factor 6 gives the same 21 gtt/min rate.

 The gtt/min flow rate can be calculated for mL/hr IV orders in one step by dividing the mL/hr to be infused by the division factor of the administration set.

EXAMPLE 1 | Infuse an IV at **100 mL/hr** using a set calibrated at **10 gtt/mL**.

Determine the division factor: 60 ÷ 10 = **6**

Calculate the flow rate: 100 mL ÷ 6 = 16.6 = **17 gtt/min**

EXAMPLE 2 | Infuse an IV at **125 mL/hr** using a set calibrated at **15 gtt/mL**.

60 ÷ 15 = **4**   125 mL ÷ 4 = 31.2 = **31 gtt/min**

EXAMPLE 3 | A set calibrated at **20 gtt/mL** is used to infuse **90 mL per hr**.

$$60 \div 20 = \mathbf{3} \qquad 90 \text{ mL} \div 3 = \mathbf{30\ gtt/min}$$

The division factor is of enormous assistance in clinical practice because hospitals and clinics generally use only one size macrodrip set. This means that the same division factor can be used for all IV flow rate calculations.

PROBLEM

Calculate the flow rates in gtt/min for the following infusions using the division factor method.

1. A rate of 110 mL/hr via a set calibrated at 20 gtt/mL   _____

2. A set is calibrated at 15 gtt/mL. Infuse at 130 mL/hr.   _____

3. Infuse 150 mL/hr using a 10 gtt/mL set.   _____

4. A set calibrated at 20 gtt/mL is used to infuse 45 mL/hr.   _____

5. Infusion is ordered at 75 mL/hr with a set calibrated at 15 gtt/mL. _____

Answers   **1.** 37 gtt/min   **2.** 33 gtt/min   **3.** 25 gtt/min   **4.** 15 gtt/min   **5.** 19 gtt/min   **Note:** Answers that vary by 1–2 gtt/min may be considered correct.

All of the preceding examples and problems using the division factor method were for **macrodrip** sets. Let's now look what happens when a **microdrip** set calibrated at **60 gtt/mL** is used.

EXAMPLE | Infuse at **50 mL/hr** using a **60 gtt/mL** microdrip.

$$60 \div 60 = \mathbf{1} \qquad 50 \text{ mL} \div 1 = \mathbf{50\ gtt/min}$$

Because the set calibration is 60, and the division factor is based on a 60-min (1 hr) time, the division factor is 1. So, **for microdrip sets the gtt/min flow rate will be identical to the mL/hr ordered**.

 When a 60 gtt/mL microdrip set is used, the flow rate in gtt/min is identical to the volume in mL/hr to be infused.

PROBLEM

What is the drip rate in gtt/min for the following infusions if a microdrip is used?

1. 120 mL/hr   _____

2. 90 mL/hr   _____

3. 100 mL/hr   _____

4. 75 mL/hr   _____

5. 80 mL/hr   _____

Answers   **1.** 120 gtt/min   **2.** 90 gtt/min   **3.** 100 gtt/min   **4.** 75 gtt/min   **5.** 80 gtt/min

The division factor method can be used to calculate the flow rate of **any volume that can be expressed in mL/hr**. Larger volumes can be divided, and smaller volumes can be multiplied and expressed in mL/hr. This does require an extra step, and if you find it confusing you may elect not to use it.

| EXAMPLE 1 | 2400 mL/24 hr = 2400 ÷ 24 = **100 mL/hr** |

| EXAMPLE 2 | 1800 mL/8 hr = 1800 ÷ 8 = **225 mL/hr** |

| EXAMPLE 3 | 10 mL/30 min = 10 × 2 (2 × 30 min) = **20 mL/hr** |

| EXAMPLE 4 | 15 mL/20 min = 15 × 3 (3 × 20 min) = **45 mL/hr** |

REGULATING FLOW RATE

Manual flow rates are regulated by **counting the number of drops falling in the drip chamber**. The standard procedure for doing this is to hold a watch next to the drip chamber and actually **count the number of drops falling**. The roller clamp is adjusted during the count until the required rate has been set. A 15-sec count is most commonly used because there is less chance of attention wandering during the count. This means that the ordered gtt/min (60 sec) rate must be divided by 4 to obtain the 15-second drip count (15 sec × 4 = 60 sec).

| EXAMPLE 1 | An IV is to run at a rate of **60 gtt/min**. What will the 15-sec count be? |

60 gtt/min ÷ 4 = **15 gtt**

Adjust the rate to 15 gtt/15 sec.

| EXAMPLE 2 | A 70 **gtt/min** IV rate is ordered. What will the 15-sec count be? |

70 gtt/min ÷ 4 = 17.5 = **18 gtt**

Adjust the rate to 18 gtt/15 sec.

| EXAMPLE 3 | Adjust an IV to a rate of **50 gtt/min** using a 15-sec count. |

50 gtt/min ÷ 4 = **13 gtt**

Adjust the rate to 13 gtt/15 sec.

PROBLEM

Answer the following questions about 15-second drip rates.

1. The 15-second count of an IV flow rate is 7 gtt. A 29 gtt/min rate is required. Is this rate correct? _____

2. You are to regulate a newly started IV to deliver 67 gtt/min. Using a 15-second count, how would you set the flow rate? _____

3. An IV is to run at 48 gtt/min. What must the 15-second drip rate be? _____

4. How many gtt will you count in 15 seconds if the rate is 55 gtt/min? _____

5. An IV is to run at 84 gtt/min. What will the 15-second rate be? _____

Answers **1.** Yes **2.** 17 gtt/15 sec **3.** 12 gtt/15 sec **4.** 14 gtt/15 sec **5.** 21 gtt/15 sec **Note:** Answers that vary by 1 gtt/min may be considered correct.

Individual hospitals and/or states/provinces may require a 30- or 60-sec (1 min) count. When a 60-sec count is required, particular care must be taken not to let your attention wander during the count, which can easily happen in this longer time frame. A 60-sec count will require a full min count, whereas a 30-sec count will require the gtt/min rate to be divided by 2 (60 sec ÷ 2 = 30 sec).

EXAMPLE 1 | An IV is to be infused at 56 gtt/min. What is the 30-sec rate?

56 gtt/min ÷ 2 = 28 gtt

Adjust the rate to 28 gtt/30 sec.

EXAMPLE 2 | A rate of 72 gtt/min has been ordered. What will the 30 sec count be?

72 gtt/min ÷ 2 = 36 gtt

Adjust the rate to 36 gtt/30 sec.

PROBLEM

Calculate the 30-sec count for the following IVs.

1. An IV is to be run at a rate of 48 gtt/min. Calculate a 30-sec count. _____

2. An IV is ordered to infuse at 52 gtt/min. _____

Answers   **1.** 24 gtt/30 sec   **2.** 26 gtt/30 sec

CORRECTING OFF-SCHEDULE RATES

Because a patient's positional changes can alter the rate slightly, IVs occasionally infuse ahead of or behind schedule. When this occurs, the usual procedure is to **recalculate the flow rate using the volume and time remaining** and to **adjust the rate accordingly**. However, each situation must be individually evaluated, especially if the discrepancy is large. If too much fluid has infused, immediately assess the patient's response to the increased intake and take appropriate action. If too little fluid has infused, it will first be necessary to assess the patient's ability to tolerate an increased rate and, secondly, to consider the type of fluid/medication involved. Some medications and fluids have restrictions on rate of administration. Both of these factors must be considered before rates can be increased to "catch up." In addition, **many hospitals will have specific policies to cover over or under infusion due to altered flow rates, and you will be responsible for knowing these**.

The following are some examples of how the rate can be recalculated. Because IVs are usually checked hourly, the focus will first be on recalculation using exact hours. Some recalculations have also been included using fractions of hours, rounded to the nearest quarter hour: 15 min = 0.25 hr, 30 min = 0.5 hr, and 45 min = 0.75 hr. These equivalents are close enough for uncomplicated infusions, because the exact time of completion is not totally predictable. IVs needing exact infusion would hopefully be monitored by electronic infusion devices.

16

EXAMPLE 1

An IV of **1000 mL** was ordered to infuse over **10 hr** at a rate of **25 gtt/min**. The set calibration is **15 gtt/mL**. After **5 hr** a total of 650 mL have infused instead of the **500 mL** ordered. Recalculate the new gtt/min flow rate to complete the infusion on schedule.

Time remaining 10 hr − 5 hr = **5 hr**

Volume remaining 1000 mL − 650 mL = **350 mL**

350 mL ÷ 5 hr = **70 mL/hr**

Set calibration is **15 gtt/mL**.

70 ÷ 4 (division factor) = 17.5 = **18 gtt/min**

Slow the rate from 25 gtt/min to 18 gtt/min.

EXAMPLE 2

An IV of **800 mL** was to infuse over **8 hr** at 20 gtt/min. After **4 hr 15 min** only **300 mL** have infused. Recalculate the **gtt/min** rate to complete on schedule. The set calibration is **15 gtt/mL**.

Time remaining 8 hr − 4.25 hr = **3.75 hr**

Volume remaining 800 mL − 300 mL = **500 mL**

500 mL ÷ 3.75 hr = 133.3 = **133 mL/hr**

Set calibration is **15 gtt/mL**.

133 ÷ 4 (division factor) = 33.2 = **33 gtt/min**

Increase the rate to 33 gtt/min.

EXAMPLE 3

An IV of **500 mL** is infusing at **28 gtt/min**. It was to complete in **3 hr**, but after 1½ hr only **175 mL** have infused. Recalculate the **gtt/min** rate to complete the infusion on schedule. Set calibration is **10 gtt/mL**.

Time remaining 3 hr − 1.5 hr = **1.5 hr**

Volume remaining 500 mL − 175 mL = **325 mL**

325 mL ÷ 1.5 hr = 216.6 = **217 mL/hr**

Set calibration is **10 gtt/mL**.

217 ÷ 6 (division factor) = 36.1 = **36 gtt/min**

Increase the rate to 36 gtt/min.

EXAMPLE 4

A volume of **250 mL** was to infuse **56 gtt/min** in **1½ hr** using a set calibrated at **20 gtt/mL**. After **30 min 175 mL** have infused. Recalculate the flow rate.

Time remaining 1.5 hr − 30 min = **1 hr**

Volume remaining 250 mL − 175 mL = **75 mL**

Set calibration is **20 gtt/mL**.

75 ÷ 3 (division factor) = **25 gtt/min**

Decrease the rate to 25 gtt/min.

PROBLEM

Recalculate the following IV rates so that the infusions will complete on schedule.

1. An IV of 500 mL was ordered to infuse in 3 hr using a 15 gtt/mL set. With 1½ hr remaining you discover that only 150 mL is left in the bag. At what rate will you need to reset the flow? _____

2. An IV of 1000 mL was scheduled to run in 12 hr. After 4 hr only 220 mL have infused. The set calibration is 20 gtt/mL. Recalculate the rate for the remaining solution. _____

3. An IV of 1000 mL was ordered to infuse in 8 hr. With 3 hr of infusion time left you discover that 600 mL have infused. The set delivers 20 gtt/mL. Recalculate the drip rate and indicate how many drops you will count in 15 sec to set the new rate.

   _____ _____

4. An IV of 750 mL was ordered to run over 6 hr with a set calibrated at 10 gtt/mL. After 2 hr you notice that 300 mL have infused. Recalculate the flow rate, and indicate how many drops you will count in 15 sec to reset the rate.

   _____ _____

5. An IV of 800 mL was started at 9 a.m. to infuse in 4 hr. At 10 a.m. 150 mL have infused. The set is calibrated at 15 gtt/mL. Recalculate the flow rate in gtt/min. _____

Answers **1.** 24 gtt/min **2.** 33 gtt/min **3.** 44 gtt/min; 11 gtt/15 sec **4.** 19 gtt/min; 4–5 gtt/15 sec **5.** 54 gtt/min **Note:** Answers that vary by 1–2 gtt/min may be considered correct.

Summary

This concludes the chapter on IV flow rate calculation and monitoring. The important points to remember from this chapter are:

- IVs are ordered as mL/hr or mL/min to be administered.

- Manual flow rates are counted in gtt/min.

- IV tubings are calibrated in gtt/mL.

- Macrodrip IV sets will have a calibration of 10, 15, or 20 gtt/mL.

- Mini or microdrip sets have a calibration of 60 gtt/mL.

● The formula for calculating flow rates is

$$\frac{Volume \ \times \ Set \ Calibration}{Time \ (in \ min)}$$

● The division factor method can only be used to calculate flow rates if the volume to be administered is specified in mL/hr (60 min).

● The division factor is obtained by dividing 60 by the set calibration.

● Flow rate by the division factor method is determined by dividing the mL/hr to be administered by the division factor.

● Because micro/minidrip sets have a calibration of 60 gtt/mL, their division factor is 1, and the flow rate in gtt/min is the same as the mL/hr ordered.

● If an IV runs ahead of or behind schedule, a possible procedure is to use the time and mL remaining to calculate a new flow rate.

● If a rate must be increased to compensate for running behind schedule, the type of fluid being infused and the patient's ability to tolerate an increased rate must be assessed.

● If an IV is determined to have infused ahead of schedule immediate assessment of the patient's tolerance to the excess fluid is required, and appropriate action taken.

Summary Self-Test

Answer the following questions as briefly as possible.

1. Determine the division factor for the following IV sets.

   a) 60 gtt/mL   _____

   b) 15 gtt/mL   _____

   c) 20 gtt/mL   _____

   d) 10 gtt/mL   _____

2. How is the flow rate determined in the division factor method?   _____

3. The division factor method can only be used if the volume to be administered is expressed in   _____

4. An IV is to infuse at 50 gtt/min. How will you set it using a 15-sec count?   _____

5. You are to adjust an IV at a rate of 60 gtt/min. What will the 15-sec count be?   _____

Calculate the flow rate in gtt/min for each of the following IV solutions and medications. Don't let the types of solutions confuse you. Concentrate on locating the information you need for your calculations.

6. D5W 2000 mL has been ordered to run 16 hr. Set calibration is 10 gtt/mL.   _____

7. The order is for 500 mL of normal saline in 8 hr. The set is calibrated at 15 gtt/mL.   _____

8. Administer 150 mL of sodium chloride 0.45% over 3 hr.
   A microdrip is used.   _____

9. 1500 mL D5W with 40 mEq KCl/L has been ordered to run over
   12 hr. Set calibration is 20 gtt/mL.   _____

10. An IV medication of 30 mL is to be administered over 30 min
    using a 15 gtt/mL set.   _____

11. Administer 100 mL of 0.9% NaCl in 1 hr using a 15 gtt/mL set.   _____

12. Infuse 500 mL of intralipids IV in 6 hr. Set calibration is
    10 gtt/mL.   _____

13. The doctor orders a liter of D5W to infuse over 10 hr. At the end
    of 8 hr you notice that there are 500 mL left in the bag. What
    would the new flow rate be if the set calibration is 10 gtt/mL?   _____

14. An IV was started at 9 a.m. with orders to infuse 500 mL over
    6 hr. At 12 noon the IV infiltrated with 350 mL left in the bag. At
    1 p.m. the IV was restarted. The set calibration is 20 gtt/mL.
    Calculate the new flow rate to deliver the fluid on time.   _____

15. A 50 mL piggyback IV is to infuse over 15 min. The set
    calibration is 15 gtt/mL. After 5 minutes the IV contains 40 mL.
    Calculate the flow rate to deliver the volume on time.   _____

16. An IV of 1000 mL D5 1/4 NaCl with 20 mEq KCl is ordered to
    run at 25 mL/hr using a microdrip set.   _____

17. Ringer's lactate 800 mL has been ordered to run in 5 hr. Set
    calibration is 10 gtt/mL.   _____

18. Administer 1500 mL of D5 lactated Ringer's solution over 8 hr
    using a set calibrated at 20 gtt/mL.   _____

19. The order is for D5 1/2 NaCl 750 mL to run in 6 hr. Set calibra-
    tion is 15 gtt/mL.   _____

20. An IV of 1000 mL was ordered to run in 8 hr. After 4 hr only
    250 mL have infused. The set calibration is 20 gtt/mL.
    Recalculate the rate for the remaining solution.   _____

21. The order is to infuse 50 mL of a piggyback antibiotic over 1 hr.
    The set calibration is a microdrip.   _____

22. An IV of 500 mL D5W is to infuse over 6 hr. You will be using a
    set calibration of 10 gtt/mL.   _____

23. Infuse 120 mL gentamicin via IVPB over 1 hr. Set calibration is
    10 gtt/mL.   _____

24. Administer 12 mL of an IV medication in 22 min using a
    microdrip set.   _____

25. A patient is to receive 3000 mL of D5W in 20 hr. Set is
    calibrated at 20 gtt/mL.   _____

26. Infuse 1 liter of D5W in 5 hr using a set calibration of 15 gtt/mL.   _____

27. A hyperalimentation solution of 1180 mL is to infuse in 12 hr
    using a set calibration of 20 gtt/mL.   _____

28. 150 mL of an antibiotic solution is to infuse in 30 min. At the end of 20 min you discover that 100 mL have infused. The set calibration is 10 gtt/mL. Should the flow rate be adjusted? If so, what is the new rate? _____ _____

29. Two 500 mL units of whole blood are ordered. Both units are to be completed in 5 hr. The set calibration is 20 gtt/mL. _____

30. Infuse 15 mL of IV medication in the next 14 min using a 20 gtt/mL set. _____

31. The patient is to receive 1000 mL 0.9% NaCl in 10 hr using a 20 gtt/mL calibration. _____

32. A minidrip is used to administer 12 mL in 17 min. _____

33. Infuse 2750 mL in 20 hr using a 10 gtt/mL set. _____

34. D5W 1800 mL is to infuse in the next 15 hr with a 15 gtt/mL set. _____

35. Infuse 600 mL of intralipids IV in 6 hr with a 10 gtt/mL set. _____

36. Administer 22 mL of an IV antibiotic solution in 18 min using a minidrip set. _____

37. 1800 mL of D5W with 30 mEq of KCl per liter have been ordered to infuse in 10 hr. Set calibration is 20 gtt/mL. _____

38. Infuse 8 mL in 9 min using a minidrip. _____

39. A patient is to receive 4000 mL D5W IV in the next 20 hr. A 20 gtt/mL set is used. _____

40. An IV of 500 mL D5W that was to infuse in 2 hr is discovered to have only 150 mL left after 30 min. Recalculate the flow rate. Set calibration is 15 gtt/mL. _____

Answers						
1. a) 1 b) 4 c) 3	**7.** 16 gtt/min	**17.** 27 gtt/min	**27.** 33 gtt/min	**35.** 17 gtt/min
d) 6	**8.** 50 gtt/min	**18.** 63 gtt/min	**28.** No, rate is	**36.** 73 gtt/min
2. mL/hr ÷	**9.** 42 gtt/min	**19.** 31 gtt/min	correct at	**37.** 60 gtt/min
division factor	**10.** 15 gtt/min	**20.** 63 gtt/min	50 gtt/min	**38.** 53 gtt/min
3. mL/hr	**11.** 25 gtt/min	**21.** 50 gtt/min	**29.** 67 gtt/min	**39.** 67 gtt/min
(mL/60 min)	**12.** 14 gtt/min	**22.** 14 gtt/min	**30.** 21 gtt/min	**40.** 25 gtt/min
4. 13 gtt/15 sec	**13.** 42 gtt/min	**23.** 20 gtt/min	**31.** 33 gtt/min	
5. 15 gtt/15 sec	**14.** 58 gtt/min	**24.** 33 gtt/min	**32.** 42 gtt/min	
6. 21 gtt/min	**15.** 60 gtt/min	**25.** 50 gtt/min	**33.** 23 gtt/min	
	16. 25 gtt/min	**26.** 50 gtt/min	**34.** 30 gtt/min	

Note: Consider answers that vary by 1–2 gtt/min accurate.

Calculating IV Infusion and Completion Times

The three main reasons for calculating IV infusion times are: (1) to know when a particular solution bag will be completed so that any additional solutions ordered can be prepared in advance and ready to hang; (2) to discontinue an IV when it has completed; and (3) to label an IV bag with the start, progress, and completion times so that the infusion can be monitored and adjusted as necessary to keep it on schedule. Knowing the infusion time is also important because laboratory studies are sometimes made before, during, or after specified amounts of IV solutions have infused. The infusion time may be calculated in hours and/or minutes, depending on the amount and type of solution and individual patient needs.

CALCULATING FROM VOLUME AND HOURLY RATE ORDERED

Most IV orders are written specifying the total volume to be infused and the hourly rate of administration, for example, 2000 mL at 100 mL per hr. The largest IV solution bag is 1000 mL, so this 2000 mL volume (or any volume) may require a combination of several 1000 mL, 500 mL, or 250 mL bags.

Because most large-volume IVs take several hours to infuse, the unit of time being calculated is most often hours (hr). An easy one-step calculation is used to obtain the infusion time. To use it you will divide the **total volume to be infused** by the **mL/hr rate** of infusion.

 IV infusion time is calculated by dividing the total volume to be infused by the mL/hr flow rate.

EXAMPLE 1   Calculate the infusion time for an IV of **500 mL** D5W ordered to infuse at **50 mL/hr**.

Infusion Time = total volume ÷ mL/hr rate

$$= 500 \text{ mL} \div 50 \text{ mL/hr} = \textbf{10 hr}$$

The infusion time for an IV of 500 mL infusing at 50 mL/hr is 10 hr.

Objectives

The learner will calculate IV infusion times using:

1. volume and hourly rate of infusion

2. volume, gtt/min rate of infusion and set calibration

3. start time and infusion time to determine completion times

4. an IV solution bag tape to label the start, progress, and completion times

EXAMPLE 2 | The order is to infuse **1000 mL** of D5NS at **75 mL/hr**. Calculate the infusion time.

1000 mL ÷ 75 mL/hr = **13.33 hr**

In this example, the 13 represents hr, whereas the **.33 represents the fraction of an additional hr**.

 Fractional hr are converted to min by multiplying 60 min by the fraction obtained.

Calculate the min by multiplying 60 min by the fractional hr.

60 min × .33 = 19.8 = **20 min**

The total infusion time is 13 hr 20 min.

EXAMPLE 3 | An IV of **1000 mL** D5W is infusing at **90 mL/hr**. How long will it take to complete?

1000 mL ÷ 90 mL/hr = **11.11 hr**

Remember that .11 represents the fraction of an additional hr. Convert this to minutes by multiplying 60 min by .11.

60 min × .11 = 6.6 = **7 min**

The total infusion time is 11 hr 7 min.

EXAMPLE 4 | Calculate the infusion time for an IV of **750 mL** RL ordered at a rate of **80 mL/hr**.

750 mL ÷ 80 mL/hr = **9.38 hr**

60 min × .38 = 22.8 = **23 min**

The infusion time is 9 hr 23 min.

EXAMPLE 5 | A rate of **75 mL/hr** is ordered for a total volume of **500 mL** D5W. Calculate the infusion time.

500 mL ÷ 75 mL/hr = **6.67 hr**

60 min × .67 = 40.2 = **40 min**

The infusion time is 6 hr 40 min.

PROBLEM

Calculate infusion times for the following IVs.

1. An IV of 900 mL RL ordered to infuse at 80 mL/hr   _____

2. A volume of 250 mL is to be infused at 30 mL/hr   _____

3. An infusion of 180 mL of NS to run at a rate of 25 mL/hr   _____

4. A volume of 1000 mL D5W ordered at a rate of 60 mL/hr   _____

5. An IV of 150 mL ordered to infuse at 80 mL/hr   _____

Answers **1.** 11 hr 15 min **2.** 8 hr 20 min **3.** 7 hr 12 min **4.** 16 hr 40 min **5.** 1 hr 53 min   **Note:** Answers may vary due to rounding or calculator setting, so variations of 1–2 min may be considered correct.

CALCULATING INFUSION TIME FROM gtt/min RATE AND SET CALIBRATION

In some instances, the only information you may have to calculate the infusion time is the gtt/min rate at which the IV is infusing, the set calibration, and the total volume to be infused. The first step is to use the gtt/min flow rate and gtt/mL set calibration to calculate the mL/min and the mL/hr rate.

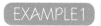 **EXAMPLE 1** | Calculate the infusion time for an IV of **1000 mL** of D5W running at **25 gtt/min** on a set calibrated at **10 gtt/mL**.

- **Convert gtt/min to mL/min.**

  10 gtt : 1 mL = 25 gtt : X mL   or $\dfrac{10 \text{ gtt}}{1 \text{ mL}} = \dfrac{25 \text{ gtt}}{X \text{ mL}}$ = **2.5 mL/min**

  X = **2.5 mL/min**

- **Convert mL/min to mL/hr.**

  60 min × 2.5 mL/min = **150 mL/hr.**

- **Calculate the infusion time by dividing the total volume to be infused by the mL/hr rate you have just obtained.**

  1000 mL ÷ 150 mL/hr = **6.67 hr**

- **Multiply 60 min by the .67 hr fraction to obtain the min of infusion.**

  60 min × .67 = 40.2 = **40 min**

The total infusion time is 6 hr 40 min.

EXAMPLE 2 | A volume of 750 mL D5RL is running at **12 gtt/min** on a set calibrated at **10 gtt/mL**. Calculate the infusion time.

- **Convert gtt/min to mL/min.**

  10 gtt : 1 mL = 12 gtt : X mL   or $\dfrac{10\ \text{gtt}}{1\ \text{mL}} = \dfrac{12\ \text{gtt}}{X\ \text{mL}}$ = **1.2 mL/min**
  X = **1.2 mL/min**

- **Convert mL/min to mL/hr.**

  60 min × 1.2 mL/min = **72 mL/hr**

- **Calculate the infusion time in hr and min.**

  750 mL ÷ 72 mL/hr = **10.42 hr**

  60 min × .42 = 25.2 = **25 min**

The infusion time is 10 hr 25 min.

EXAMPLE 3 | Determine the infusion time for **100 mL** D5NS infusing at a rate of **40 gtt/min** using a **microdrip set**.

- **Convert gtt/min to mL/min.**

  60 gtt : 1 mL = 40 gtt : X mL   or $\dfrac{60\ \text{gtt}}{1\ \text{mL}} = \dfrac{40\ \text{gtt}}{X\ \text{mL}}$ = **0.67 mL/min**
  X = **0.67 mL/min**

- **Convert mL/min to mL/hr.**

  60 min × .67 mL/min = 40.2 = **40 mL/hr**

- **Calculate the infusion time in hr and min.**

  100 mL ÷ 40 mL/hr = **2.5 hr**

  60 min × .5 = **30 min**

The infusion time is 2 hr 30 min.

EXAMPLE 4 | Calculate the infusion time for a volume of **150 mL** infusing at a rate of **20 gtt/min** on a **15 gtt/mL** calibrated set.

- **Convert gtt/min to mL/min.**

  15 gtt : 1 mL = 20 gtt : X mL   or $\dfrac{15\ \text{gtt}}{1\ \text{mL}} = \dfrac{20\ \text{gtt}}{X\ \text{mL}}$ = **1.3 mL/min**
  X = 1.33
  = **1.3 mL/min**

- **Convert mL/min to mL/hr.**

  60 min × 1.3 mL/min = **78 mL/hr**

- **Calculate the infusion time in hr and min.**

  150 mL ÷ 78 mL/hr = **1.92 hr**

  60 min × .92 = 55.2 = **55 min**

The infusion time is 1 hr 55 min.

EXAMPLE 5 | A volume of **1100 mL** hyperalimentation solution is infusing at a flow rate of **10 gtt/min** on a set calibrated at **10 gtt/mL**. Calculate the infusion time.

- **Convert gtt/min to mL/min.**

$$10 \text{ gtt} : 1 \text{ mL} = 10 \text{ gtt} : X \text{ mL} \qquad \text{or} \qquad \frac{10 \text{ gtt}}{1 \text{ mL}} = \frac{10 \text{ gtt}}{X \text{ mL}} = \textbf{1 mL/min}$$
$$X = \textbf{1 mL/min}$$

- **Convert mL/min to mL/hr.**

$$60 \text{ min} \times 1 \text{ mL/min} = \textbf{60 mL/hr}$$

- **Calculate the infusion time in hr and min.**

$$1100 \text{ mL} \div 60 \text{ mL/hr} = \textbf{18.33 hr}$$

$$60 \text{ min} \times .33 = 19.8 = \textbf{20 min}$$

The infusion time is 18 hr 20 min.

PROBLEM

Determine the infusion times for the following IVs.

1. An IV of 1 L of D5W to infuse at a flow rate of 33 gtt/min using a set calibrated at 15 gtt/mL   _____

2. An IV of 250 mL of D5RL infusing at 25 gtt/min using a 10 gtt/mL calibrated set   _____

3. A volume of 100 mL to infuse at 10 gtt/min using a 10 gtt/mL set   _____

4. A volume of 900 mL running at a rate of 30 gtt/min using a 20 gtt/mL calibrated set   _____

5. An IV of 200 mL infusing at 18 gtt/min on a set calibrated at 15 gtt/mL   _____

Answers **1.** 7 hr 35 min **2.** 1 hr 40 min **3.** 1 hr 40 min **4.** 10 hr **5.** 2 hr 47 min   **Note:** Consider amounts that vary by 1–2 min correct.

CALCULATING SMALL-VOLUME INFUSION TIMES OF LESS THAN 1 hr

Many small-volume infusions will complete in less than 1 hr. Because the infusion time being calculated is **min**, the calculation will be shorter. Calculate the **mL/min** rate first, then **divide** the **total volume** by the **mL/min** rate.

EXAMPLE 1 | An IV medication with a volume of **40 mL** is ordered to infuse at **45 gtt/min**. A microdrip set calibrated at **60 gtt/mL** is being used. Calculate the infusion time.

- **Calculate the mL/min infusing first.**

$$60 \text{ gtt} : 1 \text{ mL} = 45 \text{ gtt} : X \text{ mL} \qquad \text{or} \qquad \frac{60 \text{ gtt}}{1 \text{ mL}} = \frac{45 \text{ gtt}}{X \text{ mL}} = \textbf{0.75 mL/min}$$
$$X = \textbf{0.75 mL/min}$$

- **Divide the total volume by the mL/min rate.**

    40 mL ÷ 0.75 mL/min = 53.3 = **53 min**

The infusion time is 53 min.

 An IV medication of **60 mL** is to infuse at **50 gtt/min** using a set calibrated at **10 gtt/mL**. How long will it take to infuse?

- **Calculate the mL/min infusing.**

    10 gtt : 1 mL = 50 gtt : X mL   or $\dfrac{10\ \text{gtt}}{1\ \text{mL}} = \dfrac{50\ \text{gtt}}{X\ \text{mL}}$ = **5 mL/min**
    X = **5 mL/min**

- **Divide the total volume by the mL/min rate.**

    60 mL ÷ 5 mL/min = **12 min**

The infusion time is 12 min.

 An IV medication with a volume of **20 mL** is to infuse at a rate of **30 gtt/min** using a **15 gtt/mL** infusion set. Calculate the infusion time.

- **Calculate the mL/min infusing.**

    15 gtt : 1 mL = 30 gtt : X mL   or $\dfrac{15\ \text{gtt}}{1\ \text{mL}} = \dfrac{30\ \text{gtt}}{X\ \text{mL}}$ = **2 mL/min**
    X = **2 mL/min**

- **Divide the total volume by the mL/min rate.**

    20 mL ÷ 2 mL/min = **10 min**

The infusion time is 10 min.

PROBLEM

Calculate the infusion time for the following IV medications.

1. A medication with a volume of 25 mL to infuse at 30 gtt/min using a 60 gtt/mL (microdrip) set   _____

2. A 35 mL volume of IV medication to run at 25 gtt/min using a 15 gtt/mL set   _____

3. A rate of 40 gtt/min ordered for a 70 mL volume of medication using a 20 gtt/mL set   _____

4. A volume of 55 mL to infuse with a set calibrated at 10 gtt/mL at 45 gtt/min   _____

5. A 10 mL volume to infuse at 40 gtt/min using a microdrip   _____

Answers. **1.** 50 min **2.** 21 min **3.** 35 min **4.** 12 min **5.** 15 min **Note:** Consider answers that vary by 1–2 min correct.

DETERMINING INFUSION COMPLETION TIME

The reason for calculating infusion times is to know when an IV solution or medication will be completely infused. To obtain the **completion time** for an IV, you must now **add the infusion time** you calculated **to the start time**. This is not complicated; it just requires the same care you have been using for the other calculations in this text. The safest way to calculate the completion time is to **add the minutes first**. With them out of the way, only the hours are left to add; much less confusing. It's also safer to **write the times down** as you calculate them. So, do that in the following examples and problems. Only the first example will show calculation for military time (0–2400), because these calculations are simple additions.

 An IV started at **1450** has an infusion time of **3 hr 40 min**. What is the completion time?

- **Add the minutes first.**

    50 min + 40 min = **90 min**

Use 60 min of the 90 min total to change the 14 (hr) to 15; add the additional 30 min for a total of **1530**.

- **Now add the hr.**

    1530 + 3 hr = **1830**

Completion time = 1830

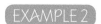 An IV medication will infuse in **20 minutes**. It is now **6:14 p.m.** When will it be complete?

- **Add the minutes.**

    6:14 p.m. + **20 min** = **6:34 p.m.**

Completion time = 6:34 p.m.

Minutes alone are easy to add, even if the answer crosses the a.m./p.m. time change.

 An IV is calculated to infuse in **2 hr 33 min**. It is now **4:43 p.m.** When will it complete?

- **Add the minutes first.**

    4:43 p.m. + **33 min** = **5:16 p.m.**

Now that the minutes are out of the way you only have to add 2 hours; much safer.

- **Add the hr.**

    5:16 p.m. + **2 hr** = **7.16 p.m.**

The infusion will complete at 7:16 p.m.

An IV infusion time is **13 hr 20 min**. What is its completion time if it was started at **10:45 a.m.**?

> • **Add the minutes first.**
>
> 10:45 a.m. + **20 min** = **11:05 a.m.**

You must now **add** the **13 hours** to the **11:05 a.m.** you just calculated. Count whichever way you prefer.

> • **Add the hr.**
>
> 11:05 a.m. + **13 hr** = **12:05 a.m.**
>
> **The completion time will be 12:05 a.m.**

 A IV with an infusion time of **10 hr 7 min** is started at **9:42 a.m.** When will it complete?

> • **Add the min.**
>
> 9:42 a.m. + **7 min** = **9:49 a.m.**
>
> • **Add the hr.**
>
> 9:49 a.m. + **10 hr** = **7:49 p.m.**
>
> **The completion time will be 7:49 p.m.**

EXAMPLE 6 | An IV with an infusion time of **12 hr 30 min** is started at **2:10 a.m.** When will it complete?

> • **Add the min.**
>
> 2:10 a.m. + **30 min** = **2:40 a.m.**
>
> • **Add the hr.**
>
> 2:40 a.m. + **12 hr** = **2:40 p.m.**
>
> **The completion time will be 2:40 p.m.**

PROBLEM

Calculate the completion times for the following infusions.

1. An IV started at 0440 that has an infusion time of 9 hr 42 min. Use military time. _____

2. An IV medication started at 7:30 a.m. that has an infusion time of 45 min. _____

3. An IV with an infusion time of 7 hr 7 min that was restarted at 10:42 a.m. _____

4. An IV with a restart time of 9:07 p.m. has an infusion time of 6 hr 27 min. _____

5. An IV with an infusion time of 3 hr 30 min was started at 11:49 p.m. _____

Answers **1.** 1422 **2.** 8:15 a.m. **3.** 5:49 p.m. **4.** 3:34 a.m. **5.** 2:19 a.m. **Note:** Consider answers that vary by 1–2 min correct.

LABELING SOLUTION BAGS WITH INFUSION AND COMPLETION TIMES

IV bags/bottles are calibrated so that the amount of fluid remaining can be checked at any time. In the majority of hospitals, it is routine to label bags when they are hung with start, progress, and finish times to provide a visual reference of the status of the infusion. Commercially prepared labels are available for this purpose; however, you can prepare one using any opaque tape available.

Refer to Figure 17-3 on page 247, where you can see close-up calibrations on a 1000 mL bag. Notice that each 50 mL is calibrated, but that only the 100 mL calibrations are numbered: 1, 2, 3 (for 100, 200, 300), etc. Notice also that the calibrations on the IV bag are not all the same width: they are somewhat wider at the bottom, because gravity and the pressure of the solution force more fluid to the bottom of the bag. On an uncomplicated infusion these differences in calibration are relatively unimportant.

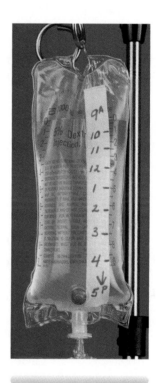

The tape on the IV solution bag in Figure 17-1 is for an 8-hour infusion, from 9 a.m. to 5 p.m. The 9A represents the start time of 9 a.m., and the 5P at the bottom represents the completion time of 5 p.m. An 8-hr infusion time for 1000 mL means that 125 mL are to be infused per hour (1000 mL ÷ 8 hr = 125 mL/hr). Each 125 mL is labeled on the calibrated scale along with the hour the IV should be at this level. This tape can be read by everyone who cares for this patient and allows for constant monitoring of the IV. No matter what your responsibility for a patient is you must be aware of IV drip rates and develop the habit of reading IV labeling, particularly if you have been giving personal care that involves the patient moving around.

Let's look at an example of how you could label an IV that is just being started. You may use a commercial time tape provided by your instructor, or copy the calibrations from one of the photos in this text to make up your own scale on scratch paper.

Figure 17-1

 EXAMPLE 1 | An IV of **1000 mL** has been ordered to run at **150 mL/hr**. It was started at **1:40 p.m.** Tape the bag with start, progress, and completion times.

Add the tape to the bag/bottle so that it is near but does not cover the calibrations. Enter the start time as 1:40 p.m. at the 1000 mL level. Next, mark each 150 mL from top to bottom with the successive hours the IV will run.

1000 mL − 150 mL = 850 mL		Label 850 mL for 2:40 p.m.
850 mL − 150 mL = 700 mL		Label 700 mL for 3:40 p.m.
700 mL − 150 mL = 550 mL		Label 550 mL for 4:40 p.m.
550 mL − 150 mL = 400 mL		Label 400 mL for 5:40 p.m.
400 mL − 150 mL = 250 mL		Label 250 mL for 6:40 p.m.
250 mL − 150 mL = 100 mL		Label 100 mL for 7:40 p.m.

Calculate the infusion time for the remaining 100 mL.

$$100 \text{ mL} \div 150 \text{ mL/hr} = 0.66 = \textbf{0.67 hr}$$

$$60 \text{ min} \times 0.67 = 40.2 = \textbf{40 min}$$

7:40 p.m. + **40 min** = **8:20 p.m.**

The completion time is 8:20 p.m.

EXAMPLE 2 | An infiltrated IV with **625 mL** remaining is restarted at **5:30 p.m.** to run at **150 mL/hr**. Relabel the bag with the new start, progress, and completion times.

Label the 625 mL level with the 5:30 p.m. restart time.

625 mL − 150 mL = 475 mL	Label 475 mL for 6:30 p.m.
475 mL − 150 mL = 325 mL	Label 325 mL for 7:30 p.m.
325 mL − 150 mL = 175 mL	Label 175 mL for 8:30 p.m.
175 mL − 150 mL = 25 mL	Label 25 mL for 9:30 p.m.

Calculate the infusion time for the remaining 25 mL.

$$25 \text{ mL} \div 150 \text{ mL/hr} = 0.166 = \textbf{0.17 hr}$$

$$60 \text{ min} \times 0.17 = 10.2 = \textbf{10 min}$$

9:30 p.m. + **10 min** = **9:40 p.m.**

The completion time is 9:40 p.m.

EXAMPLE 3 | An infiltrated IV with **340 mL** remaining is restarted at **4:15 a.m.** to run at **70 mL/hr**. Relabel the bag with the new start, progress, and completion times.

Label the 340 mL level with the 4:15 a.m. restart time.

340 mL − 70 mL = 270 mL	Label 270 mL for 5:15 a.m.
270 mL − 70 mL = 200 mL	Label 200 mL for 6:15 a.m.
200 mL − 70 mL = 130 mL	Label 130 mL for 7:15 a.m.
25 mL − 70 mL = 60 mL	Label 60 mL for 8:15 a.m.

Calculate the infusion time for the remaining 60 mL.

$$60 \text{ mL} \div 70 \text{ mL/hr} = 0.857 = \textbf{0.86 hr}$$

$$60 \text{ min} \times 0.86 = 51.6 = \textbf{52 min}$$

8:15 a.m. + **52 min** = **9:17 a.m.**

The completion time is 9:17 a.m.

PROBLEM

Calculate the infusion and completion times for the IVs pictured. Label the IV bags provided with start, progress, and completion times. Have your instructor check your labeling.

1. The IV in Figure 17-2 of 1000 mL was started at 0710 to run at 75 mL/hr.

   Infusion time _____   Completion time _____

2. The 1000 mL IV in Figure 17-3 has an ordered rate of 125 mL/hr. It was started at 6:30 p.m.

   Infusion time _____   Completion time _____

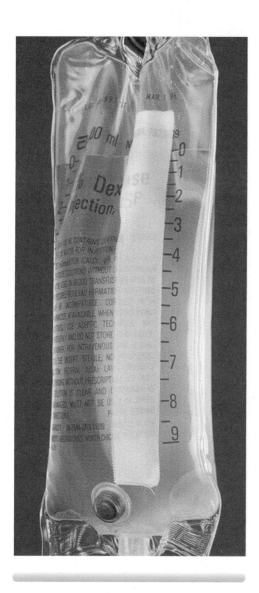

Figure 17-2

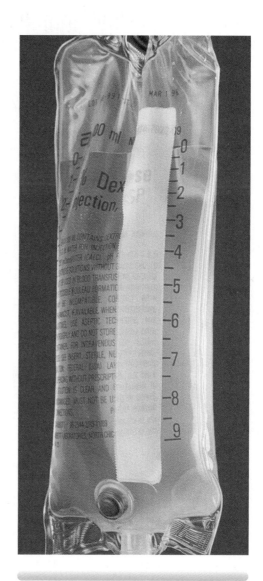

Figure 17-3

3. The IV in Figure 17-4 of 1000 mL has an ordered rate of 80 mL/hr. It was started at 5:40 a.m.

Infusion time _____   Completion time _____

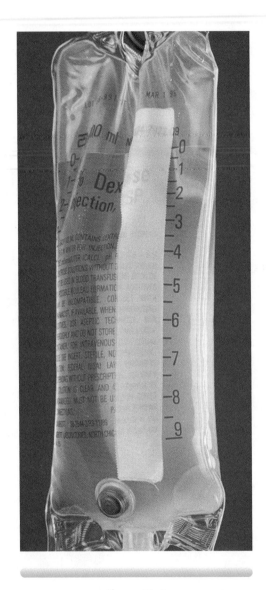

Figure 17-4

Summary

This concludes the chapter on calculation of infusion and completion times and labeling of IV bags with start, progress, and completion times. The important points to remember from this chapter are:

- The infusion time is the time necessary for an IV bag to infuse completely.

- The infusion time is calculated by dividing the total volume to infuse by the mL/hr rate ordered.

- Infusion times also may be calculated using the volume of the bag being hung, the mL/hr or gtt/min rate ordered, and set calibration.

- The completion time is calculated by adding the infusion time to the start time.

- When adding the infusion time to the start time it is safer to add the minutes first, then the hours.

- When the total min are 60 or more, an additional hr is added, and 60 min are subtracted from the total min.

- Calculating infusion and completion times provides an opportunity to plan ahead and have the next solution ordered ready to hang, or to discontinue the IV when it is completed.

- It is routine in many hospitals to label IV solutions with start, finish, and progress times to provide a visual record of the infusion status.

Summary Self-Test

Calculate the infusion and completion times for the following IVs. Don't let the solution abbreviations confuse you; concentrate on locating the information you need for your calculations.

1. The order is for 50 mL D5W to infuse at 50 gtt/min using a microdrip. The infusion was started at 10:10 a.m.

   Infusion time _____   Completion time _____

2. An infusion of 1150 mL of hyperalimentation is ordered to run at 80 mL/hr. It was started at 8:02 a.m.

   Infusion time _____   Completion time _____

3. A total of 280 mL of D10W remain in an IV bag. The flow rate is 70 mL/hr. It is now 11:03 a.m.

   Infusion time _____   Completion time _____

4. The order is to infuse 500 mL of whole blood at 90 mL/hr. The transfusion was started at 2:40 p.m.

   Infusion time _____   Completion time _____

5. An infiltrated IV with 850 mL of D5W remaining is restarted at 10 a.m. at a rate of 150 mL/hr.

   Infusion time _____   Completion time _____

6. At 4:04 a.m. an IV of 500 mL of intralipids is started at a rate of 50 mL/hr.

        Infusion time _____   Completion time _____

7. An IV medication with a volume of 50 mL is started at 1:45 p.m. to infuse at 30 gtt/min using a set calibrated at 15 gtt/mL.

        Infusion time _____   Completion time _____

8. An IV of 520 mL of RL is restarted at 0420 at a rate of 125 mL/hr.

        Infusion time _____   Completion time _____

9. It is 12.00 p.m. and an IV of 900 mL D10NS is infusing at a rate of 100 mL/hr.

        Infusion time _____   Completion time _____

10. An antibiotic of 150 mL is started at 7:10 a.m. to infuse at 33 gtt/min with a set calibrated at 10 gtt/mL.

        Infusion time _____   Completion time _____

11. An infusion of 250 mL of normal saline is started at 11:20 a.m. to infuse at a rate of 20 mL/hr.

        Infusion time _____   Completion time _____

12. The flow rate ordered for 1 L of D5W is 80 mL/hr. It was started at 8:07 p.m.

        Infusion time _____   Completion time _____

13. One unit of packed cells with a 250 mL volume is started at 3:40 p.m. to be infused at 30 gtt/min using a 20 gtt/mL set.

        Infusion time _____   Completion time _____

14. A medication volume of 100 mL is started at 4:00 p.m. to infuse at 42 gtt/min using a microdrip.

        Infusion time _____   Completion time _____

15. At 11:00 p.m. 200 mL of D5W remain in an IV. The rate is 20 gtt/min and set calibration is 10 gtt/mL.

        Infusion time _____   Completion time _____

16. An infusion of 350 mL of RL is restarted to run at 50 gtt/min using a 10 gtt/mL set. It is now 9:47 a.m.

        Infusion time _____   Completion time _____

17. An IV medication of 25 mL is started at 8:17 a.m. using a microdrip to run at 25 gtt/min.

        Infusion time _____   Completion time _____

18. An IV of 425 mL of D5 1/4NaCl is restarted at 0814 to infuse at 15 gtt/min using a 10 gtt/mL set.

        Infusion time _____   Completion time _____

19. At 10:30 p.m. there are 180 mL left in an IV of D5 0.45%NaCl that is infusing at 25 mL/hr.

        Infusion time _____   Completion time _____

20. At 2 p.m. 500 mL of D5NS is started to run at a rate of 20 gtt/min using a 20 gtt/mL set.

        Infusion time _____   Completion time _____

21. An infusion of 250 mL of NS is started at 3:04 a.m. to run at 50 gtt/min using a 15 gtt/mL set.

        Infusion time _____   Completion time _____

22. With 525 mL of D10W remaining a rate change to 35 gtt/min is ordered. It is 2:10 a.m. and a 10 gtt/mL set is being used.

        Infusion time _____   Completion time _____

23. A liter of D5 1/4NaCl with 10 U of Regular insulin is started at 8:42 a.m. at a rate of 22 gtt/min using a set calibrated at 20 gtt/mL.

        Infusion time _____   Completion time _____

24. An infusion of 1000 mL of sodium chloride 0.9% is to run at 200 mL/hr. It is started at 6:40 p.m.

        Infusion time _____   Completion time _____

25. An IV medication of 100 mL is started at 7:50 a.m. to run at 33 gtt/min using a 10 gtt/mL set.

        Infusion time _____   Completion time _____

26. A volume of 500 mL of RL is started at 4:04 p.m. at a rate of 50 gtt/min using a microdrip.

        Infusion time _____   Completion time _____

27. An IV of 950 mL NS is restarted at 2:10 a.m. at 25 gtt/min using a 15 gtt/mL set.

        Infusion time _____   Completion time _____

28. An IV medication of 30 mL is started at 0915 at a rate of 10 gtt/min using a 10 gtt/mL set.

        Infusion time _____   Completion time _____

29. A medication volume of 90 mL was started at 6:15 a.m. to be infused at 30 gtt/min using a 20 gtt/mL set.

        Infusion time _____   Completion time _____

30. A set calibrated at 15 gtt/mL is used at 4:20 p.m. to infuse a medication with a volume of 100 mL. The rate ordered is 45 gtt/min.

        Infusion time _____   Completion time _____

31. A 20 gtt/mL set is used for a restart of 750 mL of D5W at 3:03 p.m. at a rate of 32 gtt/min.

        Infusion time _____   Completion time _____

Answers

1. 60 min; 11:10 a.m.	**9.** 9 hr; 9 p.m.	**16.** 1 hr 10 min; 10:57 a.m.	**25.** 30 min; 8:20 a.m.
2. 14 hr 23 min; 10:25 p.m.	**10.** 45 min; 7:55 a.m.	**17.** 60 min; 9:17 a.m.	**26.** 10 hr; 2:04 a.m.
3. 4 hr; 3:03 p.m.	**11.** 12 hr 30 min;	**18.** 4 hr 43 min; 1257	**27.** 9 hr 19 min; 11:29 a.m.;
4. 5 hr 34 min; 8.14 p.m.	11:50 a.m.	**19.** 7 hr 12 min; 5:42 a.m.	or 9 hr 29 min;
5. 5 hr 40 min; 3:40 p.m.	**12.** 12 hr 30 min; 8:37 a.m.	**20.** 8 hr 20 min; 10:20 p.m.	11:39 a.m.
6. 10 hr; 2:04 p.m.	**13.** 2 hr 47 min; 6:27 p.m.	**21.** 1 hr 15 min; 4:19 a.m.	**28.** 30 min; 0945
7. 25 min; 2:10 p.m.	**14.** 143 min or 2 hr 23 min;	**22.** 2 hr 30 min; 4:40 a.m.	**29.** 60 min; 7:15 a.m.
8. 4 hr 10 min; 0830	6:23 p.m.	**23.** 15 hr 9 min; 11:51 p.m.	**30.** 33 min; 4:53 p.m.
	15. 1 hr 40 min; 12:40 a.m.	**24.** 5 hr; 11:40 p.m.	**31.** 7 hr 48 min; 10:51 p.m.

Note: Answers may vary slightly due to rounding.

Label the following solution bags for the times and rates indicated. Have your instructor check your labeling.

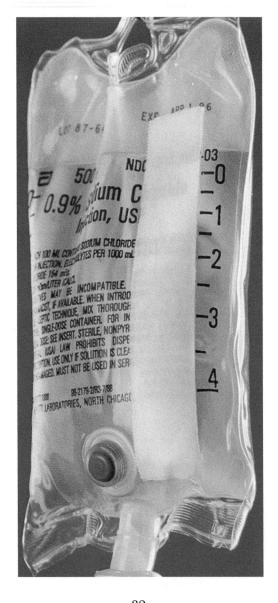

32.
Started: 10:47 a.m.
Rate: 80 mL/hr

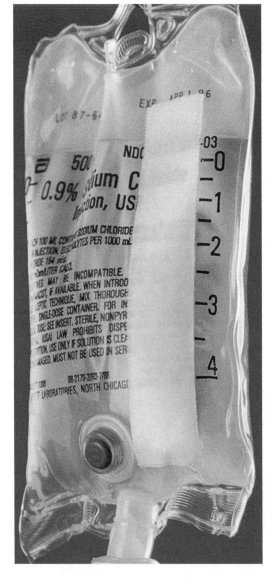

33.
Started: 1315
Rate: 100 mL/hr

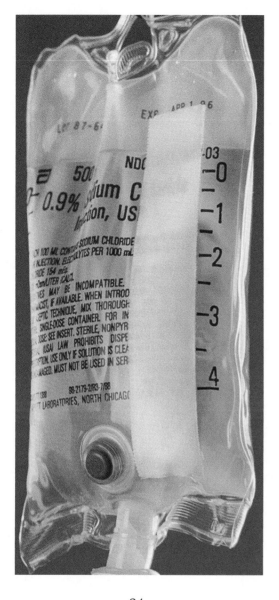

34.
Started: 2:10 p.m.
Rate: 90 mL/hr

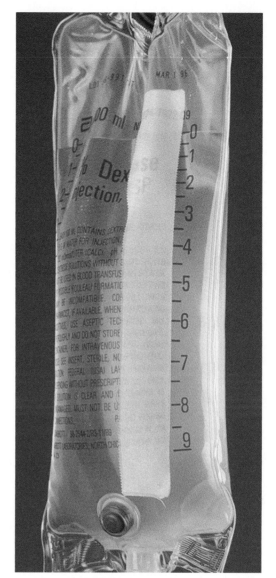

35.
Started: 0440
Rate: 75 mL/hr

17

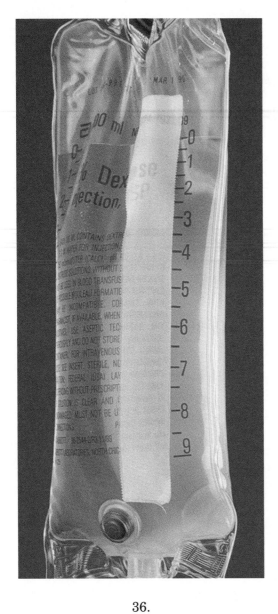

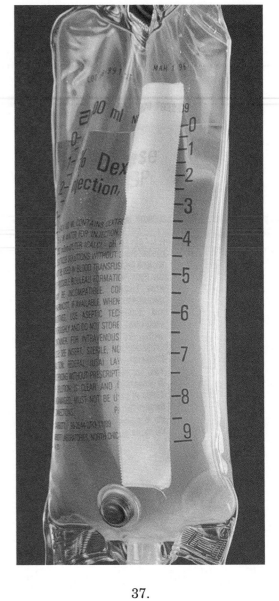

36.
Started: 0730
Rate: 50 mL/hr

37.
Started: 6:20 p.m.
Rate: 25 mL/hr

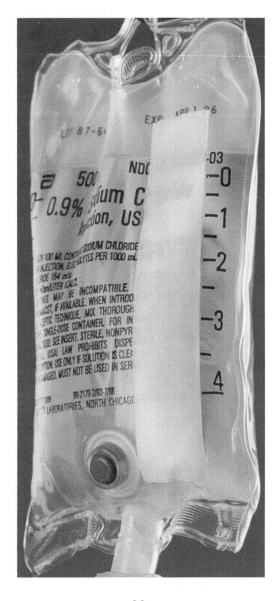

38.
Started: 3:03 a.m.
Rate: 50 mL/hr

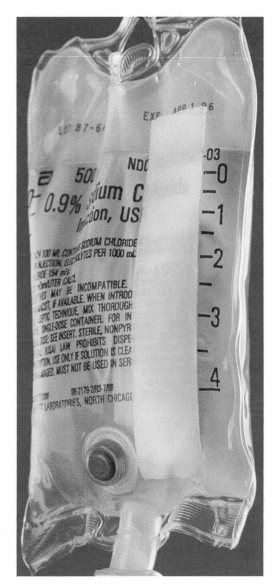

39.
Started: 0744
Rate: 125 mL/hr

40.
Started: 2140
Rate: 100 mL/hr

IV Medication and Titration Calculations

Objectives

The learner will calculate:

1. flow rates to infuse ordered dosages

2. dosages and flow rates based on kg body weight

3. dosage infusing from flow rate and solution strength

4. dosage and flow rate ranges for titrated medications

Many IV drugs are used in critical and life-threatening situations to alter or maintain vital physiologic functions, for example, heart rate, cardiac output, blood pressure, respiration, and renal function. In general, these drugs have a very rapid action and short duration. They may be administered by IV push or bolus but also diluted in 250–500 mL of IV solution, most commonly D5W.

Intravenous medications may be ordered by dosage (mcg/mg/U per min/hr), or based on a patient's weight (mcg/mg/U per kg per min/hr). They may also be ordered to infuse within a specific dosage range, for example, 1–3 mcg/min, to elicit a measurable physiologic response; an example would be to maintain a systolic BP above 100 mm Hg. This adjustment of rate is called **titration**, and dosage increments are made within the ordered range until the desired response has been established. Most IV drugs require close and continuous monitoring. When available, an electronic infusion device (EID), either volumetric pump or syringe pump, is used for their administration. If an EID is not available, a microdrip set calibrated at 60 gtt/mL, or dosage controlled Soluset/Buretrol/Volutrol burette, is routinely used. All calculations in this chapter are for an EID or microdrip, and the mL/hr and gtt/min rates are therefore interchangeable.

The calculations in this chapter include: (1) converting ordered dosages to the flow rates necessary to administer them, and (2) using flow rates to calculate the dosage infusing at any given moment. A patient's weight is often a critical factor in IV dosages, and its use in calculations will also be covered. A variety of EIDs display dosage and flow rate equivalents, but you must know how to do these calculations yourself, because you are likely to encounter situations in which you will have to do so. IV drugs that alter a basic physiologic function generally have narrow margins of safety, and accuracy is imperative in their calculation. Double-checking of math is both mandatory and routine. As a general rule, dosages are calculated to the nearest tenth, and flow rates are rounded to the nearest gtt or mL.

All calculations in this chapter assume the use of an EID or microdrip infusion set; therefore, the mL/hr and gtt/min rates are identical and interchangeable.

CALCULATING mL/hr RATE FROM DOSAGE ORDERED

One of the most common IV drug calculations is to determine the mL/hr flow rate for a specific drug dosage ordered. So let's start by looking at some examples of these.

 EXAMPLE 1 | A solution of Cardizem **125 mg/100 mL** D5W is to infuse at a rate of **20 mg/hr**. Calculate the **mL/hr** flow rate.

- **Use the solution strength available to calculate the mL/hr rate for 20 mg/hr.**

$$125 \text{ mg} : 100 \text{ mL} = 20 \text{ mg} : X \text{ mL} \quad \text{or} \quad \frac{125 \text{ mg}}{100 \text{ mL}} = \frac{20 \text{ mg}}{X \text{ mL}} = \mathbf{16 \text{ mL/hr}}$$
$$125X = 100 \times 20$$
$$X = \mathbf{16 \text{ mL/hr}}$$

To infuse 20 mg/hr set the flow rate at 16 mL/hr.

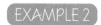 **EXAMPLE 2** | A maintenance dose of Levophed **2 mcg/min** has been ordered using an **8 mg in 250 mL** of D5W solution. Calculate the **mL/hr** flow rate.

- **Calculate the dosage per hr first.**

  2 mcg/min $\times$ 60 min = **120 mcg/hr**

The solution strength is in mg, so a mcg to mg conversion is now needed.

- **Convert 120 mcg to mg, to match the mg solution strength.**

  120 mcg = **0.12 mg**

- **Use the solution strength available to calculate the mL/hr rate.**

$$8 \text{ mg} : 250 \text{ mL} = 0.12 \text{ mg} : X \text{ mL} \quad \text{or} \quad \frac{8 \text{ mg}}{250 \text{ mL}} = \frac{0.12 \text{ mg}}{X \text{ mL}} = \mathbf{4 \text{ mL/hr}}$$
$$8X = 250 \times 0.12$$
$$X = 3.75 = \mathbf{4 \text{ mL/hr}}$$

To infuse 2 mcg/min set the flow rate at 4 mL/hr.

 Metric conversions may be made in either direction: solution strength to dosage ordered, or dosage ordered to solution strength.

EXAMPLE 3 | Neosynephrine **50 mg in 250 mL** of D5W is used to infuse a dosage of **200 mcg/min**. Calculate the flow rate in **mL/hr**.

- **Calculate the dosage per hr.**

  200 mcg/min $\times$ 60 min = **12,000 mcg/hr**

- **Convert 12,000 mcg to mg to match the mg solution strength.**

    12,000 mcg = **12 mg**

- **Calculate the mL/hr flow rate.**

    50 mg : 250 mL = 12 mg : X mL   or $\dfrac{50\ \text{mg}}{250\ \text{mL}} = \dfrac{12\ \text{mg}}{X\ \text{mL}}$ **60 mL/hr**

               $50X = 250 \times 12$

                  $X = $ **60 mL/hr**

To infuse 200 mcg/min set the flow rate at 60 mL/hr.

EXAMPLE 4   Isuprel has been ordered for a cardiac patient at the rate of **3 mcg/min** using a **1 mg/250 mL** D5W solution. Calculate the **mL/hr** flow rate.

- **Calculate the dosage per hr.**

    3 mcg/min $\times$ 60 min = **180 mcg/hr**

- **Convert 180 mcg to mg to match the solution strength.**

    180 mcg = **0.18 mg**

- **Calculate the mL/hr flow rate.**

    1 mg : 250 mL = 0.18 mg : X mL   or $\dfrac{1\ \text{mg}}{250\ \text{mL}} = \dfrac{0.18\ \text{mg}}{X\ \text{mL}} = $ **45 mL/hr**

               $X = 250 \times 0.18$

               $X = $ **45 mL/hr**

To infuse 3 mcg/min set the flow rate at 45 mL/hr.

EXAMPLE 5   A **500 mL** D5W solution with **2 g** Pronestyl is to be infused at a rate of **1 mg/min** via volumetric pump. Calculate the **mL/hr** flow rate.

- **Calculate the dosage per hr.**

    1 mg/min $\times$ 60 min = **60 mg/hr**

- **Convert g to mg in the solution strength.**

    2 g = **2000 mg**

- **Calculate the mL/hr rate.**

    2000 mg : 500 mL = 60 mg : X mL   or $\dfrac{2000\ \text{mg}}{500\ \text{mL}} = \dfrac{60\ \text{mg}}{X\ \text{mL}} = $ **15 mL/hr**

               $2000X = 500 \times 60$

                 $X = $ **15 mL/hr**

Set the pump at 15 mL/hr to infuse 1 mg/min.

PROBLEM

Calculate the mL/hr flow rates to administer the following IV dosages. Round answers to the nearest mL.

1. Trandate 20 mg/hr is ordered using a 100 mg/100 mL solution. _____

2. Levophed is ordered at the rate of 3 mcg/min. The solution strength is 8 mg Levophed in 250 mL of D5W. _____

3. A solution of 2 g Pronestyl in 500 mL of D5W is used to administer a dosage of 2 mg/min. _____

4. Isuprel 2 mcg/min is ordered. The solution strength is 1 mg/250 mL. _____

5. An initial dose of Cardizem 25 mg/hr is ordered. The solution strength is 125 mg/100 mL. _____

Answers **1.** 20 mL/hr **2.** 6 mL/hr **3.** 30 mL/hr **4.** 30 mL/hr **5.** 20 mL/hr

CALCULATING mL/hr RATE FROM DOSAGE PER kg ORDERED

Many drug dosages are calculated based on a patient's weight, for example, 5 mg/kg/hr. **Body weight, to the nearest tenth kg**, is used for these calculations. **A preliminary step** of calculating the dosage for the patient based on her/his weight is necessary before the flow rate can be calculated.

All of the following rates are for mL/hr pump or syringe pump infusion (the gtt/min microdrip rate will be identical). **Express fractional dosage answers to the nearest tenth and the mL rates to the nearest whole mL.**

 EXAMPLE 1 | Dopamine is ordered at the rate of **3 mcg/kg/min** for a patient weighing **95.9 kg**. The solution strength is **400 mg** dopamine in **250 mL** of D5W. Calculate the **mL/hr** flow rate.

- **Calculate the dosage per min first.**

  3 mcg/kg/min × 95.9 kg = **287.7 mcg/min**

- **Convert mcg/min to mcg/hr.**

  287.7 mcg/min × 60 min = **17,262 mcg/hr**

- **Convert mcg/hr to mg/hr.**

  17,262 mcg/hr = 17.26 = **17.3 mg/hr**

- **Calculate the flow rate.**

  400 mg : 250 mL = 17.3 mg : X mL   or $\dfrac{400 \text{ mg}}{250 \text{ mL}} = \dfrac{17.3 \text{ mg}}{X \text{ mL}}$

      400X = 250 × 17.3

          X = 10.8 = **11 mL/hr**   = 10.8 = **11 mL/hr**

To infuse 3 mcg/kg/min set the rate at 11 mL/hr.

Esmolol **2.5 g in 250 mL** of D5W has been ordered at a rate of **100 mcg/kg/min** for a patient weighing **104.6 kg**. Calculate the **mL/hr** flow rate

- **Calculate the dosage per min.**

    100 mcg/kg/min $\times$ 104.9 kg = **10,460 mcg/min**

- **Convert mcg/min to mg/min.**

    10,460 mcg $\div$ 1000 = 10.46 = **10.5 mg/min**

- **Convert mg/min to mg/hr.**

    10.5 mg/min $\times$ 60 min = **630 mg/hr**

- **Calculate the flow rate.**

    2500 mg : 250 mL = 630 mg : X mL   or $\dfrac{2500 \text{ mg}}{250 \text{ mL}} = \dfrac{630 \text{ mg}}{X \text{ mL}} = $ **63 mL/hr**
    2500X = 250 $\times$ 630
    X = **63 mL/hr**

To infuse 100 mcg/kg/min set the rate at 63 mL/hr.

 Nipride has been ordered at **4 mcg/kg/min** from a solution of **50 mg** in **250 mL** of D5W. The patient weighs **107.3 kg**. Calculate the **mL/hr** flow rate.

- **Calculate the dosage per min.**

    4 mcg/kg/min $\times$ 107.3 kg = **429.2 mcg/min**

- **Convert mcg/min to mcg/hr.**

    429.2 mcg/min $\times$ 60 min = **25,752 mcg/hr**

- **Convert mcg/hr to mg/hr.**

    25,752 $\div$ 1000 = 25.75 = **25.8 mg/hr**

- **Calculate the flow rate.**

    50 mg : 250 mL = 25.8 mg : X mL   or $\dfrac{50 \text{ mg}}{250 \text{ mL}} = \dfrac{25.8 \text{ mg}}{X \text{ mL}} = $ **129 mL/hr**
    50X = 250 $\times$ 25.8
    X = **129 mL/hr**

To infuse 4 mcg/kg/min set the rate at 129 mL/hr.

 Dobutrex **5 mcg/kg/min** has been ordered using a **500 mg/250 mL** of D5W strength solution. The patient weighs **99.4 kg**. Calculate the **mL/hr** flow rate.

- **Calculate the dosage per min.**

    5 mcg/kg/min $\times$ 99.4 kg = **497 mcg/min**

- **Convert mcg/min to mcg/hr.**

  497 mg/min $\times$ 60 min = **29,820 mcg/hr**

- **Convert mcg/hr to mg/hr.**

  29,820 mcg $\div$ 1000 = 29.82 = **29.8 mg/hr**

- **Calculate the flow rate.**

  $$500 \text{ mg} : 250 \text{ mL} = 29.8 \text{ mg} : X \text{ mL} \quad \text{or} \quad \frac{500 \text{ mg}}{250 \text{ mL}} = \frac{29.8 \text{ mg}}{X \text{ mL}} = \textbf{15 mL/hr}$$
  $$500X = 250 \times 29.8$$
  $$X = 14.9 = \textbf{15 mL/hr}$$

To infuse 5 mcg/kg/min set the rate at 15 mL/hr.

 Brevibloc **100 mcg/kg/min** has been ordered using a **5 g/500 mL** of D5W solution. The patient weighs **77.6 kg**. Calculate the **mL/hr** flow rate.

- **Calculate the dosage per min.**

  100 mcg/kg/min $\times$ 77.6 kg = **7760 mcg/min**

- **Convert mcg/min to mg/min.**

  7760 mcg $\div$ 1000 = 7.76 = **7.8 mg/min**

- **Convert mg/min to mg/hr.**

  7.8 mg/min $\times$ 60 min = **468 mg/hr**

- **Calculate the flow rate.**

  $$5000 \text{ mg} : 500 \text{ mL} = 468 \text{ mg} : X \text{ mL} \quad \text{or} \quad \frac{5000 \text{ mg}}{500 \text{ mL}} = \frac{468 \text{ mg}}{X \text{ mL}}$$
  $$5000X = 500 \times 468$$
  $$X = 46.8 = \textbf{47 mL/hr} \qquad\qquad = 46.8 = \textbf{47 mL/hr}$$

To infuse 100 mcg/kg/min set the rate at 47 mL/hr.

PROBLEM

Calculate the dosage per min, and mL/hr flow rate for the following infusions.

1. Nipride 3 mcg/kg/min has been ordered for an 87.4 kg patient. The solution has a strength of 50 mg in 250 mL of D5W.   _____   _____

2. Dopamine has been ordered at 4 mcg/kg/min using a 400 mg/250 mL of D5W solution. The patient weighs 92.4 kg.   _____   _____

3. Dobutamine 2.5 mcg/kg/min has been ordered. The solution is 500 mg/250 mL of D5W. The patient weighs 80.7 kg.   _____   _____

4. Esmolol 150 mcg/kg/min has been ordered for a 92.1 kg patient. The solution strength is 2.5 g/250 mL of D5W.   _____ _____

5. Propofol 5 mcg/kg/min is ordered for an 80.3 kg patient. The solution strength is 1 g/100 mL of D5W.   _____ _____

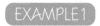 **1.** 262.2 mcg/min; 79 mL/hr **2.** 369.9 mcg/min; 14 mL/hr **3.** 201.8 mcg/min; 6 mL/hr **4.** 13,815 mcg or 13.8 mg/min; 83 mL/hr **5.** 401.5 mcg/min; 2 mL/hr

CALCULATING DOSAGE INFUSING FROM FLOW RATE

It is possible to calculate the dosage being administered at any moment from the **flow rate infusing** and the **solution concentration**.

EXAMPLE 1 | **500 mL** of D5W containing dopamine **800 mg** is infusing at a rate of **25 mL/hr**. Calculate the dosage infusing in **mg/hr** and **mcg/min**.

• **Calculate the mg/hr infusing first.**

$$500 \text{ mL} : 800 \text{ mg} = 25 \text{ mL} : X \text{ mg} \quad \text{or} \quad \frac{500 \text{ mL}}{800 \text{ mg}} = \frac{25 \text{ mL}}{X \text{ mg}} = \textbf{40 mg/hr}$$
$$500X = 800 \times 25$$
$$X = \textbf{40 mg/hr}$$

• **Convert mg/hr to mcg/hr.**

40 mg/hr = **40,000 mcg/hr**

• **Convert mcg/hr to mcg/min.**

40,000 mcg ÷ 60 min = 666.6 = **667 mcg/min**

A dosage of 40 mg/hr, or 667 mcg/min, is infusing.

EXAMPLE 2 | A postop cardiac bypass patient has Nipride infusing at **30 gtt/min** (30 mL/hr). The solution strength is **100 mg** Nipride in **500 mL** of D5W. Calculate the **mg/hr** and **mcg/min** infusing.

• **Calculate the mg/hr infusing.**

$$500 \text{ mL} : 100 \text{ mg} = 30 \text{ mL} : X \text{ mg} \quad \text{or} \quad \frac{500 \text{ mL}}{100 \text{ mg}} = \frac{30 \text{ mL}}{X \text{ mg}} = \textbf{6 mg/hr}$$
$$500X = 100 \times 30$$
$$X = \textbf{6 mg/hr}$$

• **Convert mg/hr to mcg/hr.**

6 mg/hr = **6000 mcg/hr**

• **Convert mcg/hr to mcg/min.**

6000 mcg ÷ 60 min = **100 mcg/min**

A dosage of 6 mg/hr, or 100 mcg/min, is infusing.

EXAMPLE 3 | A patient with ventricular ectopi is receiving a continuous lidocaine infusion at a flow rate of **15 mL/hr**. The solution strength is **2 g** lidocaine in **500 mL** of D5W. Calculate the **mg/hr** and **mg/min** being infused. The average dosage of lidocaine is **1–4 mg/min**. Is the dosage within normal range?

- **Convert the g to mg first.**

  2 g = **2000 mg**

- **Calculate the mg/hr infusing.**

  500 mL : 2000 mg = 15 mL : X mg   or $\dfrac{500\ \text{mL}}{2000\ \text{mg}} = \dfrac{15\ \text{mL}}{X\ \text{mg}}$ = **60 mg/hr**
  $500X = 2000 \times 15$
  $X =$ **60 mg/hr**

- **Calculate the mg/min infusing.**

  60 mg ÷ 60 min = **1 mg/min**

A dosage of 60 mg/hr, or 1 mg/min, is infusing. This dosage is within the normal 1–4 mg/min range.

EXAMPLE 4 | A solution of **5 g (5000 mg)** Brevibloc in **500 mL** of D5W is infusing at **30 mL/hr**. Calculate the **mg/min** infusing.

- **Calculate the mg/hr infusing.**

  500 mL : 5000 mg = 30 mL : X mg   or $\dfrac{500\ \text{mL}}{5000\ \text{mg}} = \dfrac{30\ \text{mL}}{X\ \text{mg}}$ = **300 mg/hr**
  $500X = 5000 \times 30$
  $X =$ **300 mg/hr**

- **Calculate the mg/min infusing.**

  300 mg/hr ÷ 60 min = **5 mg/min**

A dosage of 5 mg/min is infusing.

PROBLEM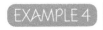

Calculate the dosages indicated in the following problems. Express dosages to the nearest tenth.

1. A continuous infusion of Isuprel is ordered for a newly admitted patient in cardiogenic shock. The solution strength is 2 mg in 500 mL of D5W, and the rate of infusion is 40 mL/hr. Calculate the mcg/min infusing. _____

   Is this within the normal 1–5 mcg/min range? _____

2. The order is to infuse dobutamine 500 mg in 250 mL at a rate of 7 mL/hr. Calculate the mg/hr and mcg/min the patient will receive. _____ _____

3. Pronestyl 2 g in 500 mL of D5W is ordered for a patient with frequent PVCs, to run at 30 mL/hr. Calculate the number of mg/min the patient is receiving. _____

   The normal dosage range for this drug is between 1 and 6 mg/min. Is the dosage within these limits? _____

4. A patient has an order for nitroglycerine 6 mL/hr by volumetric pump. The solution strength is 50 mg/250 mL. How many mcg/min are being infused? _____

5. Esmolol is ordered to control the ventricular rate of a patient during surgery. The solution available has a strength of 2.5 g in 250 mL of D5W. The order is to infuse at 32 mL/hr. Calculate the mg/hr and mg/min being infused. _____ _____

Answers **1.** 2.7 mcg/min; yes **2.** 14 mg/hr; 233.3 mcg/min **3.** 2 mg/min; yes **4.** 20 mcg/min **5.** 320 mg/hr; 5.3 mg/min

TITRATION OF INFUSIONS

Titration refers to the adjustment of dosage within a specific range to obtain a measurable physiologic response, for example, Levophed 2–4 mcg/min to maintain systolic BP >100. The dosage is increased or decreased within the ordered range until the desired response is obtained. The **lowest dosage is set first** and adjusted upwards and downwards as necessary. The **upper dosage is never exceeded** unless a new order is obtained.

EIDs (pumps or syringe pumps) are most often used for administration. Flow rates are calculated in mL/hr for the lowest and highest dosage ordered and adjusted within this range to elicit the desired physiologic response. Let's look at some examples.

 Levophed **2–4 mcg/min** has been ordered to maintain systolic BP >100 mm. The solution being titrated has **8 mg** Levophed in **250 mL** of D5W. Calculate the flow rate for the **2–4 mcg range**.

The **lower** 2 mcg/min flow rate is calculated first.

- **Convert mcg/min to mcg/hr.**

  2 mcg/min × 60 min = **120 mcg/hr**

- **Convert mcg/hr to mg/hr.**

  120 mcg = **0.12 mg/hr**

- **Calculate the lower mL/hr flow rate.**

  $$8 \text{ mg} : 250 \text{ mL} = 0.12 \text{ mg} : X \text{ mL} \quad \text{or} \quad \frac{8 \text{ mg}}{250 \text{ mL}} = \frac{0.12 \text{ mg}}{X \text{ mL}}$$
  $$8X = 250 \times 0.12$$
  $$X = 3.75 = \textbf{4 mL/hr} \qquad\qquad = 3.75 = \textbf{4 mL/hr}$$

The flow rate for the lower 2 mcg/min dosage is 4 mL/hr.

The **upper** 4 mcg/min flow rate is calculated next.

- **Convert mcg/min to mcg/hr.**

  4 mcg/min × 60 min = **240 mcg/hr**

- **Convert mcg/hr to mg/hr.**

  240 mcg/hr = **0.24 mg/hr**

- **Calculate the upper mL/hr flow rate.**

  8 mg : 250 mL = 0.24 mg : X mL   or $\dfrac{8\ mg}{250\ mL} = \dfrac{0.24\ mg}{X\ mL}$

  8X = 250 × 0.24

  X = 7.5 − **8 mL/hr**   − 7.5 = **8 mL/hr**

The flow rate for the upper 4 mcg/min dosage is 8 mL/hr.

The flow rate range to titrate a dosage of 2–4 mcg/min is 4–8 mL/hr.

Note: Because the range of dosage was 2–4 mcg/min, or exactly double, the calculations could have been done for only the lower 2 mcg/min dosage and simply doubled to obtain the 4 mcg/min rate.

Let's assume that several changes in mL/hr have been made, and that the BP has now stabilized using a flow rate of **5 mL/hr**. Look how simple it is to determine how many **mcg/min** (or per hr) the patient is now receiving.

- **Calculate the dosage infusing at 5 mL/hr.**

  250 mL : 8 mg = 5 mL : X mg   or $\dfrac{250\ mL}{8\ mg} = \dfrac{5\ mL}{X\ mg}$ = **0.16 mg/hr**

  250X = 8 × 5

  X = **0.16 mg/hr**

- **Convert mg/hr to mcg/hr.**

  0.16 mg/hr = **160 mcg/hr**

- **Convert mcg/hr to mcg/min infusing.**

  160 mcg/hr ÷ 60 min = 2.67 = **2.7 mcg/min**

At a flow rate of 5 mL/hr the patient is now receiving 2.7 mcg/min.

 Inocor is to be titrated between **415 and 830 mcg/min** to maintain diastolic BP <90 mm. The solution concentration is **100 mg** in **40 mL** NS. Calculate the **mL/hr** flow rate range.

The **lower 415** mcg/min flow rate is calculated first.

- **Convert mcg/min to mcg/hr.**

  415 mcg/min × 60 min = **24,900 mcg/hr**

- **Convert mcg/hr to mg/hr.**

  24,900 mcg/hr = **24.9 mg/hr**

- **Calculate the lower mL/hr flow rate.**

$$100 \text{ mg} : 40 \text{ mL} = 24.9 \text{ mg} : X \text{ mL} \quad \text{or} \quad \frac{100 \text{ mg}}{40 \text{ mL}} = \frac{24.9 \text{ mg}}{X \text{ mL}}$$
$$100X = 40 \times 24.9$$
$$X = 9.96 = \textbf{10 mL/hr} \qquad\qquad = 9.96 = \textbf{10 mL/hr}$$

The **upper** 830 mcg/min dosage is exactly double the lower 415 mcg/min dosage, so the flow rate range for the upper dosage will be double that of the lower.

- **Calculate the upper dosage flow rate.**

$$10 \text{ mL/hr} \times 2 = \textbf{20 mL/hr}$$

A dosage of 415–830 mcg/min requires a flow rate of 10–20 mL/hr.

The rate is adjusted several times, and the IV is now infusing at **14 mL/hr**. How many **mcg/min** are now infusing?

- **Calculate the mg/hr infusing.**

$$40 \text{ mL} : 100 \text{ mg} = 14 \text{ mL} : X \text{ mL} \quad \text{or} \quad \frac{40 \text{ mL}}{100 \text{ mg}} = \frac{14 \text{ mL}}{X \text{ mg}} = \textbf{35 mg/hr}$$
$$40X = 100 \times 14$$
$$X = \textbf{35 mg/hr}$$

- **Convert mg/hr to mcg/hr.**

$$35 \text{ mg/hr} = \textbf{35,000 mcg/hr}$$

- **Convert mcg/hr to mcg/min infusing.**

$$35,000 \text{ mcg/hr} \div 60 \text{ min} = 583.33 = \textbf{583.3 mcg/min}$$

A 14 mL/hr flow rate will infuse 583.3 mcg/min.

 EXAMPLE 3 | A patient weighing **103.1 kg** has orders for Nipride to be titrated between **0.3 and 3 mcg/kg/min** to sustain BP >100 mm. The solution concentration is **50 mg in 250 mL** of D5W.

The **dosage range for this weight** is calculated first.

- **Calculate the lower dosage per min.**

$$0.3 \text{ mcg/kg/min} \times 103.1 \text{ kg} = 30.93 = \textbf{30.9 mcg/min}$$

- **Calculate the upper dosage per min.**

$$3 \text{ mcg/kg/min} \times 103.1 \text{ kg} = \textbf{309.3 mcg/min}$$

The dosage range for this 103.1 kg patient is 30.9 to 309.3 mcg/min.

The flow rate for the **lower** 30.9 mcg/min dosage is now calculated.

- **Convert mcg/min to mcg/hr.**

$$30.9 \text{ mcg/min} \times 60 \text{ min} = \textbf{1854 mcg/hr}$$

- **Convert mcg/hr to mg/hr.**

  1854 mcg/hr = **1.9 mg/hr**

- **Calculate the lower mL/hr flow rate.**

  $$50 \text{ mg} : 250 \text{ mL} = 1.9 \text{ mg} : X \text{ mL} \quad \text{or} \quad \frac{50 \text{ mg}}{250 \text{ mL}} = \frac{1.9 \text{ mg}}{X \text{ mL}}$$
  $$50X = 250 \times 1.9$$
  $$X = 9.5 = \textbf{10 mL/hr} \qquad\qquad\qquad = 9.5 = \textbf{10 mL/hr}$$

The flow rate for the **upper** 309.3 mcg/min dosage is now calculated.

- **Convert mcg/min to mcg/hr.**

  309.3 mcg/min × 60 min = **18,558 mcg/hr**

- **Convert mcg/hr to mg/hr.**

  18,558 mcg/hr = 18.55 = **18.6 mg/hr**

- **Calculate the flow rate.**

  $$50 \text{ mg} : 250 \text{ mL} = 18.6 \text{ mg} : X \text{ mL} \quad \text{or} \quad \frac{50 \text{ mg}}{250 \text{ mL}} = \frac{18.6 \text{ mg}}{X \text{ mL}} = \textbf{93 mL/hr}$$
  $$50X = 250 \times 18.6$$
  $$X = \textbf{93 mL/hr}$$

To deliver 0.3–3 mcg/kg/min to this 103.1 kg patient, the flow rate must be titrated between 10 and 93 mL/hr.

If after several titrations the patient's BP has stabilized using a flow rate of **22 mL/hr**, how many **mcg/min** will be infusing?

- **Calculate the mg/hr infusing.**

  $$250 \text{ mL} : 50 \text{ mg} = 22 \text{ mL} : X \text{ mL} \quad \text{or} \quad \frac{250 \text{ mL}}{50 \text{ mg}} = \frac{22 \text{ mL}}{X \text{ mg}} = \textbf{4.4 mg/hr}$$
  $$250X = 50 \times 22$$
  $$X = \textbf{4.4 mg/hr}$$

- **Convert mg/hr to mcg/hr.**

  4.4 mg/hr × 1000 = **4400 mcg/hr**

- **Convert mcg/hr to mcg/min infusing.**

  4400 mcg/hr ÷ 60 min = **73.3 mcg/min**

A flow rate of 22 mL/hr will infuse 73.3 mcg/min.

EXAMPLE 4 | Nipride has been ordered to titrate at **3–6 mcg/kg/min**. The solution strength is **50 mg in 250 mL**. Calculate the flow rate range for a **72.4 kg** patient.

The **dosage range for this weight** is calculated first.

- **Calculate the lower dosage per min.**

  3 mcg/kg/min × 72.4 kg = **217.2 mcg/min**

The **upper** dosage of 6 mcg/kg/min is exactly double the lower rate, so multiply the lower rate by 2 to obtain the upper dosage range.

- **Calculate the upper dosage per min.**

  217.2 mcg/min $\times$ 2 = **434.4 mcg/min**

The dosage range for this patient is 217.2–434.4 mcg/min.

The flow rate for the **lower** dosage is now calculated.

- **Convert mcg/min to mcg/hr.**

  217.2 mcg/min $\times$ 60 min = **13,026 mcg/hr**

- **Convert mcg/hr to mg/hr.**

  13,026 mcg/hr = **13 mg/hr**

- **Calculate the lower mL/hr flow rate.**

$$50 \text{ mg} : 250 \text{ mL} = 13 \text{ mg} : X \text{ mL} \quad \text{or} \quad \frac{50 \text{ mg}}{250 \text{ mL}} = \frac{13 \text{ mg}}{X \text{ mL}} = \textbf{65 mL/hr}$$
$$50X = 250 \times 13$$
$$X = \textbf{65 mL/hr}$$

The **upper flow rate** will be exactly double the lower.

- **Calculate the upper flow rate.**

  65 mL/hr $\times$ 2 = **130 mL/hr**

To deliver 3–6 mcg/kg/min to this 72.4 kg patient, the flow rate must be titrated between 65 and 130 mL/hr.

If after several adjustments upwards the flow rate is stabilized at **75 mL/hr**, what will the **mcg/min** dosage be?

- **Calculate the mg/hr infusing.**

$$250 \text{ mL} : 50 \text{ mg} = 75 \text{ mL} : X \text{ mL} \quad \text{or} \quad \frac{250 \text{ mL}}{50 \text{ mg}} = \frac{75 \text{ mL}}{X \text{ mg}} = \textbf{15 mg/hr}$$
$$250X = 50 \times 75$$
$$X = \textbf{15 mg/hr}$$

- **Convert mg/hr to mcg/hr.**

  15 mg/hr = **15,000 mcg/hr**

- **Convert mcg/hr to mcg/min infusing.**

  15,000 mcg $\div$ 60 min = **250 mcg/min**

An infusion rate of 75 mL/hr will deliver Nipride 250 mcg/min.

PROBLEM

Calculate the dosage range, mL/hr flow rate, and stabilizing dosages as indicated for the following titrations. Express fractional dosages to the nearest tenth.

1. A 2 g in 500 mL of D5W solution of bretylium is ordered to titrate at 1–2 mg/min for ventricular arrythmias. After several titrations the rate is stabilized at 18 mL/hr.

   Flow rate range _____   Stabilizing dosage/min _____

2. Isuprel is ordered to titrate between 1 and 3 mcg/min to sustain heart rate at a minimum of 64/min. The solution strength is 1 mg per 250 mL of D5W. The patient is stabilized at 35 mL/hr.

   Flow rate range _____   Stabilizing dosage/min _____

3. A stabilizing dosage of Inocor is established is at a rate of 14 mL/hr. The dosage range being titrated is 5–8 mcg/kg/min. The patient weighs 103.7 kg, and the solution strength is 100 mg in 40 mL of NS.

   Dosage range mcg/min _____   Flow rate range mL/hr _____

   Stabilizing dosage/min _____

4. Esmolol is to titrate between 50 and 100 mcg/kg/min. The patient weighs 78.7 kg, and the solution strength is 2500 mg in 250 mL of D5W. After several titrations the rate is stabilized at 30 mL/hr.

   Dosage range mcg/min _____   Flow rate range mL/hr _____

   Stabilizing dosage/min _____

5. A patient weighing 73.2 kg has a Dobutrex solution of 500 mg in 250 mL of D5W ordered to titrate between 3 and 10 mcg/kg/min. After many adjustments, the rate is stabilized at 27 mL/hr.

   Dosage range mcg/min _____   Flow rate range mL/hr _____

   Stabilizing dosage/min _____

Answers   **1.** 15–30 mL/hr; 1.2 mg/min   **2.** 15–45 mL/hr; 2.3 mcg/min   **3.** 518.5–829.6 mcg/min; 12–20 mL/hr; 583.3 mcg/min   **4.** 3935–7870 mcg/min; 24–47 mL/hr; 5000 mcg/min   **5.** 219.6–732 mcg/min; 7–22 mL/hr; 900 mcg/min

Summary

This concludes the chapter on titration of IV medications. The important points to remember about these medications are:

- They have a rapid action and short duration.

- They have a narrow margin of safety, and continuous patient monitoring is required in their use.

- They are frequency titrated within a specific dosage/flow rate to elicit a measurable physiologic response.

- When titrated they are initiated at the lowest dosage ordered and increased or decreased slowly to obtain the desired response.

- They are infused using an EID or 60 gtt/mL microdrip set.

- The mL/hr flow rate for EIDs and the gtt/min microdrip rate are identical and interchangeable.

- Because they alter vital functions, calculations for dosage and flow rates must be double-checked.

Summary Self-Test

Read each question thoroughly, and calculate only the dosages and flow rates indicated.

1. Dobutrex 6 mcg/kg/min is ordered to infuse IV to sustain the blood pressure of a patient weighing 75.4 kg. The solution available is 500 mg in 250 mL of D5W.

   mcg/min dosage _____ mL/hr flow rate _____

2. The order is to infuse a Nipride solution of 50 mg in 250 mL of DSW at 0.8 mcg/kg/min. Calculate the flow rate in mL/hr for a 65.9 kg patient.

   mcg/min dosage _____ mL/hr flow rate _____

3. A patient with aspiration pneumonia has an order for aminophylline 250 mg in 500 mL of D5W to infuse between 0.5 and 0.7 mg/kg/hr. The patient weighs 82.4 kg. He stabilizes at 75 mL/hr.

   mg/hr dosage range _____ mL/hr flow rate range _____

   Stabilizing dosage/hr _____

4. A solution of 400 mg dopamine HCl in 250 mL of D5W is infusing at 20 gtt/min.

   mcg/min dosage _____

5. Pronestyl 1–6 mg/min is ordered. The solution strength is 2 g/500 mL. The patient stabilizes at a rate of 80 mL/hr.

   mL/hr flow rate range _____

   Stabilizing dosage mg/min _____

6. A patient with bigeminy has orders for an infusion of 2 g lidocaine in 500 mL of D5W at 60 mL/hr. Is this dosage within the normal 1–4 mg/min range?

   mg/min dosage _____ mg/hr dosage _____

   Normal range? _____

7. A patient with terminal cancer has orders for continuous morphine sulfate IV. The solution available is 25 mg in 50 mL. The order is to infuse at 8 mg/hr.

   mL/hr flow rate _____

8. A solution of amrinone lactate 100 mg in 40 mL of NS is ordered to infuse at 5 mcg/kg/min for a patient weighing 77.1 kg.

   mL/hr flow rate _____

9. A patient in heart block has Isuprel ordered at 4 mcg/min. The solution available is 1 mg in 250 mL of D5W.

mL/hr flow rate _____

10. A patient weighing 80 kg has an order for Intropin to infuse at 8 mcg/kg/min. The solution strength is 800 mg Intropin in 500 mL of D5W.

mcg/min dosage _____ mL/hr flow rate _____

11. Dopamine 400 mg is added to 250 mL of D5W and infused at 45 gtt/min. Calculate the mcg/min and mg/hr infusing.

mcg/min dosage _____ mg/hr dosage _____

12. A patient with tetanus has orders for IV Thorazine 1 mg/min. The solution strength is 250 mg in 250 mL of D5W.

mL/hr flow rate _____

13. A patient weighing 77.9 kg is to receive Esmolol 80 mcg/kg/min. The solution strength is 2.5 g in 250 mL of D5W.

mcg/min dosage _____ mL/hr flow rate _____

14. Levophed 4 mcg/min has been ordered using an 8 mg in 250 mL of D5W solution.

mL/hr flow rate _____

15. A patient who weighs 81.7 kg has orders for dopamine 8–10 mcg/kg/min. The solution strength is 400 mg dopamine in 250 mL of D5W. The IV is infusing at 25 mL/hr.

mcg/min dosage range _____ mcg/min infusing _____

Within ordered range? _____

16. Nitroprusside 6 mcg/kg/min has been ordered for a 90.7 kg patient. The solution strength is 50 mg nitroprusside in 250 mL of D5W.

mcg/min dosage _____ mL/hr flow rate _____

17. Dopamine 5 mcg/kg/min is ordered. The solution available is 400 mg dopamine in 250 mL of D5W. The patient's weight is 70.7 kg.

mcg/min dosage _____ mL/hr flow rate _____

18. Pronestyl 3 mg/min is ordered. The solution strength is 2 g in 500 mL of D5W.

mL/hr flow rate _____

19. A nitroglycerine solution of 50 mg/250 mL of D5W is infusing at 15 gtt/min.

mcg/min infusing _____

20. Bretylol 2 g in 500 mL of D5W is to infuse at a rate of 2 mg/min.

mL/hr flow rate _____

21. A patient whose weight is 102.4 kg is to receive Nembutal 2 mg/kg/hr. The solution strength is 1 g in 500 mL of D5W.

mg/hr dosage _____ mL/hr flow rate _____

22. Deprovan 1 g in 100 mL of D5W is to infuse at a rate of 15 mcg/kg/min. The patient's weight is 94.4 kg.

          mcg/min dosage _____ mL/hr flow rate _____

23. A patient with severe hypotension is receiving 4 gtt/min of a solution of Levophed that contains 8 mg in 250 mL of D5W. Is this within the normal range of 2–4 mcg/min?

          mcg/min infusing _____ Normal range? _____

24. Inocor is ordered to titrate between 5 and 10 mcg/kg/min. The patient's weight is 97.1 kg, and the solution strength is 100 mg/40 mL of NS. The stabilizing flow rate is 17 mL/hr.

          mcg/min range _____ mL/hr flow rate range _____

          mcg/min stabilizing dosage _____

25. Dobutrex 500 mg in 250 mL of D5W is ordered for a 101.2 kg patient to titrate between 3 and 10 mcg/kg/min. The patient stabilizes at 23 mL/hr.

          mcg/min dosage range _____ mL/hr flow rate range _____

          mcg/min stabilizing dosage _____

26. An infusion of dobutamine 500 mg in 250 mL of D5W has a stabilizing rate of 14 mL/hr.

          mcg/min infusing _____

27. Amrinone 5–10 mcg/kg/min is to be titrated for a patient weighing 79.6 kg. The solution strength is 100 mg in 40 mL of NS. The patient stabilizes at 12 mL/hr.

          mcg/min dosage range _____ mL/hr flow rate range _____

          mcg/min stabilizing dosage _____

28. Dopamine 400 mg in 250 mL of D5W is to be titrated at 2–20 mcg/kg/min to maintain systolic BP >110. The patient's weight is 62.3 kg. The BP stabilizes at 32 mL/hr.

          mcg/min dosage range _____ mL/hr flow rate range _____

          mcg/min stabilizing dosage _____

29. Dobutamine has been ordered for a patient weighing 84.9 kg to titrate at 2.5–10 mcg/kg/min. The solution strength is 500 mg dobutamine in 250 mL of D5W. The patient stabilizes at a rate of 18 mL/hr.

          mcg/min dosage range _____ mL/hr flow rate range _____

          mcg/min stabilizing dosage _____

30. Lidocaine is ordered at a rate of 1–4 mg/min. The solution strength is 2 g in 500 mL of D5W.

          mL/hr flow rate range _____

31. A 10 mcg/min dosage of Levophed is ordered using an 8 mg/250 mL of D5W solution.

          mL/hr flow rate _____

32. Pronestyl 2 g in 500 mL of DSW is to infuse at 3 mg/min.
    A microdrip is used.

    mL/hr flow rate _____

33. A 250 mL of D5W solution with 1 mg Isuprel is to be infused at
    5 mcg/min.

    mL/hr flow rate _____

34. A 4 mcg/min maintenance dosage of Isuprel is ordered. The
    solution is 250 mL of D5W with 8 mg Isuprel.

    mL/hr flow rate _____

35. Pronestyl 2 g in 500 mL of D5W is ordered to infuse at a rate of
    6 mg/min.

    mL/hr flow rate _____

36. A 2 g in 500 mL of D5W solution of Pronestyl is ordered to infuse
    at 4 mg/min.

    mL/hr flow rate _____

37. A 12 mcg/min dosage of Levophed from an 8 mg in 250 mL of
    D5W solution is ordered.

    mL/hr flow rate _____

38. A 40 mg/hr dosage of Trandate from a 100 mg in 100 mL of D5W
    solution is ordered.

    mL/hr flow rate _____

39. The order is to infuse Isuprel 4 mcg/min from a 250 mL solution
    of D5W containing 1 mg of Isuprel.

    mL/hr flow rate _____

40. Cardizem 10 mg/hr from a 125 mg/100 mL of D5W solution has
    been ordered.

    mL/hr flow rate _____

Answers

1. 452.4 mcg/min;
   14 mL/hr
2. 52.7 mcg/min; 16 mL/hr
3. 41.2–57.7 mg/hr;
   82–115 mL/hr;
   37.5 mg/hr
4. 533.3 mcg/min
5. 15–90 mL/hr;
   5.3 mg/min
6. 4 mg/min; 240 mg/hr;
   yes
7. 16 mL/hr
8. 9 mL/hr
9. 60 mL/hr
10. 640 mcg/min; 24 mL/hr

11. 1200 mcg/min; 72 mg/hr
12. 60 mL/hr
13. 6232 mcg/min; 37 mL/hr
14. 8 mL/hr
15. 653.6–817 mcg/min;
    666.7 mcg/min; yes
16. 544.2 mcg/min;
    163 mL/hr
17. 353.5 mcg/min;
    13 mL/hr
18. 45 mL/hr
19. 50 mcg/min
20. 30 mL/hr
21. 204.8 mg/hr; 102 mL/hr
22. 1416 mcg/min; 9 mL/hr
23. 2.1 mcg/min; yes

24. 485.5–971 mcg/min;
    12–23 mL/hr;
    708.3 mcg/min
25. 303.6–1012 mcg/min;
    9–30 mL/hr;
    766.7 mcg/min
26. 466.7 mcg/min
27. 398–796 mcg/min;
    10–19 mL/hr;
    500 mcg/min
28. 124.6–1246 mcg/min;
    5–47 mL/hr;
    853.3 mcg/min
29. 212.3–849 mcg/min;
    6–25 mL/hr;
    600 mcg/min

30. 15–60 mL/hr
31. 19 mL/hr
32. 45 mL/hr
33. 75 mL/hr
34. 8 mL/hr
35. 90 mL/hr
36. 60 mL/hr
37. 23 mL/hr
38. 40 mL/hr
39. 60 mL/hr
40. 8 mL/hr

Heparin Infusion Calculations

Heparin is an anticoagulant drug that inhibits new blood clot formation or the extension of already existing clots. Heparin dosages are expressed in USP units (U), and are commonly administered intravenously. Dosages may be ordered on the basis of U/hr, or, if a standard concentration of IV solution is used, by mL/hr flow rate. Heparin dosages are ordered on a very individualized basis, and blood tests to monitor coagulation times are essential.

 The normal heparinizing dosage for adults is 20,000–40,000 U every 24 hours.

This means that the average patient will receive a daily dosage that falls within these 20,000 U to 40,000 U parameters. Dosages larger or smaller may be ordered based on a patient's coagulation time, but dosages markedly different from the average may need to be questioned.

In this chapter you will be introduced to several of the commercially prepared IV solutions containing heparin, as well as to heparin vial labels, which you will use to calculate the preparation of a variety of IV heparin solution strengths using standard solutions. You will also practice calculating heparin flow rates; calculating hourly dosage being administered; and assessing the accuracy of prescribed heparin dosages. The calculations are identical to those you have already practiced in previous chapters except that heparin is measured in units (U). Heparin is most frequently administered using a microdrip and/or a volumetric pump, but the examples and exercises that follow will provide practice in calculations using all IV set calibrations: 10, 15, 20, and 60 gtt/mL as well as mL/hr rates.

READING HEPARIN LABELS AND PREPARING IV SOLUTIONS

Commercially prepared IV solutions containing heparin are available in several strengths. Refer to the IV bag labeling in Figure 19-1, and notice the blue "Heparin Sodium 1,000 units in 0.9% Sodium Chloride Injection" on this 500 mL bag, and the additional red dosage labeling "Heparin 1,000 units (2 units/mL)." The red dosages draw particular attention to the fact that

Objectives

The learner will calculate the:

1. amount of heparin to be added to prepare IV solutions

2. mL/hr flow rates for an EID

3. gtt/min flow rates for microdrip and macrodrip sets

4. hourly dosage infusing from mL/hr and gtt/min rates

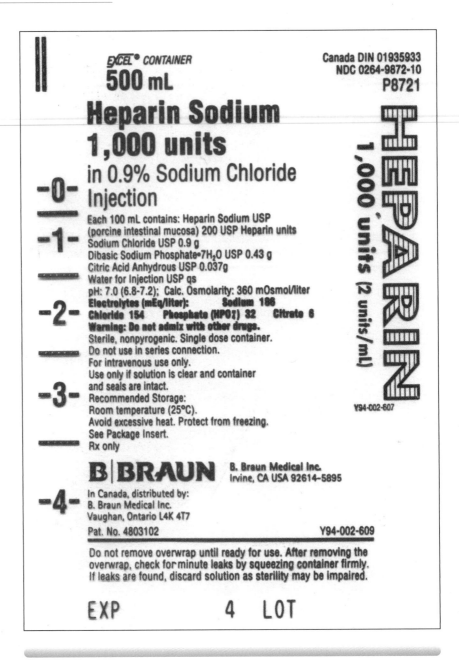

EXCEL® CONTAINER
500 mL

Heparin Sodium 1,000 units
in 0.9% Sodium Chloride Injection

Canada DIN 01935933
NDC 0264-9872-10
P8721

-0-
-1-

Each 100 mL contains: Heparin Sodium USP (porcine intestinal mucosa) 200 USP Heparin units
Sodium Chloride USP 0.9 g
Dibasic Sodium Phosphate•7H$_2$O USP 0.43 g
Citric Acid Anhydrous USP 0.037g
Water for Injection USP qs
pH: 7.0 (6.8-7.2); Calc. Osmolarity: 360 mOsmol/liter
Electrolytes (mEq/liter):   Sodium 186

-2-

Chloride 154   Phosphate (HPO$_4$) 32   Citrate 6
Warning: Do not admix with other drugs.
Sterile, nonpyrogenic. Single dose container.
Do not use in series connection.
For intravenous use only.
Use only if solution is clear and container and seals are intact.

-3-

Recommended Storage:
Room temperature (25°C).
Avoid excessive heat. Protect from freezing.
See Package Insert.
Rx only

B|BRAUN B. Braun Medical Inc.
Irvine, CA USA 92614-5895

-4-

In Canada, distributed by:
B. Braun Medical Inc.
Vaughan, Ontario L4K 4T7
Pat. No. 4803102   Y94-002-609

Do not remove overwrap until ready for use. After removing the overwrap, check for minute leaks by squeezing container firmly. If leaks are found, discard solution as sterility may be impaired.

EXP   4 LOT

HEPARIN
1,000 units
(2 units/mL)
Y94-002-607

Figure 19-1

these bags contain heparin to make the bags instantly recognizable. They serve as an important safety factor in solution identification.

If a commercially prepared heparin dosage strength that you require is not available, you may be required to prepare the solution yourself from **a number of available vial dosage strengths**. Let's stop and look at several vial labels now, so that you can refresh your memory with some typical calculations.

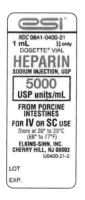

Figure 19-2

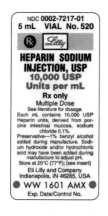

Figure 19-3

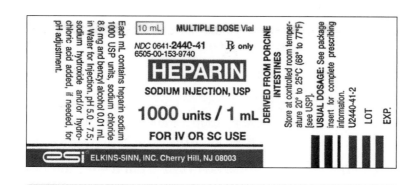

Figure 19-4

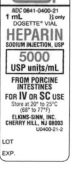

Figure 19-5

Figure 19-6

PROBLEM

Read the heparin labels provided and determine how many mL of heparin will be necessary to prepare the solutions indicated.

1. Refer to the label in Figure 19-2 and determine how many mL will be required to add 20,000 U to an IV solution. _____

2. Refer to the label in Figure 19-3 and determine how many mL will be required to add 30,000 U to an IV solution. _____

3. Refer to the label in Figure 19-4 and determine how many mL will be required to add 20,000 U to an IV solution. _____

4. Refer to the label in Figure 19-5 and determine how many mL of heparin will be required to add 25,000 U to an IV solution. _____

5. Refer to the label in Figure 19-6 and determine how many mL will be required to add 10,000 U to an IV solution. _____

Answers **1.** 4 mL **2.** 3 mL **3.** 2 mL **4.** 5 mL **5.** 10 mL

CALCULATING mL/hr FLOW RATE FROM U/hr ORDERED

Because heparin is most frequently ordered in U/hr to be administered, for example, 1000 U/hr, and infused using an EID, a common calculation will be the mL/hr flow rate. Let's look at these calculations first, keeping in mind that the mL/hr flow rate for an EID is identical to the gtt/min rate for a microdrip.

 The order is to infuse heparin **1000 U/hr** from a solution of **20,000 U in 500 mL** of D5W.

• **Calculate the mL/hr flow rate.**

$$20,000 \text{ U} : 500 \text{ mL} = 1000 \text{ U} : X \text{ mL} \quad \text{or} \quad \frac{20,000 \text{ U}}{500 \text{ mL}} = \frac{1000 \text{ U}}{X \text{ mL}} = \textbf{25 mL/hr}$$
$$20{,}000X = 500 \times 1000$$
$$X = \textbf{25 mL/hr}$$

The flow rate to infuse 1000 U/hr from a solution of 20,000 U in 500 mL is 25 mL/hr.

 The order is for heparin **800 U/hr**. The solution available is **40,000 U in 1000 mL** of D5W.

• **Calculate the mL/hr flow rate.**

$$40,000 \text{ U} : 1000 \text{ mL} = 800 \text{ U} : X \text{ mL} \quad \text{or} \quad \frac{40,000 \text{ U}}{1000 \text{ mL}} = \frac{800 \text{ U}}{X \text{ mL}} = \textbf{20 mL/hr}$$
$$40{,}000X = 1000 \times 800$$
$$X = \textbf{20 mL/hr}$$

The flow rate to infuse 800 U/hr from a solution of 40,000 U in 1000 mL is 20 mL/hr.

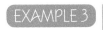 The order is to infuse heparin **1100 U/hr** from a solution of **60,000 U in 1 L** of D5W.

• **Calculate the mL/hr flow rate.**

$$60,000 \text{ U} : 1000 \text{ mL} = 1100 \text{ U} : X \text{ mL} \quad \text{or} \quad \frac{60,000 \text{ U}}{1000 \text{ mL}} = \frac{1100 \text{ U}}{X \text{ mL}}$$
$$60{,}000X = 1000 \times 1100$$
$$X = 18.3 = \textbf{18 mL/hr} \qquad = 18.3 = \textbf{18 mL/hr}$$

The flow rate to infuse 1100 U/hr from a solution of 60,000 U in 1 L is 18 mL/hr.

PROBLEM

Calculate the mL/hr flow rates for the following heparin infusions.

1. The order is to infuse 1000 U heparin per hour from an available solution strength of 25,000 U in 500 mL of D5W. _____

2. A patient with deep vein thrombosis has orders for heparin 2500 U per hour. The solution strength is 50,000 U in 1000 mL of D5W. _____

3. The order is to infuse 1100 U per hour from a 15,000 U in 1 L of D5W solution.   _____

4. A newly admitted patient has orders for 50,000 U of heparin in 1000 mL of D5W to infuse at a rate of 2000 U per hour.   _____

5. Administer 1500 U per hour of heparin from an available strength of 40,000 U in 1 L.   _____

 Answers **1.** 20 mL/hr **2.** 50 mL/hr **3.** 73 mL/hr **4.** 40 mL/hr **5.** 38 mL/hr

CALCULATING gtt/min FLOW RATE FROM U/hr ORDERED

When a gtt/min rate is calculated for a 10, 15, 20, or 60 gtt/mL set, the calculation will include the set calibration.

EXAMPLE 1 | A heparin solution with a strength of **40,000 U per 1000 mL** of D5W is ordered to infuse at a rate of **1000 U/hr**. A **15 gtt/mL** set is used.

• **Calculate the mL/hr to be infused first.**

$$40,000 \text{ U} : 1000 \text{ mL} = 1000 \text{ U} : X \text{ mL} \quad \text{or} \quad \frac{40,000 \text{ U}}{1000 \text{ mL}} = \frac{1000 \text{ U}}{X \text{ mL}} = \textbf{25 mL/hr}$$
$$X = \textbf{25 mL/hr}$$

• **Calculate the flow rate in gtt/min.**

The division factor for a 15 gtt/mL set is 4 (60 ÷ 15).

$$25 \div 4 = 6.2 = \textbf{6 gtt/min}$$

To infuse 1000 U/hr from a 40,000 U/1000 mL solution using a 15 gtt/mL set, the rate will be 6 gtt/min.

EXAMPLE 2 | A solution of heparin **20,000 U in 500 mL** of D5W is ordered to infuse at a rate of **800 U** per hour using a **10 gtt/mL** set.

• **Calculate the mL/hr to be infused.**

$$20,000 \text{ U} : 500 \text{ mL} = 800 \text{ U} : X \text{ mL} \quad \text{or} \quad \frac{20,000 \text{ U}}{500 \text{ mL}} = \frac{800 \text{ U}}{X \text{ mL}} = \textbf{20 mL/hr}$$
$$X = \textbf{20 mL/hr}$$

• **Calculate the flow rate in gtt/min.**

The division factor for a 10 gtt/mL set is 6 (60 ÷ 10).

$$20 \div 6 = 3.3 = \textbf{3 gtt/min}$$

To infuse 800 U/hr from a 20,000 U in 500 mL solution using a 10 gtt/mL set, the rate will be 3 gtt/min.

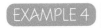 EXAMPLE 3 The order is for heparin to infuse at **1200 U per hour**. The solution strength is **60,000 U in 1 L** of D5W. A **20 gtt/mL** set is used.

- **Calculate the mL/hr to be infused.**

$$60{,}000 \text{ U} : 1000 \text{ mL} = 1200 \text{ U} : X \text{ mL} \quad \text{or} \quad \frac{60{,}000 \text{ U}}{1000 \text{ mL}} = \frac{1200 \text{ U}}{X \text{ mL}} = \textbf{20 mL/hr}$$
$$X = \textbf{20 mL/hr}$$

- **Calculate the flow rate in gtt/min.**

The division factor for a 20 gtt/mL set is 3 (60 ÷ 20).

$$20 \div 3 = 6.6 = \textbf{7 gtt/min}$$

To infuse 1200 U/hr from a 60,000 U in 1 L solution using a 20 gtt/mL set, the rate will be 7 gtt/min.

EXAMPLE 4 An IV of **500 mL** of D5W with **25,000 U** of heparin is to infuse at **1500 U/hr** using a **microdrip**.

- **Calculate the mL/hr to be infused.**

$$25{,}000 \text{ U} : 1000 \text{ mL} = 1500 \text{ U} : X \text{ mL} \quad \text{or} \quad \frac{25{,}000 \text{ U}}{500 \text{ mL}} = \frac{1500 \text{ U}}{X \text{ mL}} = \textbf{30 mL/hr}$$
$$X = \textbf{30 mL/hr}$$

- **Calculate the flow rate in gtt/min.**

The division factor for a 60 gtt/mL set is 1 (60 ÷ 60).

$$30 \div 1 = 6.6 = \textbf{30 gtt/min}$$

To infuse 1500 U/hr from a 25,000 U in 500 mL solution using a microdrip, the rate will be 30 gtt/min.

PROBLEM

Calculate the gtt/min flow rates to administer the following heparin dosages.

1. A solution of 25,000 U of heparin in 500 mL of D5W is to infuse at a rate of 1000 U per hour using a 10 gtt/mL set. _____

2. Heparin 2500 U per hour using a 20 gtt/mL set; the solution strength is 50,000 U in 1000 mL of D5W. _____

3. A solution strength of heparin 15,000 U per 1 L is to infuse at 1100 U/hr using a 15 gtt/mL set. _____

4. Heparin 2000 U per hour using a 20 gtt/mL set; the solution strength is 50,000 U in 1000 mL of D5W. _____

5. A 30,000 U in 500 mL of heparin solution is to infuse at 1500 U/hr with a 10 gtt/mL set. _____

6. A 500 mL D5W with 20,000 U of heparin is to infuse at 1000 U/hr using a microdrip. _____

Answers   **1.** 3 gtt/min   **2.** 17 gtt/min   **3.** 18 gtt/min   **4.** 13 gtt/min   **5.** 4 gtt/min   **6.** 25 gtt/min

CALCULATING U/hr INFUSING FROM mL/hr INFUSING

If a heparin order specifies infusion at a predetermined mL/hr flow rate, the doctor has already calculated the dosage per hour/day the patient is to receive. However, it remains a nursing responsibility to double-check dosages to determine if they are within **the normal heparinizing range of 20,000–40,000 U per day**. Here's how you would do this.

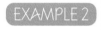 An IV of **1000 mL** of D5W containing **40,000 U** of heparin has been ordered to infuse at **30 mL/hr**.

- **Calculate the U/hr infusing first.**

$$1000 \text{ mL} : 40,000 \text{ U} = 30 \text{ mL} : X \text{ U} \quad \text{or} \quad \frac{1000 \text{ mL}}{40,000 \text{ U}} = \frac{30 \text{ mL}}{X \text{ U}} = \textbf{1200 U/hr}$$
$$X = \textbf{1200 U/hr}$$

An IV of 1000 mL containing 40,000 U of heparin infusing at 30 mL/hr is administering 1200 U/hr.

- **Assess for heparinizing range.**

1200 U/hr $\times$ 24 hr = **28,800 U/24 hr**

This dosage is within the 20,000 to 40,000 U in 24 hr heparinizing range.

 The order is to infuse a solution of heparin **20,000 U** to **1 L** of D5W at **80 mL/hr**. Calculate the **U/hr** infusing and assess the accuracy of the order.

- **Calculate the U/hr infusing first.**

$$1000 \text{ mL} : 20,000 \text{ U} = 80 \text{ mL} : X \text{ U} \quad \text{or} \quad \frac{1000 \text{ mL}}{20,000 \text{ U}} = \frac{80 \text{ mL}}{X \text{ U}} = \textbf{1600 U/hr}$$
$$X = \textbf{1600 U/hr}$$

An IV of 1 L containing 20,000 U of heparin infusing at 80 mL/hr is administering 1600 U/hr.

- **Assess for heparinizing range.**

1600 U/hr $\times$ 24 hr = **38,400 U/24 hr**

This dosage is within the 20,000 to 40,000 U in 24 hr heparinizing range.

EXAMPLE 3 An IV of D5W **500 mL** with **10,000 U** of heparin is infusing at **30 mL/hr**. Calculate the **U/hr** dosage and determine if this dose is within the normal range.

- **Calculate the U/hr infusing first.**

$$500 \text{ mL} : 10,000 \text{ U} = 30 \text{ mL} : X \text{ U} \quad \text{or} \quad \frac{500 \text{ mL}}{10,000 \text{ U}} = \frac{30 \text{ mL}}{X \text{ U}} = \textbf{600 U/hr}$$
$$X = \textbf{600 U/hr}$$

An IV of 500 mL containing 10,000 U of heparin infusing at 30 mL/hr is administering 600 U/hr.

• **Assess for heparinizing range.**

600 U/hr × 24 hr = **14,400 U/day**

This dosage less than the 20,000 to 40,000 U in 24 hr heparinizing range, so the order should be reconfirmed.

PROBLEM

Calculate the following U/hr heparin dosages, and determine if they are within the normal daily range.

1. The order is to add 30,000 U of heparin to 750 mL of D5W and infuse at 25 mL/hr.

   U/hr _____   U/day _____   Within normal range? _____

2. A solution of 20,000 U of heparin in 500 mL of D5W is to be infused at 30 mL/hr.

   U/hr _____   U/day _____   Within normal range? _____

3. One liter of D5N5 with heparin 60,000 U is ordered to infuse at 40 mL/hr.

   U/hr _____   U/day _____   Within normal range? _____

4. The order is to add 20,000 U of heparin to 1 L of D5W and infuse at 30 mL/hr.

   U/hr _____   U/day _____   Within normal range? _____

5. A 25,000 U in 500 mL of D5W heparin solution is infusing at 30 mL/hr.

   U/hr _____   U/day _____   Within normal range? _____

Answers   **1.** 1000 U/hr; 24,000 U/day; yes   **2.** 1200 U/hr; 28,800 U/day; yes   **3.** 2400 U/hr; 57,600 U/day; high   **4.** 600 U/hr; 14,400 U/day; low   **5.** 1500 U/hr; 36,000 U/day; yes

CALCULATING U/hr INFUSING FROM SOLUTION STRENGTH, SET CALIBRATION, AND gtt/min RATE

The U/hr dosage can also be calculated from a solution ordered or infusing as gtt/min. The solution strength, gtt/min rate, and set calibration will be used for the calculation.

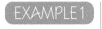 EXAMPLE 1 | An IV of **10,000 U** of heparin in **1000 mL** of D5W is infusing at **40 gtt/min** using a **20 gtt/mL** set. Calculate the **U/hr** infusing.

• **Convert gtt/min to mL/min infusing first.**

$$20 \text{ gtt} : 1 \text{ mL} = 40 \text{ gtt} : X \text{ mL} \quad \text{or} \quad \frac{20 \text{ gtt}}{1 \text{ mL}} = \frac{40 \text{ gtt}}{X \text{ mL}} = \textbf{2 mL/min}$$
$$X = \textbf{2 mL/min}$$

• **Calculate the mL/hr infusing.**

2 mL/min × 60 min = **120 mL/hr**

- **Calculate the U/hr infusing.**

$$1000 \text{ mL} : 10{,}000 \text{ U} = 120 \text{ mL} : X \text{ U} \quad \text{or} \quad \frac{1000 \text{ mL}}{10{,}000 \text{ U}} = \frac{120 \text{ mL}}{X \text{ U}} = \textbf{1200 U/hr}$$
$$X = \textbf{1200 U/hr}$$

The patient is receiving 1200 U/hr from this 10,000 U in 1000 mL heparin solution infusing at 40 gtt/min on a 20 gtt/mL set.

EXAMPLE 2 | A heparin solution with a strength of **15,000 U** in **500 mL** is infusing at a rate of **10 gtt/min** using a **10 gtt/mL** set. Calculate **U/hr** infusing.

- **Convert gtt/min to mL/min infusing.**

$$10 \text{ gtt} : 1 \text{ mL} = 10 \text{ gtt} : X \text{ mL} \quad \text{or} \quad \frac{10 \text{ gtt}}{1 \text{ mL}} = \frac{10 \text{ gtt}}{X \text{ mL}} = \textbf{1 mL/min}$$
$$X = \textbf{1 mL/min}$$

- **Calculate the mL/hr infusing.**

$$1 \text{ mL/min} \times 60 \text{ min} = \textbf{60 mL/hr}$$

- **Calculate the U/hr infusing.**

$$500 \text{ mL} : 15{,}000 \text{ U} = 60 \text{ mL} : X \text{ U} \quad \text{or} \quad \frac{500 \text{ mL}}{15{,}000 \text{ U}} = \frac{60 \text{ mL}}{X \text{ U}} = \textbf{1800 U/hr}$$
$$X = \textbf{1800 U/hr}$$

The patient is receiving 1800 U/hr from this 15,000 U in 500 mL heparin solution infusing at 10 gtt/min on a 10 gtt/mL set.

EXAMPLE 3 | A **15 gtt/mL** set is used to infuse a **20,000 U/1000 mL** heparin solution at **25 gtt/min**. Calculate **U/hr** infusing.

- **Convert gtt/min to mL/min infusing.**

$$15 \text{ gtt} : 1 \text{ mL} = 40 \text{ gtt} : X \text{ mL} \quad \text{or} \quad \frac{15 \text{ gtt}}{1 \text{ mL}} = \frac{25 \text{ gtt}}{X \text{ mL}} = \textbf{1.6 mL/min}$$
$$X = \textbf{1.6 mL/min}$$

- **Calculate the mL/hr infusing.**

$$1.6 \text{ mL/min} \times 60 \text{ min} = \textbf{96 mL/hr}$$

- **Calculate the U/hr infusing.**

$$1000 \text{ mL} : 20{,}000 \text{ U} = 96 \text{ mL} : X \text{ U} \quad \text{or} \quad \frac{1000 \text{ mL}}{20{,}000 \text{ U}} = \frac{96 \text{ mL}}{X \text{ U}} = \textbf{1920 U/hr}$$
$$X = \textbf{1920 U/hr}$$

The patient is receiving 1920 U/hr from this 20,000 U in 1000 mL heparin solution infusing at 25 gtt/min on a 15 gtt/mL set.

PROBLEM

Calculate the U/hr of heparin infusing in the following.

1. A solution strength of 40,000 U in 1000 mL infusing at a rate of 35 gtt/min using a 60 gtt/mL microdrip   _____

2. A set calibrated at 15 gtt/mL infusing a 30,000 U/1000 mL heparin solution at 8 gtt/min   _____

3. A 25,000 U in 1000 mL strength heparin solution infusing at 15 gtt/min using a 20 gtt/mL set   _____

4. An IV running at 20 gtt/min using a 20 gtt/mL set with a solution strength of heparin 10,000 U in 500 mL   _____

5. A 20,000 U/500 mL heparin solution infusing at 22 gtt/min using a 60 gtt/mL set   _____

Answers **1.** 1400 U/hr **2.** 960 U/hr **3.** 1125 U/hr **4.** 1200 U/hr **5.** 880 U/hr

Summary

This concludes the chapter on heparin administration. The important points to remember from this chapter are:

- Heparin is a potent anticoagulant that is frequently added to IV solutions.

- It is measured in USP units, abbreviated U.

- The normal heparinizing dosage is 20,000–40,000 U/day.

- The patient on heparin therapy will have frequent blood tests to check coagulation times.

- Heparin may be ordered by mL/hr flow rate, or by U/hr to infuse.

- If an EID or microdrip is used for infusion, the mL/hr and gtt/min rate will be identical.

- The gtt/min rates are calculated from set calibration, IV solution strength, and dosage ordered.

- The dosage infusing at any moment can be calculated from the flow rate, set calibration, and solution strength.

- Commercially prepared IV solutions are available for several heparin strengths.

- Additional strengths may require the preparation of heparin from a variety of available vial strengths.

Summary Self-Test

Calculate the heparin flow rates or hourly dosages as indicated in the following questions.

1. A patient is to receive heparin 1000 U/hr. The IV solution available has 25,000 U in 1 L of D5W, and a volumetric pump will be used. Flow rate _____

2. A solution of 25,000 U of heparin in 1 L of D5 1/4NS is infusing at 15 gtt/min using a 10 gtt/mL set. Dosage per hr _____

3. A solution of 35,000 U of heparin in 1 L of D5 1/2NS is to infuse via volumetric pump at 1200 U/hr. Flow rate _____

4. A patient has orders for 20,000 U of heparin in 500 mL of D5W to infuse at 40 mL/hr. Dosage per hr _____

5. A solution of 1 L of D5W with 50,000 U of heparin is to be administered at 1250 U/hr using a 15 gtt/mL set. Flow rate _____

6. A patient with pulmonary emboli has orders for 2500 U of heparin per hour. The solution strength is 40,000 U in 1 L of D5W, and a 10 gtt/mL set is used. Flow rate _____

7. Calculate the flow rate to administer heparin at a rate of 1000 U/hr using a set calibrated at 10 gtt/mL and a solution strength of 25,000 U in 1000 mL D5W. Flow rate _____

8. Calculate the U/hr of heparin infusing at 25 gtt/min from a solution strength of 40,000 U in 1 L of D5W. A microdrip is being used. Dosage per hr _____

   Within normal daily range? _____

9. Calculate the hourly heparin dosage infusing at 50 mL/hr from a 35,000 U heparin in 1 L D5W solution. Dosage per hr _____

10. A patient who had recent open heart surgery has an IV of 500 mL of D5W with 20,000 U of heparin infusing at 20 gtt/min using a microdrip. Dosage per hr _____

11. A patient is to receive 2000 U of heparin per hour from a solution of 50,000 U in 1000 mL of D5NS using a 10 gtt/mL set. Flow rate _____

12. An IV of 1000 mL of D5W with 20,000 U of heparin is infusing at 12 gtt/min using a 10 gtt/mL set. Dosage per hr _____

13. A patient with a fractured pelvis has orders for 1 L of D5 1/2NS with 60,000 U of heparin to infuse at 30 mL/hr. Dosage per hr _____

    Within normal range? _____

14. The order is for 1000 U of heparin per hour. The solution strength is 20,000 U in 500 mL of D5NS. A microdrip is used. Flow rate _____

15. A newly admitted patient has an order for 1250 U/hr of heparin from a solution strength of 15,000 U in 500 mL of D5W. A volumetric pump is used to monitor the infusion. Flow rate _____

16. Calculate the hourly dosage infusing with a 25 mL/hr rate from a 1 L D5 1/4NS with 45,000 U heparin solution. Dosage _____

17. A solution of 10,000 U of heparin in 500 mL of D5W is ordered to infuse at 1000 U/hr via a volumetric pump. Flow rate _____

18. A liter of D5W containing 15,000 U of heparin is infusing at 20 gtt/min using a 10 gtt/mL set. Dosage per hr _____

19. During morning rounds, you time a patient's IV at 20 gtt/min. The solution is heparin 25,000 U in 1 L of D5W, and the set calibration 10 gtt/mL. An hourly dosage of 1500 U was ordered. Flow rate correct? _____

20. A patient has an IV of 25,000 U of heparin in 1 L of D5W infusing at 10 gtt/min using a 15 gtt/mL set. Dosage per hr _____

21. A solution of 500 mL of D5NS with 30,000 U of heparin is infusing at 25 mL/hr. Dosage per hr _____

Within normal limits? _____

22. A patient with multiple fractures has an order for 2 L of D5 1/2NS each to contain 20,000 U of heparin to infuse at 50 mL/hr using a microdrip. Dosage per hr _____

23. A patient is receiving 500 mL of D5W with 10,000 U of heparin at 20 gtt/min using a 10 gtt/mL set. Dosage per hr _____

24. An IV of 1000 mL of D5 1/4NS with 40,000 U of heparin is to infuse at 1200 U/hr via pump. Flow rate _____

25. A patient is receiving 900 U/hr of heparin from a 500 mL D5W with 20,000 U solution. The infusion set is calibrated at 20 gtt/mL. Flow rate _____

26. The order is to infuse 500 mL of D5 1/4NS with 25,000 U of heparin at 1500 U/hr. A microdrip is used. Flow rate _____

27. A liter of D5W with 40,000 U of heparin is infusing at 25 mL/hr. Dosage per hr _____

28. A 500 mL IV with 25,000 U of heparin is infusing at 30 mL/hr. Dosage per hr _____

29. 500 mL of D5W with 30,000 U of heparin is to infuse via volumetric pump at 1500 U/hr. Flow rate _____

30. The order is to infuse 1 L of D5 1/2NS with 45,000 U of heparin at 1875 U/hr using a volumetric pump. Flow rate _____

31. The order is to infuse 1400 U/hr from a 1 L D5W with a 35,000 U heparin solution using a 15 gtt/mL set. Flow rate _____

32. A patient is receiving 1 L of D5W with 12,500 U of heparin at 30 gtt/min using a set calibrated at 20 gtt/mL. Dosage per hr _____

Answers

	8. 1400 U/hr; yes	**15.** 42 mL/hr	**21.** 1500 U/hr; yes	**29.** 25 mL/hr
1. 40 mL/hr	**9.** 1750 U/hr	**16.** 1125 U/hr	**22.** 1000 U/hr	**30.** 42 mL/hr
2. 2250 U/hr	**10.** 800 U/hr	**17.** 50 mL/hr	**23.** 2400 U/hr	**31.** 10 gtt/min
3. 34 mL/hr	**11.** 7 gtt/min	**18.** 1800 U/hr	**24.** 30 mL/hr	**32.** 1125 U/hr
4. 1600 U/hr	**12.** 1440 U/hr	**19.** No, double	**25.** 8 gtt/min	
5. 6 gtt/min	**13.** 1800 U/hr;	the dose is	**26.** 30 gtt/min	
6. 10 gtt/min	high	infusing	**27.** 1000 U/hr	
7. 7 gtt/min	**14.** 25 gtt/min	**20.** 1000 U/hr	**28.** 1500 U/hr	

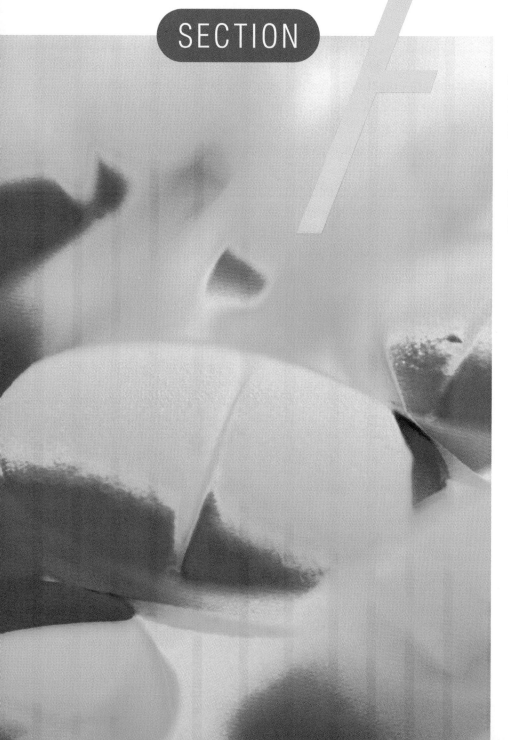

SECTION 7

Pediatric Medication Calculations

Pediatric Oral and Parenteral Medications

Objectives

The learner will:

1. explain how suspensions are measured and administered

2. calculate pediatric oral dosages

3. list the precautions of IM and s.c. injection in infants and children

4. calculate pediatric IM and s.c. dosages

Two differences between adult and pediatric dosages will be immediately apparent: **most oral drugs are prepared as liquids** because infants and small children cannot be expected to swallow tablets easily, if at all, and **dosages are dramatically smaller**. The oral route is used whenever possible, but when a child cannot swallow, or the drug is ineffective given orally, drugs will be administered by a parenteral route.

Both the subcutaneous and intramuscular routes may be used depending on the type of drug to be administered. However, the small muscle size of infants and children limits the use of the intramuscular route, as does the nature of the drug being used. For example, most antibiotics are administered intravenously rather than intramuscularly.

ORAL MEDICATIONS

Most oral pediatric drugs are prepared as liquids to facilitate ease in swallowing. If the child is old enough to cooperate these dosages may be measured in a medication cup. Solutions may also be measured using oral syringes, such as the ones shown in Figure 20-1. Notice that oral syringes have the same metric calibrations as hypodermic syringes, but also include household measures, for example, tsp. Oral syringes have different-sized tips to prevent use with hypodermic needles. On some oral syringes the tip is positioned off center (termed *eccentric*), to further distinguish them from hypodermic syringes, or they may be amber colored, as in the Figure 20-1 illustration.

If oral syringes are not available, hypodermic syringes (**without the needle**) can also be used for dosage measurement. In addition to accuracy, syringes provide an excellent method of administering oral liquid drugs to infants and small children. Some oral liquids are prepared using a calibrated medication dropper that is an integral part of the medication bottle. These may be calibrated in mL like the dropper shown in Figure 20-2, or in actual dosage, for example, 25 mg or 50 mg. Animal-shaped measures such as those shown in Figure 20-3 are also helpful in enticing reluctant toddlers to take necessary medications. In each instance the goal is to be sure the infant or child actually swallows the total dosage.

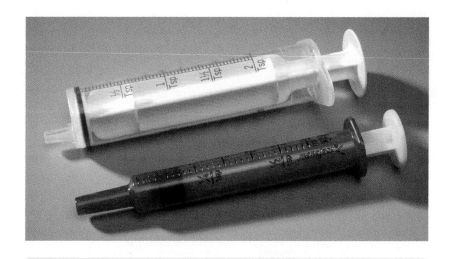

Figure 20-1

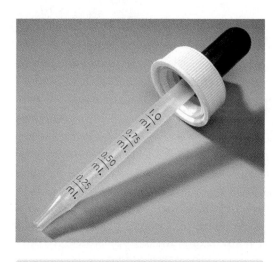

Figure 20-2

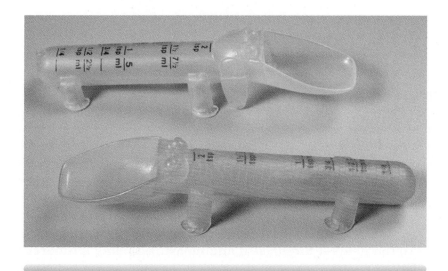

Figure 20-3

Care must be taken with liquid oral drugs to identify those prepared as **suspensions**. A **suspension consists of an insoluble drug in a liquid base** as for example in the Augmentin® suspension in Figure 20-4. The drug in a suspension settles to the bottom of the bottle between uses, and **thorough mixing immediately prior to pouring** is mandatory. Suspensions must also be administered to the child promptly after measurement to prevent the drug from settling out again and an incomplete dosage being administered.

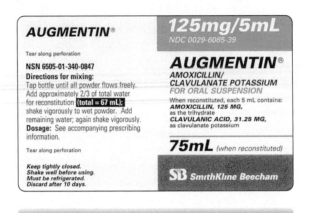

Figure 20-4

 Suspensions must be thoroughly mixed before measurement and promptly administered to prevent settling out of their insoluble drugs.

When a tablet or capsule is administered, the child's mouth must be checked to be certain it has actually been swallowed. If swallowing is a problem, some tablets can be crushed and given in a small amount of applesauce, ice cream, or juice, if the child has no dietary restrictions to contraindicate this. Keep in mind, however, that **enteric coated and timed release tablets or capsules cannot be crushed** because this would destroy the coating that allows them to function on a delayed action basis.

IM AND s.c. MEDICATIONS

The drugs most often given subcutaneously are insulin and immunizations that specifically require the subcutaneous route. Any site with sufficient subcutaneous tissue may be used, with the upper arm being the site of choice for immunizations. The intramuscular route is used most frequently for preoperative and postoperative medications for sedation and pain and for immunizations such as DPT (diphtheria, pertussis, tetanus), which must be administered deep IM. The intramuscular site of choice for infants and small children is the vastus lateralis or rectus femoris of the thigh, because the gluteal muscles do not develop until a child has learned to walk. Usually not more than 1 mL is injected per site, and sites are rotated regularly.

Dosage calculation is the same as for adults, except **dosages are sometimes calculated to the nearest hundredth and measured using a tuberculin syringe** (refer to Chapter 7 if you need to review the calibrations and use of a TB syringe). There is less margin for error in pediatric dosages, and calculations and measurements are carefully double-checked.

Summary

This concludes the introduction to pediatric oral and IM and s.c. medication administration. The important points to remember from this chapter are:

- Care must be taken when administering oral drugs to be positive that the child has actually swallowed the dosage.
- If liquid medications are prepared as suspensions, mix thoroughly prior to measurement, and administer promptly to prevent settling out of their insoluble drugs.
- Care must be taken not to confuse oral syringes, which are unsterile, with hypodermic syringes, which are sterile.
- The IM site of choice for infants and small children is the vastus lateralis or rectus femoris of the thigh.
- Usually not more than 1 mL is injected per IM or s.c. site, and sites are rotated regularly.
- Pediatric parenteral dosages are frequently calculated to the nearest hundredth and measured using a TB syringe.

Summary Self-Test

Use the pediatric medication labels provided to measure the following oral dosages. Indicate in column two if the medication is a suspension.

PART I	mL	Suspension
1. Prepare a 125 mg dosage of Augmentin.	_____	_____
2. Prepare a 125 mg dosage of Amoxil.	_____	_____

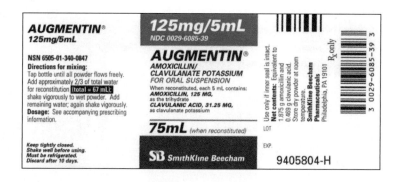

	mL	Suspension
3. Prepare a 0.1 dosage of digoxin.	_____	_____
4. Prepare 100 mg of Vantin.	_____	_____
5. Prepare 400,000 U of oral penicillin V.	_____	_____
6. Prepare 5 mg of Lomotil.	_____	_____
7. Prepare 250 mg of tetracycline.	_____	_____
8. Peri-Colace 3 tsp is ordered. How many mL will this be?	_____	_____
9. Prepare 250 mg of amoxicillin.	_____	_____
10. Prepare 120 mg of acetaminophen.	_____	_____
11. Prepare 187 mg of Ceclor.	_____	_____

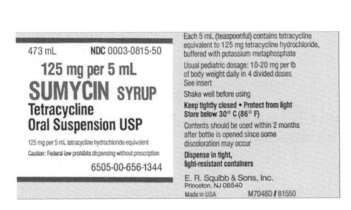

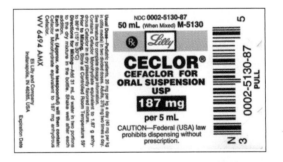

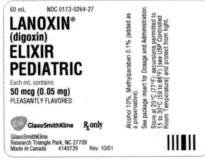

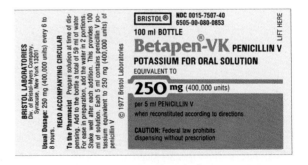

NDC 0087-0730-01
DROPS
TEMPRA®
ACETAMINOPHEN
ANALGESIC
10% SOLUTION
1/2 FL. OZ. (15 ML.)
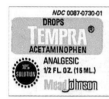
Mead Johnson

TO RELIEVE DISCOMFORT DUE TO COLDS, SIMPLE HEADACHES, MINOR ACHES AND PAINS.
Each 0.6 ml. of TEMPRA® drops contains 60 mg. (1 grain) of acetaminophen and 10% alcohol.
Your physician is the best source of counsel and guidance in illness when pain or fever is present.
KEEP THIS AND ALL MEDICATIONS OUT OF THE REACH OF CHILDREN.
Made in U.S.A.   © M.J.& Co.
MEAD JOHNSON NUTRITIONAL DIVISION
Mead Johnson & Company · Evansville, Indiana 47721 U.S.A.

AMOXIL®
125mg/5mL

125mg/5mL
NDC 0029-6008-22

Directions for mixing: Tap bottle until all powder flows freely. Add approximately 1/3 total amount of water for reconstitution (total=116 mL); shake vigorously to wet powder. Add remaining water; again shake vigorously. Each 5 ml (1 teaspoonful) will contain amoxicillin trihydrate equivalent to 125 mg amoxicillin.
Usual Adult Dosage: 250 to 500 mg every 8 hours.
Usual Child Dosage: 20 to 40 mg/kg/day in divided doses every 8 hours, depending on age, weight and infection severity. See accompanying prescribing information.

Keep tightly closed.
Shake well before using.
Refrigeration preferable but not required.
Discard suspension after 14 days.

AMOXIL®
AMOXICILLIN
FOR ORAL SUSPENSION

R only

150mL
(when reconstituted)

gsk GlaxoSmithKline

Gentle laxative and stool softener for treating temporary constipation.
Usual dose: (preferably at bedtime).
Children over 3: 1 to 3 teaspoons.
Adults: 1 to 2 tablespoons.
Warning: Not to be used when abdominal pain, nausea, or vomiting are present.
Frequent or prolonged use of this preparation may result in dependence on laxatives.

Keep this and all medication out of reach of children.

NDC 0087-0721-01
SYRUP
PERI-COLACE®
CASANTHRANOL AND DIOCTYL SODIUM SULFOSUCCINATE
LAXATIVE PLUS STOOL SOFTENER

8 FL. OZ. (1/2 PT.)

Mead Johnson

Each tablespoon (15 ml., 3 teaspoons) contains 30 mg. Peristim® (casanthranol, Mead Johnson) and 60 mg. COLACE® (dioctyl sodium sulfosuccinate, Mead Johnson).

Contains alcohol 10%.

PERI-COLACE is also available in 1-pint bottles of syrup and in bottles of 30 and 60 capsules.

Made in U.S.A.   © M. J. & Co.

Mead Johnson
PHARMACEUTICAL DIVISION
Mead Johnson & Company
Evansville, Indiana 47721 U.S.A.

R only
See package insert for dosage and complete product information.
Warning: Not for injection
Store unconstituted product at controlled room temperature 20° to 25°C (68° to 77°F) [see USPI]. Store constituted suspension in a refrigerator 2° to 8°C (36° to 46°F). Shake well before using. Keep container tightly closed. The mixture may be used for 14 days. Discard unused portion after 14 days.
Directions for mixing: Shake bottle to loosen granules. Add approximately 1/2 the total amount of distilled water required for constitution (total water = 29 mL). Shake vigorously to wet the granules. Add remaining water and shake vigorously.
Each 5 ml of suspension contains cefpodoxime proxetil equivalent to 100 mg cefpodoxime.
U.S. Patent Nos. 4,486,425; 4,409,215
Licensed from Sankyo Company, Ltd., Japan
Manufactured by
Pharmacia & Upjohn S.A.-N.V., Puurs · Belgium
For
Pharmacia & Upjohn Company
Kalamazoo, MI 49001, USA
B17 150 101
5Q5358

NDC 0009-3615-03
50 mL (when mixed)

Vantin® For Oral Suspension
cefpodoxime proxetil
for oral suspension

100 mg per 5 mL

Equivalent to 100 mg per 5 mL
cefpodoxime when constituted

Pharmacia
&Upjohn

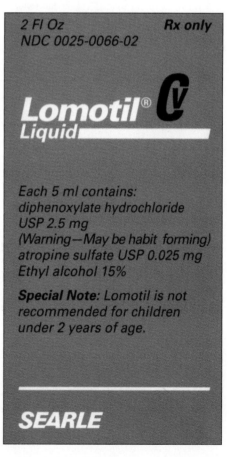

2 Fl Oz   **Rx only**
NDC 0025-0066-02

Lomotil® **C^V**
Liquid

Each 5 ml contains:
diphenoxylate hydrochloride
USP 2.5 mg
(Warning—May be habit forming)
atropine sulfate USP 0.025 mg
Ethyl alcohol 15%

Special Note: *Lomotil is not recommended for children under 2 years of age.*

SEARLE

Use the labels provided to calculate the following IM/s.c. dosages. Calculate to hundredths.

PART II

12. Prepare a 20 mg dosage of meperidine. _____

13. A dosage of morphine 10 mg has been ordered. _____

14. Prepare a 15 mg dosage of tobramycin. _____

15. Draw up a 100 mg dosage of clindamycin. _____

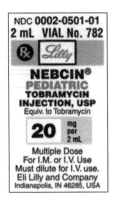

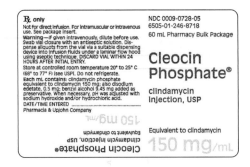

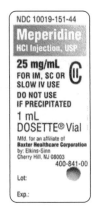

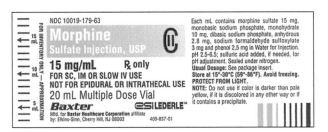

PART III

16. Prepare a 40 mg dosage of meperidine. _____

17. Draw up a 75 mg dosage of kanamycin. _____

18. A dosage of Dilantin 50 mg has been ordered. _____

19. Prepare a 6 mg dosage of morphine. _____

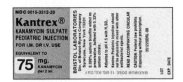

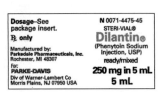

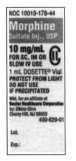

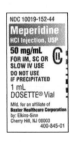

Answers
1. 5 mL; suspension	**5.** 5 mL	**10.** 1.2 mL	**15.** 0.67 mL
2. 2.5 mL; suspension	**6.** 10 mL	**11.** 5 mL; suspension	**16.** 0.8 mL
3. 2 mL	**7.** 10 mL; suspension	**12.** 0.8 mL	**17.** 2 mL
4. 5 mL; suspension	**8.** 15 mL	**13.** 0.67 mL	**18.** 1 mL
	9. 10 mL; suspension	**14.** 1.5 mL	**19.** 0.6 mL

Pediatric Intravenous Medications

Pediatric IV medication administration involves a challenge and a responsibility that is multifaceted. Infants and children, particularly under the age of 4, are incompletely developed physiologically, and drug tolerance, absorption, and excretion are ongoing concerns. In addition infants and acutely ill children can tolerate only a narrow range of hydration, making administration of IV drugs, which are diluted for administration, a critical and exact skill. Drug dilution protocols may specify a range for dilution, and on many occasions the smallest possible volume may have to be used in order not to overhydrate a child. Dosage and dilution decisions may have to be made on a day-to-day or even dose-to-dose basis and will involve the team effort of nurse, physician, and pharmacist. In addition the suitability of any flow rate calculated for administration must be made on an individual basis. For example, a calculated flow rate of 100 gtt/min for a 2-year-old child is too high a rate to administer.

The fragility of infants' and children's veins, and the irritating nature of many medications, mandate careful site inspection for signs of inflammation and infiltration. This should be done immediately before, during, and after each infusion. Signs of inflammation include redness, heat, swelling, and tenderness. Signs of infiltration include swelling, coldness, pain, and lack of blood return in the IV tubing. Either complication necessitates discontinuance of the IV and a restart at a new site.

IV medication guidelines are always used to determine drug dosages, dilutions, and administration rates. In this chapter, all examples and problems are representative of actual rates.

Let's start by looking at the different methods of IV medication administration.

METHODS OF IV MEDICATION ADMINISTRATION

Intravenous medications may be administered over a period of several hours, or on an **intermittent** basis involving several dosages in a 24-hour period. When ordered to infuse over several hours, medications are usually added to

Objectives

The learner will:

1. list the steps in preparing and administering IV medications from a solution bag

2. list the steps in preparing and administering IV medications using a calibrated burette

3. explain why a flush is included in IV medication administration

4. calculate flow rates for administration of pediatric IV medications

5. use normal daily and hourly dosage ranges to calculate and assess dosages ordered

Prerequisites

Chapters 13, 14, 15, and 16

an IV solution bag. Adding the drug to the IV bag may be a hospital pharmacy or staff nurse responsibility, but, in any event, it is not a complicated procedure. The steps for adding the drug to the solution are as follows:

STEP 1 **Locate the type and volume of IV solution ordered.**

STEP 2 **Measure the dosage of drug to be added.**

STEP 3 **Use strict aseptic technique to add the drug to the solution bag through the medication port.**

STEP 4 **Mix the drug thoroughly in the solution.**

STEP 5 **Label the IV solution bag with the name and dosage of the drug added.**

STEP 6 **Add your initials with the time and date you added the drug.**

STEP 7 **Hang the IV and set the flow rate for the infusion. Chart the administration when it has completed.**

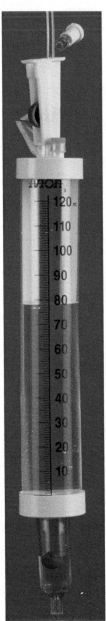

For intermittent administrations the medication may also be prepared in small-volume solution bags or using a calibrated burette, such as the one illustrated in Figure 21-1. Because the total capacity of burettes is between 100 and 150 mL, calibrated in 1 mL increments, exact measurement of small volumes is possible.

Regardless of the method of intermittent administration, the medication infusion is **routinely followed by a flush**, to make sure the medication has cleared the tubing, and that the total dosage has been administered. The volume of the flush will vary depending on the length of IV tubing from the medication source, that is, the burette or syringe, to the infusion site. If a primary line exists, the medication may be administered IVPB (IV piggy-back) via a secondary line. If no IV is infusing, a saline or heparin lock (heplock) is frequently in place and used for intermittent administration.

When IV medications are diluted for administration, it is necessary to determine hospital policy on **inclusion of the medication volume as part of the volume specified for dilution**. For example, if 20 mg has a volume of 2 mL, and it is to be diluted in 30 mL, does this mean you must add 28 mL of diluent to the burette, or 30 mL?

Hospital policies may vary, but in all examples and problems in this chapter **the drug volume will be treated as part of the total diluent volume**. The sequencing of medication and flush administration covered next for burette use is also representative of the procedure that might be followed for IVPB administrations.

Figure 21-1

MEDICATION ADMINISTRATION VIA BURETTE

When a burette is used for medication administration, the entire preparation is usually done by staff nurses. Volumetric pumps are used extensively to administer intermittent IV medications to infants and children. When these are used, the alarm will sound each time the burette empties to signal when each successive step is necessary. For example, it will alarm when the medication has infused and the flush must be started, and again when the flush is completed.

Let's look at some sample orders and go step by step through one procedure that may be used.

EXAMPLE 1

A dosage of 250 mg in **15 mL** of D5 1/2NS is to be infused over **30 minutes**. It is to be followed with a 5 mL D5 1/2NS flush. A volumetric pump will be used, and the tubing is a **microdrip** burette.

STEP 1 | **Read the drug label and determine what volume the 250 mg dosage is contained in. Let's assume this is 1 mL.**

STEP 2 | **The dilution is to be 15 mL. Run a total of 14 mL of D5 1/2NS into the burette, then add the 1 mL containing the dosage of 250 mg. This gives the ordered volume of 15 mL. Roll the burette between your hands to mix the drug thoroughly with the solution.**

STEP 3 | **Calculate the flow rate for this microdrip.**

Total volume = **15 mL**   Infusion time = **30 min**

Use ratio or proportion to calculate mL/hr rate.

$$15 \text{ mL} : 30 \text{ min} = X \text{ mL} : 60 \text{ min} \quad \text{or} \quad \frac{15 \text{ mL}}{30 \text{ min}} = \frac{X \text{ mL}}{60 \text{ min}}$$
$$30X = 60 \times 15$$
$$X = \mathbf{30 \text{ mL/hr}} \qquad\qquad\qquad X = \mathbf{30 \text{ mL/hr}}$$

STEP 4 | **Set the pump to infuse 30 mL/hr.**

STEP 5 | **Label the burette to identify the drug and dosage added. Attach a label that states "medication infusing." This makes it possible for others to know the status of the administration if you are not present when the infusion is complete and the pump alarms.**

STEP 6 | **When the medication has infused add the 5 mL D5 1/2NS flush. Remove the "medication infusing" label and attach a "flush infusing" label. Continue to infuse at the 30 mL/hr rate until the burette empties for the second time.**

STEP 7 | **When the flush has been completed, restart the primary IV, or disconnect from the saline/heparin lock. Remove the "flush infusing" label. Chart the dosage and time.**

EXAMPLE 2

An antibiotic dosage of **125 mg in 1 mL** is to be **diluted in 20 mL** of D5 1/4NS and infused over **30 min**. A **flush of 15 mL** D5 1/4NS is to follow. A volumetric pump will be used.

STEP 1   **125 mg has a volume of 1 mL. Add 19 mL of D5 1/4NS to the burette, add the 1 mL of medication, and mix thoroughly.**

STEP 2   **Calculate the mL/hr flow rate.**

Total volume = **20 mL**   Infusion time = **30 min**

$$20 \text{ mL} : 30 \text{ min} = X \text{ mL} : 60 \text{ min} \quad \text{or} \quad \frac{20 \text{ mL}}{30 \text{ min}} = \frac{X \text{ mL}}{60 \text{ min}}$$
$$30X = 60 \times 20$$
$$X = \textbf{40 mL/hr} \qquad\qquad\qquad X = \textbf{40 mL/hr}$$

STEP 3   **Set the pump to infuse 40 mL/hr.**

STEP 4   **Label the burette with the drug and dosage, and attach a "medication infusing" label.**

STEP 5   **When the medication has infused, start the 15 mL flush. Remove the "medication infusing" label and add the "flush infusing" label.**

STEP 6   **When the flush has completed, restart the primary IV or disconnect from the saline lock. Remove the "flush infusing" label. Chart the dosage and time.**

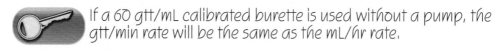 If a 60 gtt/mL calibrated burette is used without a pump, the gtt/min rate will be the same as the mL/hr rate.

EXAMPLE 3

An antibiotic dosage of **50 mg** has been ordered diluted in **20 mL** of D5W to infuse over **20 min**. A **15 mL flush** of D5W is to follow. A **microdrip** will be used, but an infusion control device will not be used.

STEP 1   **Read the medication label to determine what volume contains 50 mg. You determine that 50 mg is contained in 2 mL.**

STEP 2   **Run 18 mL of D5W into the burette and add the 2 mL containing 50 mg of drug. Roll between your hands to mix thoroughly.**

STEP 3   **Calculate the flow rate in gtt/min necessary to deliver the medication.**

Total volume = **20 mL**   Infusion time = **20 min**

$$20 \text{ mL} : 20 \text{ min} = X \text{ mL} : 60 \text{ min} \quad \text{or} \quad \frac{20 \text{ mL}}{20 \text{ min}} = \frac{X \text{ mL}}{60 \text{ min}}$$
$$20X = 20 \times 60$$
$$X = \textbf{60 mL/hr} \qquad\qquad\qquad X = \textbf{60 mL/hr}$$

STEP 4 The mL/hr and gtt/min rates are identical for a microdrip. Set the rate at 60 gtt/min.

STEP 5 Label the burette with drug name and dosage, and attach a "medication infusing" label.

STEP 6 When the medication has cleared the burette, add the 15 mL D5W flush. Continue to run at 60 gtt/min. Remove the "medication infusing" label and replace with a "flush infusing" label.

STEP 7 When the burette empties for the second time, restart the primary IV, or disconnect from the saline lock. Remove the "flush infusing" label. Chart the dosage and time administered.

EXAMPLE 4

An IV medication dosage of 100 mcg has been ordered diluted in **35 mL** of NS and infused in **50 min**. A **10 mL** flush is to follow. A **microdrip** burette will be used.

STEP 1 Read the medication label to determine what volume contains 100 mcg: 100 mcg = 1.5 mL.

STEP 2 Run 33.5 mL of NS into the burette, and add the 1.5 mL of medication. Roll the burette between your hands to mix thoroughly.

STEP 3 Calculate the gtt/min flow rate.

Total volume = **35 mL**   Infusion time = **50 min**

$$35 \text{ mL} : 50 \text{ min} = X \text{ mL} : 60 \text{ min} \qquad \text{or} \qquad \frac{35 \text{ mL}}{50 \text{ min}} = \frac{X \text{ mL}}{60 \text{ min}}$$

$$50X = 35 \times 60 \qquad\qquad\qquad\qquad\qquad$$
$$X = \mathbf{42 \text{ mL/hr}} \qquad\qquad\qquad X = \mathbf{42 \text{ mL/hr}}$$
$$= \mathbf{42 \text{ gtt/min}} \qquad\qquad\qquad = \mathbf{42 \text{ gtt/min}}$$

STEP 4 Set the flow rate at 42 gtt/min.

STEP 5 Label the burette with the drug name and dosage and "medication infusing" label.

STEP 6 When the medication has cleared the burette, add the 10 mL flush. Continue to run at 42 gtt/min. Replace the "medication infusing" label with the "flush infusing" label.

STEP 7 When the burette empties of the flush solution, restart the primary IV, or disconnect from the saline lock. Remove the "flush infusing" label, and chart the dosage and time administered.

21

PROBLEM

Determine the volume of solution that must be added to the burette to mix the following IV drugs. Then calculate the flow rate in gtt/min for each administration using a microdrip, and indicate the mL/hr setting for a pump.

1. An IV medication of 75 mg in 3 mL is ordered diluted to 55 mL to infuse over 45 min.

   Dilution volume _____ gtt/min _____ mL/hr _____

2. A dosage of 100 mg in 2 mL is diluted to 30 mL of D5W to infuse in 20 min.

   Dilution volume _____ gtt/min _____ mL/hr _____

3. The volume of a 10 mg dosage of medication is 1 cc. Dilute to 40 mL and administer over 50 min.

   Dilution volume _____ gtt/min _____ mL/hr _____

4. A dosage of 15 mg with a volume of 3 mL is to be diluted to 70 mL and administered in 50 min.

   Dilution volume _____ gtt/min _____ mL/hr _____

5. A medication of 1 g in 4 mL is to be diluted to 60 mL and infused over 90 min.

   Dilution volume _____ gtt/min _____ mL/hr _____

Answers **1.** 52 mL; 73 gtt/min; 73 mL/hr **2.** 28 mL; 90 gtt/min; 90 mL/hr **3.** 39 mL; 48 gtt/min; 48 mL/hr **4.** 67 mL; 84 gtt/min; 84 mL/hr **5.** 56 mL; 40 gtt/min; 40 mL/hr

COMPARING IV DOSAGES ORDERED WITH AVERAGE DOSAGES

Knowing how to compare dosages ordered with average dosages for a particular medication is a nursing responsibility.

 Dosages of IV medications are calculated on the basis of body weight, or BSA.

Average dosages may be listed in terms of mg, mcg, or U per day, or per hour. BSA in m² is most often used to calculate chemotherapeutic drugs, which are administered only by certified nursing staff. The following examples will demonstrate how to use average dosage to check dosages ordered.

 EXAMPLE 1

A child weighing **22.6 kg** has an order for **500 mg** of medication in 100 mL of D5W **q.12.h.** The normal dosage range is **40–50 mg/kg/day**. Determine if the dosage ordered is within the normal range.

STEP 1 | **Calculate the normal daily dosage range for this child.**

$$40 \text{ mg/day} \times 22.6 \text{ kg} = \textbf{904 mg}$$
$$50 \text{ mg/day} \times 22.6 \text{ kg} = \textbf{1130 mg}$$

STEP 2 | **Calculate the dosage infusing in 24 hr.**

500 mg in 12 hr = **1000 mg in 24 hr**

STEP 3 | **Assess the accuracy of the dosage ordered.**

The 500 mg in 12 hr is within the 904–1130 mg/day dosage range.

EXAMPLE 2

A child with a body weight of **18.4 kg** is to receive a medication with a dosage range of **100–150 mg/kg/day**. The order is for **600 mg** in 75 mL of D5W **q.6.h.** Determine if the dosage is within normal range.

STEP 1 | **Calculate the normal daily dosage range.**

100 mg/day $\times$ 18.4 kg = **1840 mg/day**
150 mg/day $\times$ 18.4 kg = **2760 mg/day**

STEP 2 | **Calculate the daily dosage ordered.**

The dosage ordered is 600 mg q.6.h. (4 doses).
600 mg $\times$ 4 = **2400 mg/day**

STEP 3 | **Assess the accuracy of the dosage ordered.**

The dosage ordered, 2400 mg/day, is within the normal range of 1840–2760 mg/day.

EXAMPLE 3

A child weighing **17.7 kg** is receiving an IV of **250 mL** of D5W containing **2000 U** of heparin, which is to infuse at **50 mL/hr**. The dosage range of heparin is **10–25 U/kg/hr**. Assess the accuracy of this dosage.

STEP 1 | **Calculate the dosage range per hour.**

10 U/kg/hr $\times$ 17.7 kg = **177 U/hr**
25 U/kg/hr $\times$ 17.7 kg = **442.5 U/hr**

STEP 2 | **Calculate the dosage infusing per hour.**

$$2000\ U : 250\ mL = X\ U : 50\ mL \qquad \text{or} \qquad \frac{2000\ U}{250\ mL} = \frac{X\ U}{50\ mL}$$
$$250X = 2000 \times 50$$
$$X = \textbf{400 U/hr} \qquad\qquad\qquad\qquad X = \textbf{400 U/hr}$$

STEP 3 | **Assess the accuracy of the dosage ordered.**

The IV is infusing at a rate of 50 mL per hour, which is 400 U/hr. The normal dosage range is 177–442.5 U/hr. The dosage is within normal range.

EXAMPLE 4

A child weighing **32.7 kg** has an IV of **250 mL** of D5 1/4S containing **400 mcg** of medication to infuse over **5 hours**. The normal range for this drug is **1–3 mcg/kg/hr**. Determine if this dosage is within the normal dosage range.

STEP 1 | **Calculate the hourly dosage range.**

1 mcg/kg/hr × 32.7 kg = **32.7 mcg/hr**
3 mcg/kg/hr × 32.7 kg = **98.1 mcg/hr**

STEP 2 | **Calculate the dosage infusing per hour.**

400 mcg ÷ 5 hr = **80 mcg/hr**

STEP 3 | **Assess the accuracy of the dosage ordered.**

The dosage of 80 mcg/hr infusing is within the normal range of 32.7–98.1 mcg/hr.

PROBLEM

Calculate the normal dosage range to the nearest tenth and the dosage being administered for the following medications. Assess the dosages ordered.

1. A child weighing 24.4 kg has an IV of 250 mL of D5W containing 2500 U of a drug. The dosage range for this drug is 15–25 U/kg/hr. The pump is set to deliver 50 mL/hr.

    Dosage range per hr _____ Dosage infusing per hr _____

    Assessment _____

2. A solution of D5W containing 25 mg of a drug is to infuse in 30 min. The dosage range is 4–8 mg/kg/day, q.6.h. The child weighs 18.7 kg.

    Dosage range per day _____ Daily dosage ordered _____

    Assessment _____

3. An IV solution containing 125 mg of medication is infusing. The dosage range is 5–10 mg/kg/dose, and the child weighs 14.2 kg.

    Dosage range per dose _____ Assessment _____

4. A child weighing 14.3 kg is to receive an IV drug with a dosage range of 50–100 mcg/kg/day in two divided doses. An infusion of 50 mL of D5W containing 400 mcg to run 30 min has been ordered.

    Daily dosage range _____ Daily dosage ordered _____

    Assessment _____

5. A dosage of 4 mg (4000 mcg) of drug in 500 mL of D5 1/2S is to infuse over 4 hours. The dosage range of the drug is 24–120 mcg/kg/hr, and the child weighs 16.1 kg.

   Dosage range per hr _____ Dosage infusing per hr _____

   Assessment _____

6. A child weighing 20.9 kg is to receive a medication with a normal dosage range of 80–160 mg/kg/day, in divided doses q.6.h. The IV ordered contains 500 mg.

   Dosage range per day _____ Daily dosage ordered _____

   Assessment _____

7. A child weighing 22.3 kg is to receive 750 mL of D5 1/45 containing 6 g of a drug, which is to run over 24 hours. The dosage range of the drug is 200–300 mg/kg/day.

   Dosage range per day _____ Assessment _____

8. An IV of 50 mL of D5W containing 55 mcg of a drug is infusing over a 30-min period. The child weighs 14.9 kg and the dosage range is 6–8 mcg/kg/day, q.12.h.

   Dosage range per day _____ Daily dosage ordered _____

   Assessment _____

9. A child weighing 27.1 kg is to receive a medication with a normal range of 0.5–1 mg/kg/dose. An IV containing 20 mg of medication has been ordered.

   Dosage per dose _____ Assessment _____

10. An IV medication of 60 mcg in 200 mL is ordered to infuse over 2 hr. The normal dosage range is 1.5–3 mcg/kg/hr. The child weighs 16.7 kg.

   Dosage range per hr _____ Dosage infusing per hr _____

   Assessment _____

Answers **1.** 366–610 U/hr; 500 U/hr; normal range **2.** 74.8–149.6 mg/day; 100 mg/day; normal range **3.** 71–142 mg/dose; normal range **4.** 715–1430 mcg/day; 800 mg; normal range **5.** 386.4–1932 mcg/hr; 1000 mcg; normal range **6.** 1672–3344 mg/day; 2000 mg; normal range **7.** 4460–6690 mg/day; normal range **8.** 89.4–119.2 mcg/day; 110 mcg; normal range **9.** 13.6–27.1 mg/dose; normal range **10.** 25.1–50.1 mcg/hr; 30 mcg; normal range

Summary

This concludes the chapter on administration of IV drugs to infants and children. The important points to remember from this chapter are:

- IV medications may be ordered to infuse over a period of several hours or minutes.

- IV medications are diluted for administration, and it is important to determine hospital policy on inclusion of the medication volume as part of the total dilution volume.

- A flush is used following medication administration to make sure the medication has cleared the tubing and the total dosage has been administered.

- The volume of flush solution on intermittent infusions will vary depending the amount needed to clear the infusion line.

- Average dosage ranges are used to assess dosages ordered.

- Pediatric IV medication administration requires constant assessment of the child's ability to tolerate dosage, dilution, and rate of administration.

- Children's veins are very fragile, and intravenous sites must be checked for inflammation and infiltration immediately before, during, and following each medication administration.

Summary Self-Test

Determine the volume of solution that must be added to a calibrated burette to mix the following IV drugs. The medication volume is included in the total dilution volume. Calculate the flow rate in gtt/min for each infusion. A microdrip with a calibration of 60 gtt/mL is used.

	Volume of diluent	gtt/min rate
1. An IV antibiotic of 750 mg in 3 mL has been ordered diluted to a total of 25 mL of D5W to infuse over 40 minutes.	_____	_____
2. A dosage of 500,000 U of a penicillin preparation with a volume of 4 mL has been ordered diluted to 50 mL D5 1/2NS to infuse in 60 min.	_____	_____
3. A dosage of 1.5 g/2 mL of an antibiotic is to be diluted to a total of 40 mL of D5W and administered over 40 min.	_____	_____
4. An antibiotic dosage of 200 mg in 4 mL is to be diluted to 50 mL and administered over 70 min.	_____	_____
5. A dosage of 20 mg in 2 mL has been ordered diluted to 30 mL, to be infused over 35 min.	_____	_____
6. A dosage of 25 mg in 5 mL has been ordered diluted to 40 mL and administered in 50 min.	_____	_____
7. A 10 mg in 2 mL dosage has been ordered diluted to 20 mL to infuse over 30 min.	_____	_____

8. A medication dosage of 800 mg in 4 mL is to be
   diluted to 60 mL and infused over 80 min.   _____ _____

9. A dosage of 0.5 g in 2 mL is to be diluted to
   40 mL and run in 30 min.   _____ _____

10. A medication of 1000 mg in 1 mL is to be diluted
    to 15 mL and administered over 20 min.   _____ _____

The following IV drugs are to be administered using a volumetric or syringe pump. Determine the amount of diluent to be added and the flow rate in mL/hr to set the pumps.

	Volume of diluent	mL/hr rate

11. A dosage of 40 mg in 4 mL is to be diluted to
    50 mL and administered in 90 min.   _____ _____

12. A 2 g in 5 mL dosage has been ordered diluted to
    a total of 90 mL and administered in 45 min.   _____ _____

13. An 80 mg dosage with a volume of 2 mL is to be
    diluted to 80 mL and administered in 60 min.   _____ _____

14. A 60 mg dosage with a volume of 4 mL is ordered
    diluted to 30 mL and run over 20 min.   _____ _____

15. A 5 mg per 2 mL dosage is to be diluted to 80 mL
    and administered in 50 min.   _____ _____

16. The dosage ordered is 0.75 g in 3 mL to be diluted
    to 30 mL. Run in over 40 min.   _____ _____

17. A medication of 100 mg in 2 mL is ordered diluted
    to 30 mL and run in 25 min.   _____ _____

18. The dosage ordered is 100 mg in 1 mL to be
    diluted to 50 mL. Run in over 45 min.   _____ _____

19. A 30 mg dosage in 1 mL has been ordered diluted
    to 10 mL to infuse in 10 min.   _____ _____

20. A dosage of 250 mg in 5 mL has been ordered
    diluted to 40 mL and infused in 60 min.   _____ _____

Calculate the normal dosage range to the nearest tenth and the dosage being administered for the following medications. Assess the dosages ordered.

21. A child weighing 15.4 kg is to receive a dosage with a range of
    5–7.5 mg/kg/dose. The solution bag is labeled 100 mg.

    Dosage range _____ Assessment _____

22. The order is for 200 U in 75 mL. The child weighs 13.1 kg and the
    dosage range is 15–20 U/kg per dose.

    Dosage range _____ Assessment _____

23. A dosage of 1.5 mg in 20 mL has been ordered. The normal dosage range is 0.1–0.3 mg/kg/day in two divided doses. The child's weight is 12.4 kg.   Dosage range per day _____

   Daily dosage ordered _____   Assessment _____

24. A dosage of 400 mg in 75 mL of medication is to be infused q.8.h. The normal range is 15–45 mg/kg/day, and the child weighs 27.9 kg.   Dosage range per day _____

   Daily dosage ordered _____   Assessment _____

25. A child weighing 15.7 kg is to receive a medication with a normal hourly range of 3–7 mcg/kg. A 250 mL solution bag containing 350 mcg is infusing at a rate of 50 mL/hr.

   Dosage range per hr _____   Dosage infusing per hr _____

   Assessment _____

26. A child weighing 19.6 kg is to receive a medication with a normal dosage range of 60–80 mg/kg/day. A 90 mL infusion containing 375 mg has been ordered q.6.h.   Dosage range per day _____

   Daily dosage ordered _____   Assessment _____

27. Two infusions of 250 mL each containing 300 mg of medication are to infuse continuously over a 24-hr period (250 mL q.12.h.). The child receiving the infusion weighs 11.7 kg, and the normal dosage range of the drug is 50–100 mg/kg/day.

   Dosage range per day _____   Daily dosage ordered _____

   Assessment _____

28. The order is for 100 mL of D5W containing 150 mg of medication to infuse q.8.h. The normal dosage range is 3–12 mg/kg/day, and the child weighs 40.1 kg.   Dosage range per day _____

   Daily dosage ordered _____   Assessment _____

29. A child has an infusion of 250 mL containing 500 U of medication to run at 50 mL/hr. The normal dosage range is 10–25 U/hr. The child weighs 10.3 kg.   Dosage range per hr _____

   Dosage infusing per hr _____   Assessment _____

30. The normal dosage range of a drug is 0.5–1.5 U/hr. A child weighing 10.7 kg has a 150 mL volume of solution containing 45 U infusing at a rate of 20 mL/hr.   Normal dosage range per hr _____

   Dosage infusing per hr _____   Assessment _____

31. A child weighing 12.5 kg is receiving an IV of 2500 U of heparin in 250 mL of D5W at 40 mL/hr. The normal dosage range for heparin is 10–25 U/kg/hr.   Normal dosage range per hr _____

   Dosage infusing per hr _____   Assessment _____

21

32. A child with a weight of 10 kg is to receive a medication with a normal dosage range of 60–80 mg/kg/day. The order is for 200 mg q.6.h.   Normal dosage range per day _____

    Daily dosage ordered _____   Assessment _____

33. Order: 0.5 g nafcillin in 100 mL of D5W q.6.h. Normal dosage range is 100–200 mg/kg/day. The child weighs 15 kg.

    Normal dosage range per day _____

    Daily dosage ordered _____   Assessment _____

34. A continuous IV of 500 mL with 20 mEq KCl is infusing at 30 mL/hr. The dosage for potassium chloride is not to exceed 40 mEq/day.   Dosage infusing per hr _____

    Dosage infusing per day _____   Assessment _____

35. A 24-kg child is receiving 116 mg per hr of rifampin IV for 3 hours. Dosage range for this drug is 10–20 mg/kg/day.

    Normal dosage range per day _____

    Dosage received after 3 hours _____   Assessment _____

36. A 25% solution of serum albumin is infusing at 15 mL/hr for a total of 6 hours. Normal dosage for children is 5–25 g/day.

    Grams infused after 6 hr _____   Assessment _____

37. The usual dosage of chloramphenicol for children is 50 mg/kg/24 hr in equally divided doses. Order: infuse 50 mL with 290 mg chloramphenicol q.6.h. The child weighs 51 lb.

    Normal dosage per day _____   Daily dosage ordered _____

    Assessment _____

38. Order: 500 mL D5RL with 30 mEq KCl to infuse at 40 mL/hr. A maximum of 10 mEq/hr of KCl should not be exceeded and the total 24-hr dosage should not exceed 40 mEq/day.

    Dosage infusing per hr _____   Dosage infusing per day _____

    Assessment _____

39. A child weighing 30 kg has an IV of 100 mL of D5W containing 600 mcg of medication to infuse over 2 hours. The normal range for this drug is 2–4 mcg/kg/hr.   Normal dosage range per hr _____

    Dosage infusing per hr _____   Assessment _____

40. 150 mL with 18 mg of medication is ordered to infuse over 10 hours. The normal range for this drug is 0.2 mg–0.6 mg/kg/hr. The child weighs 9 kg.   Normal dosage range per hr _____

    Dosage infusing per hr _____   Assessment _____

Answers

1. 22 mL; 38 gtt/min
2. 46 mL; 50 gtt/min
3. 38 mL; 60 gtt/min
4. 46 mL; 43 gtt/min
5. 28 mL; 51 gtt/min
6. 35 mL; 48 gtt/min
7. 18 mL; 40 gtt/min
8. 56 mL; 45 gtt/min
9. 38 mL; 80 gtt/min
10. 14 mL; 45 gtt/min
11. 46 mL; 33 mL/hr
12. 85 mL; 120 mL/hr
13. 78 mL; 80 mL/hr
14. 26 mL; 90 mL/hr
15. 78 mL; 96 mL/hr

16. 27 mL; 45 mL/hr
17. 28 mL; 72 mL/hr
18. 49 mL; 67 mL/hr
19. 9 mL; 60 mL/hr
20. 35 mL; 40 mL/hr
21. 77–115.5 mg/dose; normal
22. 196.5–262 U/dose; normal
23. 1.2–3.7 mg/day; 3 mg; normal
24. 418.5–1255.5 mg/day; 1200 mg; normal
25. 47.1–109.9 mcg/hr; 70 mcg; normal

26. 1176–1568 mg/day; 1500 mg; normal
27. 585–1170 mg/day; 600 mg; normal
28. 120.3–481.2 mg/day; 450 mg; normal
29. 103–257.5 U/hr; 100 U/hr; normal
30. 5.4–16.1 U/hr; 6 U/hr; normal
31. 125–312.5 U/hr; 400 U/hr; too high
32. 600–800 mg/day; 800 mg; normal
33. 1500–3000 mg/day; 2000 mg; normal

34. 1.2 mEq/hr; 28.8 mEq/day; normal
35. 240–480 mg/day; 348 mg; normal
36. 22.5 g/6 hr; normal
37. 1160 mg/day; 1160 mg; normal
38. 2.4 mEq/hr; 58 mEq/day; too high
39. 60–120 mcg/hr; 300 mcg; too high
40. 1.8–5.4 mg/hr; 1.8 mg; normal

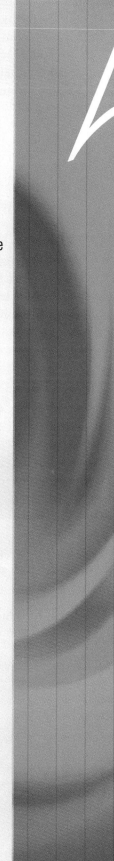

Medication Administration Records

A

In most hospitals the medications being given a patient on a continuing basis are recorded on a single record, which is often referred to by the acronym MAR (Medication Administration Record). Computer-controlled records are slowly making their appearance in many institutions, but the printed MARs are still widely enough in use to warrant their inclusion here.

The focus of this appendix is to introduce three different records, so that the similarities, rather than the differences, will become apparent. The focus will be on locating the drugs, dosage, time, and route of medications being administered on a continuing basis. Medications given intravenously or on a p.r.n. (as needed) basis and preoperative medications are sometimes recorded in a separate location or record.

MEDICATION RECORD 1

Refer to Medication Record 1. First locate on the left the list of drugs that are being given on a continuing basis. Below the first drug name, Humulin Lente, is the frequency of administration, q.a.m., and the date the drug was ordered and when administration started, 7/3. To the right of the drug name is the dosage to be given, 22 U, and the route, s.q. This record uses military time, 0–2300, but time entries omit the extra zeros; for example, 0800 is written as 08. Columns follow to allow for entry of the initials of the persons administering the medications. These columns allow for a week of entries.

Notice that the third drug on this list, Enalapril, has a contingency factor associated with administration. Enalapril lowers blood pressure; therefore, the patient's blood pressure must not only be checked, it must also be recorded before the drug is given. If the pressure falls below the ordered minimum, the drug must not be given. Another drug on the list, heparin, has been discontinued, which on this record is indicated with yellow coloring of the remaining columns to draw attention to the cancellation.

At the extreme left are areas for the recording of RN and pharmacist initials that acknowledge they have checked the orders for accuracy. Whereas the columns for the initials of the persons administering the medications are on this page, space for identification of their initials is on the opposite side, as are spaces to record p.r.n., preoperative, and IV medications.

PROBLEM

Read Medication Record 1 and list the drug, dosage, route, and time of all medications ordered.

Drug	Dosage	Route	Time
1. _____	_____	_____	_____
2. _____	_____	_____	_____
3. _____	_____	_____	_____
4. _____	_____	_____	_____
5. _____	_____	_____	_____
6. _____	_____	_____	_____

7. Which drugs were given by JBC on the evening shift on 7/3 (March 7th)? _____

Answers **1.** Humulin Lente, 22 U, s.q., 0800 **2.** Digoxin, 0.125 mg, p.o., 0900 **3.** Enalapril, 2.5 mg, p.o., 0900 **4.** Colace, 100 mg, p.o., 0900, 2100 **5.** Heparin, 5000 U, s.q., 0900 **6.** Coumadin 2 mg p.o. at 1800 **7.** Colace, 100 mg at 2100; Coumadin 2 mg at 1800

PHARMACY USE ONLY: filled by/checked by
1/ OBD 2/ OBD 3/ OBD 4/ OBD 5/ OBD 6/ OBD 7/ OBD

SCHEDULED MEDICATIONS

PHARM USE ONLY		DATE D/M/Y		TIME	1 7/31-	2 8/31-	3 9/31-	4 10/31-	5 11/31-	6 12/31-	7 13/31-
FILL QTY.	T. FKB	MEDICATION	DOSE								
1.	R.	HUMULIN LENTE	22		② adt	⑥ adt	⑱ adt				
2. 3.	√ BY RN adt	FREQUENCY & DIRECTIONS QAM	U	08							
4. 5.	√ BY PHM		ROUTE SQ								
6. 7.	Ave	ORDERED DATE 7/31-	STOP DATE / /								
FILL QTY.	T. FKB	MEDICATION	DOSE								
1.	R.	DIGOXIN	0.125	09	adt	adt	adt				
2. 3.	√ BY RN adt	FREQUENCY & DIRECTIONS QD	mg								
4. 5.	√ BY PHM		ROUTE PO								
6. 7.	Ave	ORDERED DATE 7/31-	STOP DATE / /								
FILL QTY.	T. FKB	MEDICATION	DOSE								
1.	R.	ENALAPRIL	2.5	09	adt	adt	adt				
2. 3.	√ BY RN adt	FREQUENCY & DIRECTIONS QD	mg		BP 118/90	BP 145/90	BP 138/80				
4. 5.	√ BY PHM		ROUTE PO								
6. 7.	Ave	ORDERED DATE 7/31-	STOP DATE / /								
FILL QTY.	T. FKB	MEDICATION	DOSE								
1.	R.	COLACE	100	09	adt	adt	adt				
2. 3.	√ BY RN adt	FREQUENCY & DIRECTIONS BID	mg								
4. 5.	√ BY PHM		ROUTE PO	21	JBC	JBC	JBC				
6. 7.	Ave	ORDERED DATE 7/31-	STOP DATE / /								
FILL QTY.	T. FKB	MEDICATION	DOSE								
1.	R.	HEPARIN	5000	09	adt ⑪	adt ⑤	adt ⑯			D/C	
2. 3.	√ BY RN adt	FREQUENCY & DIRECTIONS QD	U								
4. 5.	√ BY PHM		ROUTE SQ								
6. 7.	Ave	ORDERED DATE 7/31-	STOP DATE 10/31-								
FILL QTY.	T. FKB	MEDICATION	DOSE								
1.	R.	COUMADIN	2								
2. 3.	√ BY RN adt	FREQUENCY & DIRECTIONS QD	mg	18	JBC	JBC	JBC				
4. 5.	√ BY PHM		ROUTE PO								
6. 7.	Ave	ORDERED DATE 7/31-	STOP DATE / /								

LEGEND: T = TRANSCRIBED BY   R = RECOPIED BY

MEDICATION RECORD 2

The similarities of this record to Medication Record 1 are quite obvious. The main difference is in the placement of the dosage, route, and frequency of administration of continuing medications. Space is provided for recording 2 weeks of administration entries.

This record uses standard, not military, time. Notice that near the bottom the record provides space for entering preoperative and p.r.n. medications. Once again no space is provided for the identification of nurse initials, which is located elsewhere on the form. Produced by Lionville Systems, Inc., this particular record is in use in many smaller medical institutions.

PROBLEM

Read Medication Record 2 and list the drug, dosage, and route of each drug that will be administered at 6 p.m.

	Drug	Dosage	Route
1.	_____	_____	_____
2.	_____	_____	_____
3.	_____	_____	_____

Answers   Tagamet 300 mg p.o.; Nitro-Bid ung 1" topical to chest; Bactrim DS 1 p.o.

MEDICATION ADMINISTRATION RECORD - 14 DAY

Enter Here
IN PENCIL
Number of
Forms in Use

NAME
ADM. NO.

PATIENT IDENTIFICATION

IMPRINT HERE

DIAGNOSES: _____

ALLERGIC TO: _____
(Record in Red)

DIET: _____

Scheduled Medications

DATES GIVEN

OR. DATE / INITIALS	EXP. DATE / TIME	MEDICATION-DOSAGE-FREQUENCY-RT. OF ADM.	HR.	5/3	5/4	5/5	5/6	5/7	5/8	5/9	5/10	5/11	5/12	5/13	5/14	5/15	5/16
5-3 ARE		Tagamet 300 mg p.o. q.6.h.	6														
			12														
			6														
			12														
5-2 ARE	5-16 P9a	Blocadren 10 mg p.o. b.i.d.	9														
			9														
5-3 ARE		Nitro-Bid ung 1" (top) apply to chest q.6.h. while awake	6														
			12														
			6														
			12														
5-3 ARE		Dialose cap ī p.o. t.i.d.	9														
			1														
			9														
5-3 ARE		Bactrim DS ī p.o. b.i.d.	6														
			6														

Single Orders + Pre-Operatives

USE RED ASTERISK *TO INDICATE DOSES
NOT GIVEN - EXPLAIN IN NURSE'S NOTES

OR. DATE / INITIALS	MEDICATION-DOSAGE-RT. OF ADM.	TO BE GIVEN DATE	TIME	NURSE INITIAL	OR. DATE / INITIALS	MEDICATION-DOSAGE-RT. OF ADM.	TO BE GIVEN DATE	TIME	NURSE INITIAL

AGE _____ RELIGION _____ DOCTOR _____ DATE/TIME ADMITTED _____

RM. _____ NAME _____

Lionville Systems, Inc.

MEDICATION RECORD 3

The final record, Medication Record 3, also uses military time. Once again you can see the similarities with the previous records; however, this record lists both trade and generic drug names in the "Medication and Dose" column.

Military time is used for frequency of administration, once again without the extra zeros. Only 4 days of entries are provided for on the form, and there is a space designated for "Site," for the recording of parenteral medications. There is also a space on the bottom of the form to record the initials and names of persons administering the medications.

PROBLEM

Use the drug entry for Capoten on Medication Record 3 as reference to enter the following drugs, dosages, frequency, and route of administration on this form. Record your initials in the "Nurse" column to indicate you have done the transcribing, and identify your initials appropriately on the record. Have your instructor check your completed entries.

1. Coumadin (warfarin Na) 5 mg p.o. q.d. 1800

2. Pronestyl (procainamide) 1000 mg q.6.h. p.o. 0600 1200 1800 2400

3. Mefoxin (cefoxitin Na) 1.5 g q.8.h. IM 0600 1400 2200

4. Ansaid (flurbiprofen) 100 mg p.o. b.i.d. c̄ meals 0800 1800

5. Hismanal (astemizole) 10 mg p.o. q.h.s. 2200

Summary

This concludes the introduction to Medication Administration Records. The important points to remember from this appendix are:

- All the drugs the patient is receiving on a continuing basis are entered on a single medication administration record (MAR).

- Records contain columns for drug, dosage, route, frequency, and times of administration.

- Dosages are charted and initialed for each calendar day in the appropriate time slots.

- Initials of the person administering medications are identified with a full signature on each record.

- p.r.n., preoperative, and IV medications are frequently recorded on a separate page, or in a separate section of the continuing medication record (MAR).

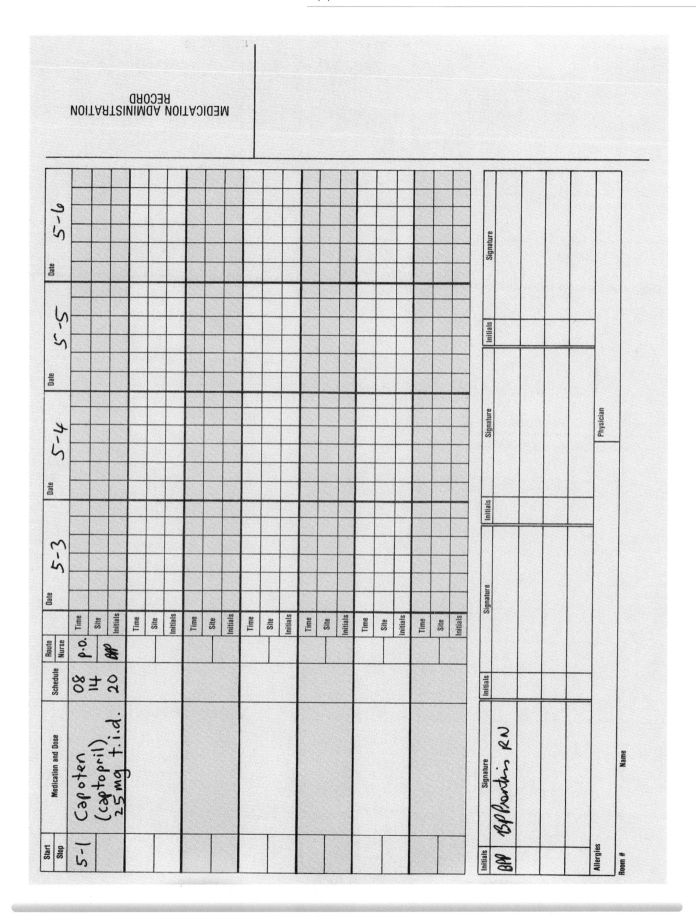

MEDICATION ADMINISTRATION
RECORD

Start Stop	Medication and Dose	Schedule	Route Nurse		Date 5-3		Date 5-4		Date 5-5		Date 5-6	
5-1	Capoten (captopril) 2.5 mg t.i.d.	08 14 20	p.o. *BM*	Time Site Initials								
				Time Site Initials								
				Time Site Initials								
				Time Site Initials								
				Time Site Initials								
				Time Site Initials								
				Time Site Initials								

Initials	Signature	Initials	Signature	Initials	Signature	Initials	Signature
BM	*BMartin RN*						

Physician	
Allergies	
Room #	Name

Index

License Agreement for Thomson Delmar Learning, a part of the Thomson Corporation

SYSTEM REQUIREMENTS

Operating system: Microsoft Windows 98, Me, NT, 4.0, 2000, XP, or newer

Processor: Pentium II processor or faster

Memory: 32–64 MB

Hard disk space: 16 MB

Monitor: SVGA-compatible color

Graphics adapter: SVGA or higher: 800×600, True Color (24-bit or 32-bit) or High Color (16-bit) modes

CD-ROM drive: $8\times$ or faster

An Internet connection and Netscape Navigator 6.2 or Microsoft Internet Explorer 5.5, or newer, are required.

Microsoft is a registered trademark, and Windows and Windows NT are trademarks of Microsoft Corporation.

SETUP INSTRUCTIONS

1. Insert disc into CD-ROM player. The program should start. If it does not, go to step 2.

2. From My Computer, double click the icon for the CD drive.

3. Double click the *index.htm* file to start the program.